Neuroethics in Principle and Praxis - Conceptual Foundations

Edited by Denis Larrivee

Published in London, United Kingdom

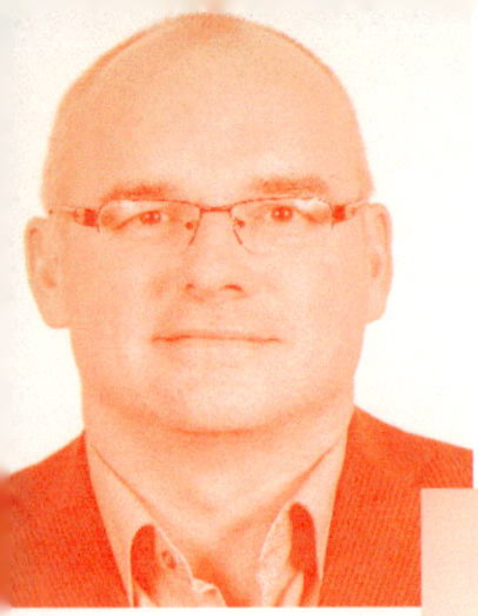
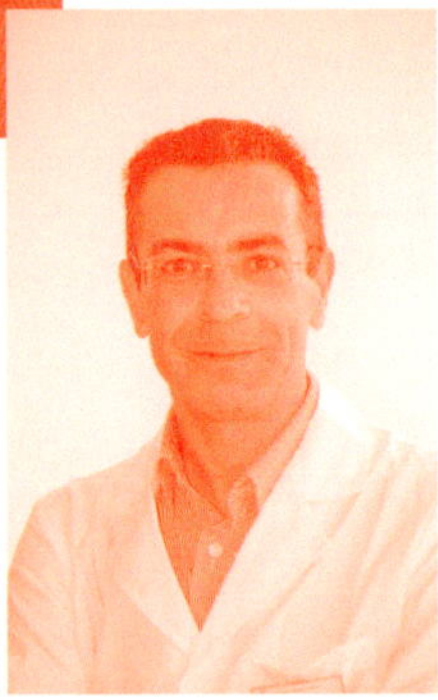
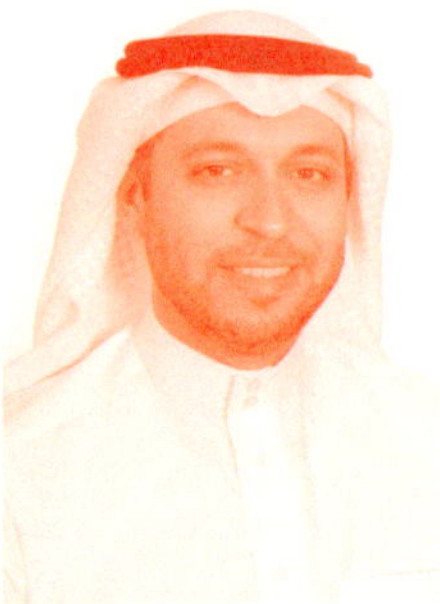
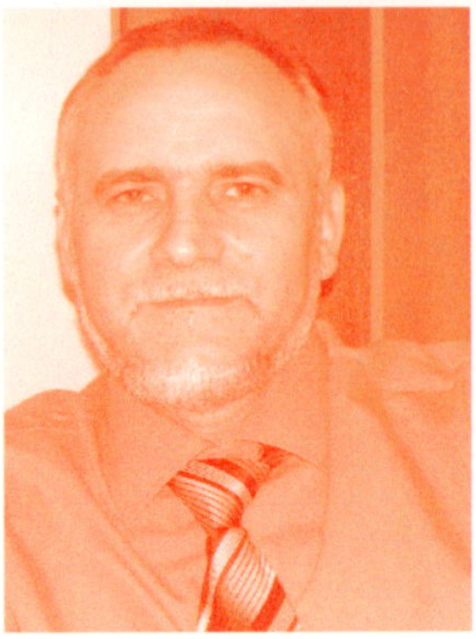
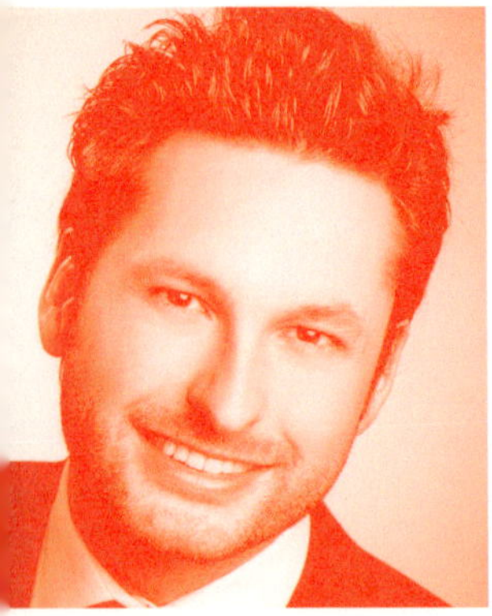
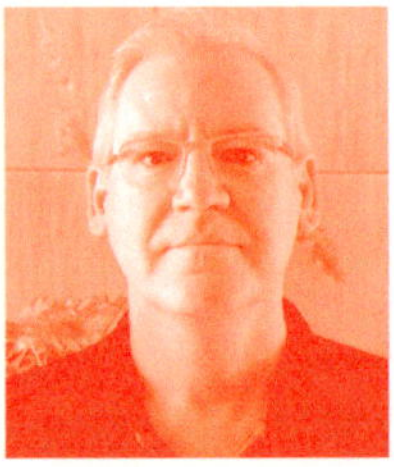
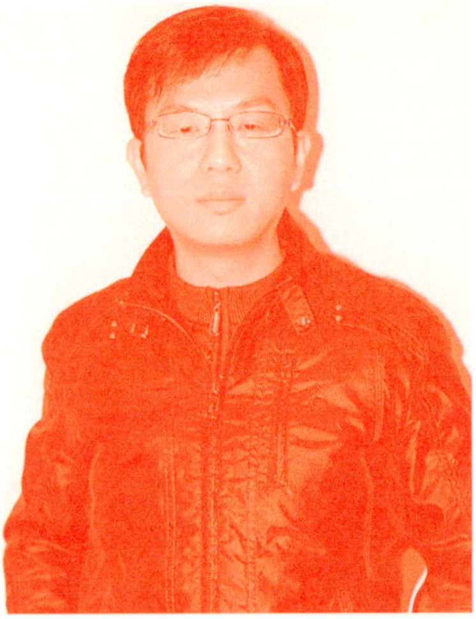

IntechOpen

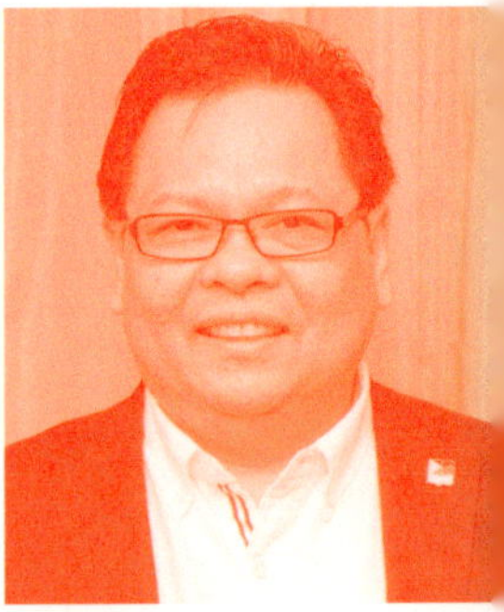
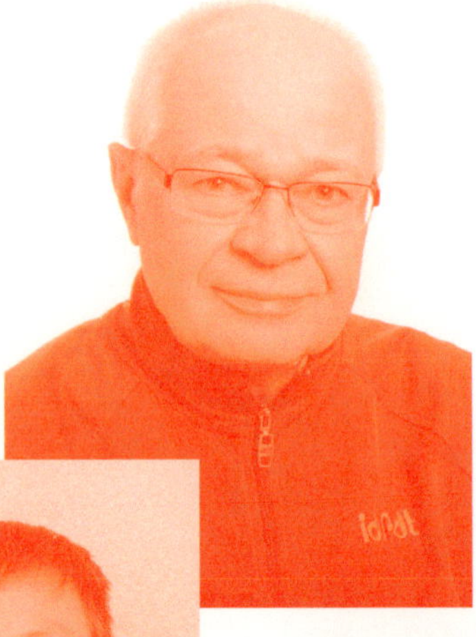
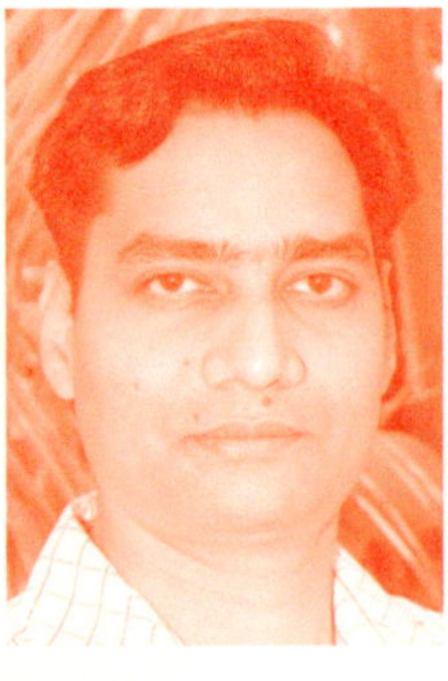
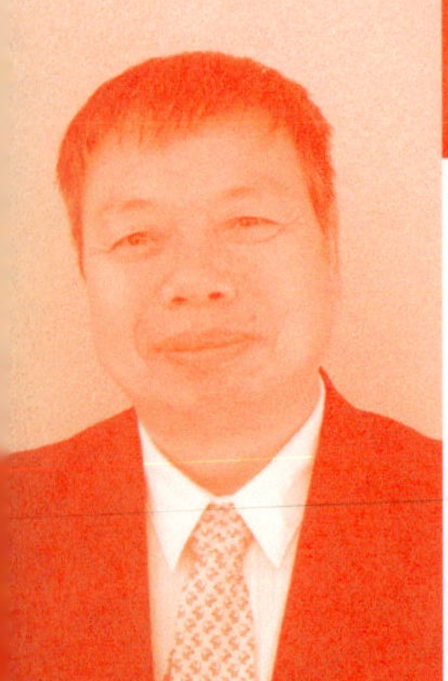
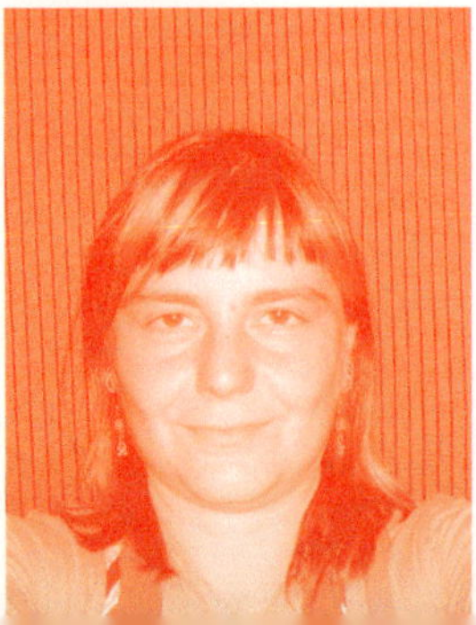
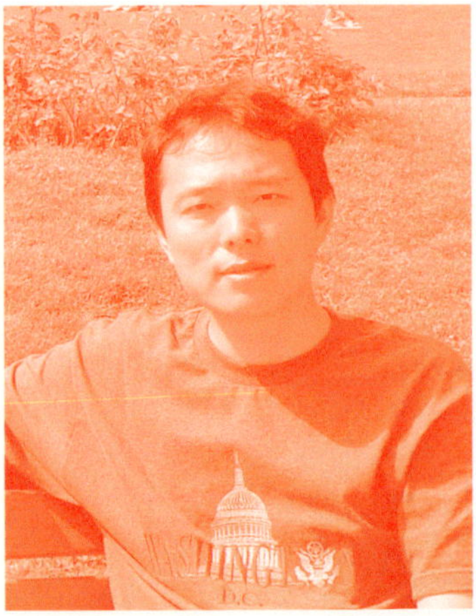

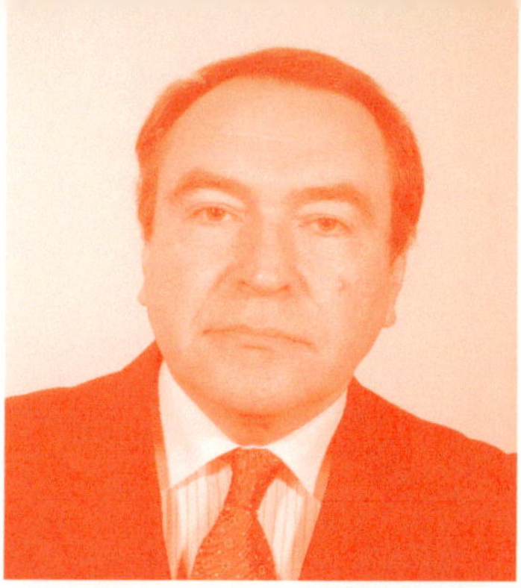
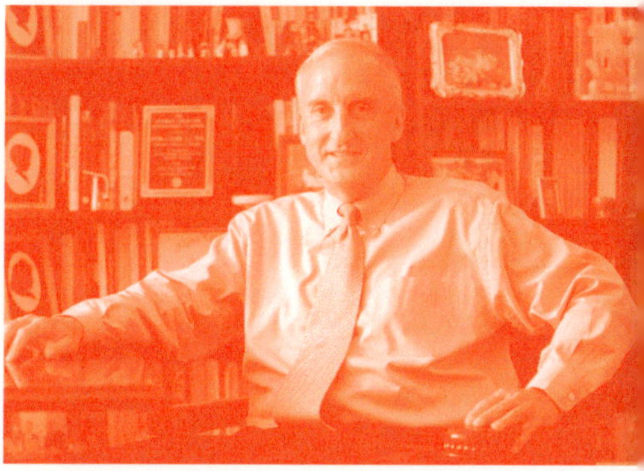
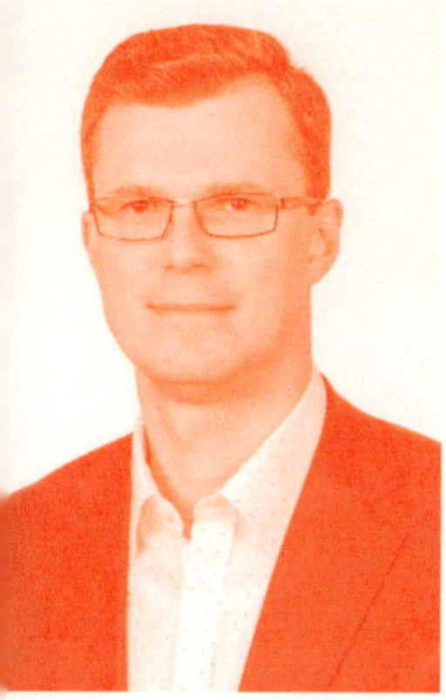
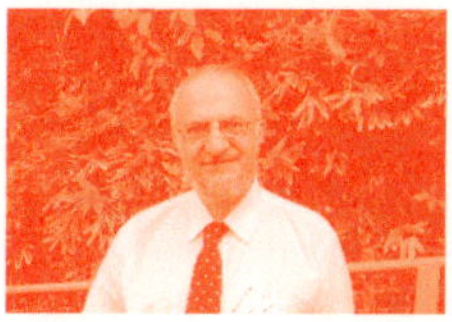
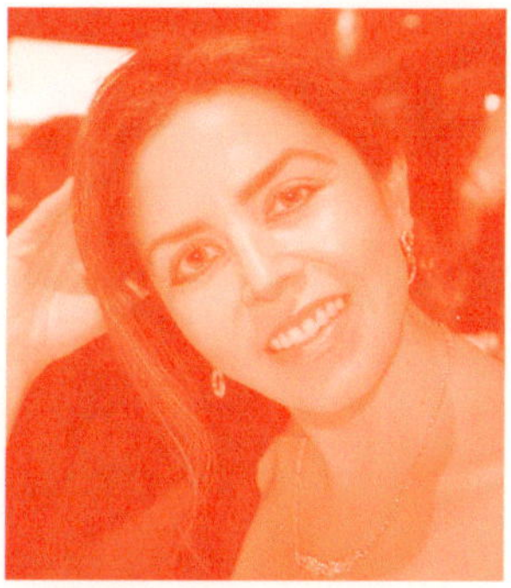

Supporting open minds since 2005

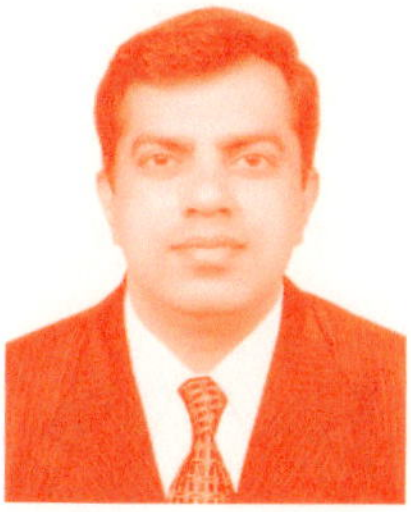
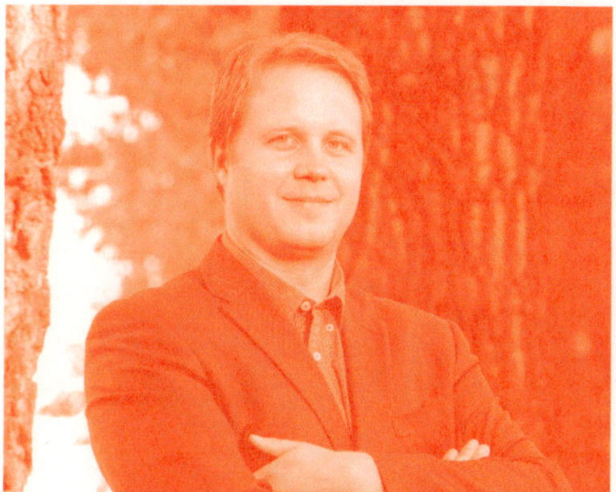
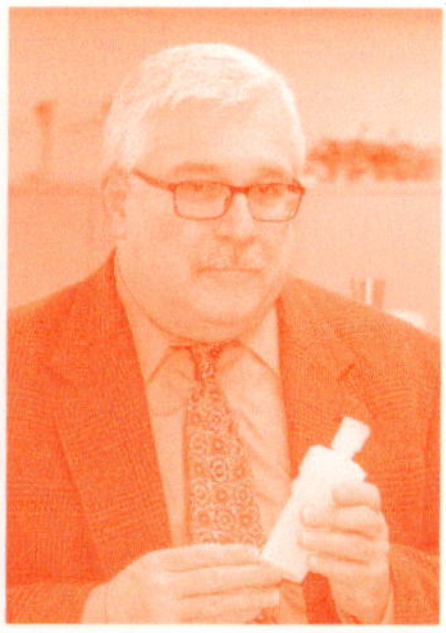
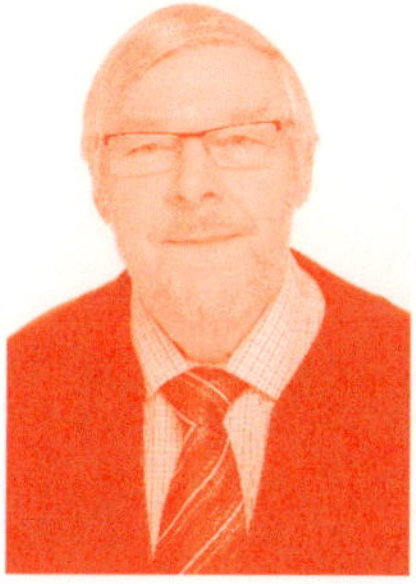
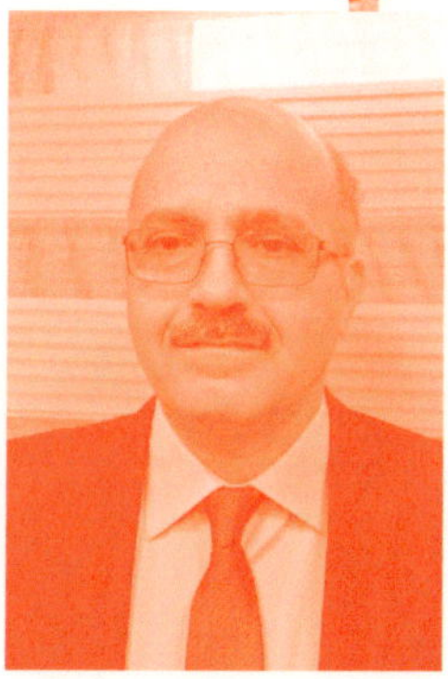
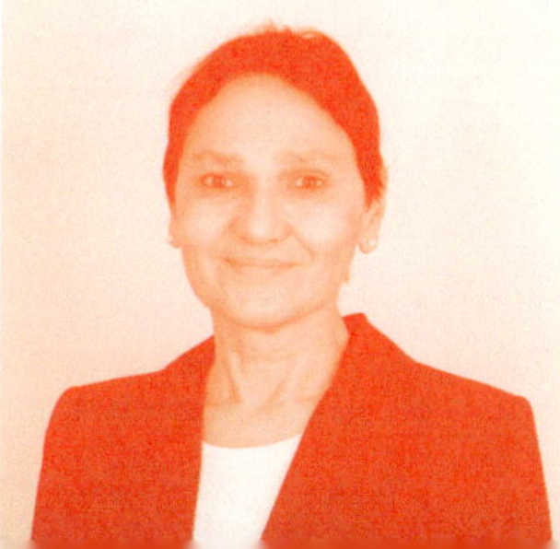
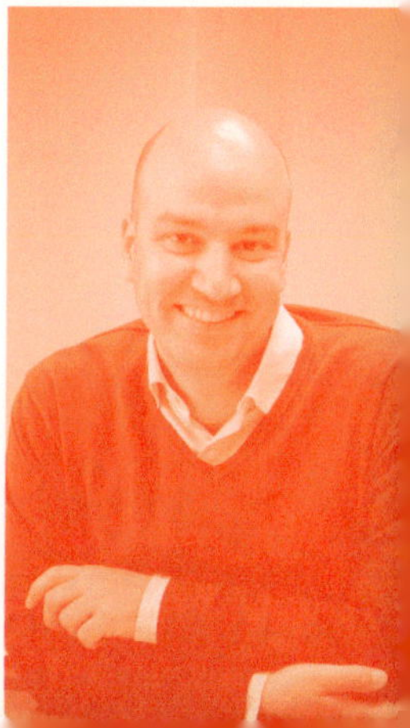

Neuroethics in Principle and Praxis - Conceptual Foundations
http://dx.doi.org/10.5772/intechopen.77614
Edited by Denis Larrivee

Contributors
James Giordano, John Shook, Ahmed Ammar, Michio Nomura, Shoichi Shiota, Simon Smith, Denis Larrivee, Juliana Dias Reis Pessalacia, Jacqueline Resende Boaventura, Ana Paula Da Silva, Luciana Ferreira Da Silva, Adriano Menis Ferreira, Larissa Da Silva Barcelos, Carlos Eduardo Pereira Furlani

First published in London, United Kingdom, 2019 by IntechOpen
IntechOpen is the global imprint of INTECHOPEN LIMITED, registered in England and Wales, registration number: 11086078, The Shard, 25th floor, 32 London Bridge Street
London, SE19SG - United Kingdom
Printed in Croatia

British Library Cataloguing-in-Publication Data
A catalogue record for this book is available from the British Library

Additional hard and PDF copies can be obtained from orders@intechopen.com

Neuroethics in Principle and Praxis - Conceptual Foundations
Edited by Denis Larrivee
p. cm.
Print ISBN 978-1-83962-644-9
Online ISBN 978-1-78984-760-4
eBook (PDF) ISBN 978-1-78984-761-1

For EU product safety concerns:
IN TECH d.o.o., Prolaz Marije Krucifikse Kozulić 3, 51000 Rijeka, Croatia, info@intechopen.com or visit our website at intechopen.com.

Meet the editor

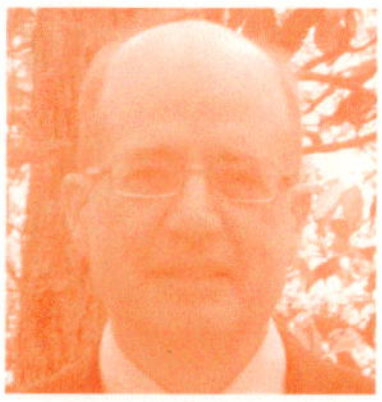

Dr. Denis Larrivee is a visiting scholar at the Mind and Brain Institute, University of Navarra Medical School and Loyola University Chicago, and has held professorships at the Weill Cornell University Medical College, NYC, and Purdue University, Indiana. A former fellow at Yale University's Medical School he received the Association for Research in Vision and Ophthalmology's first place award for studies on photoreceptor degenerative and developmental mechanisms. He is the editor of a recently released text on brain computer interfacing with IntechOpen Publishing and an editorial board member of the journals *Annals of Neurology and Neurological Sciences* (USA) and *EC Neurology* (UK). An International Neuroethics Society Expert he is the author of more than 80 papers and book chapters in such varied journals/venues as *Neurology and Neurological Sciences* (USA), *Journal of Neuroscience*, *Journal of Religion and Mental Health*, and IEEE Explore. In 2018 he was a finalist in the international Joseph Ratzinger Expanded Reason award.

Contents

Preface

Less than 50 years ago, neuroscientific understanding was in its infancy by millennial standards, with no consensus on such basic cell features as signal transduction, membrane channels, most neurotransmitters, synaptic circuits, and the like. In this early milieu there was little need for an ethical discipline that would be uniquely concerned with the nervous system. By 2013, in contrast, neuroscience has advanced well beyond single neuron functions, often touching on the global properties that emerge from central nervous system operation. This new era has seen, for example, the launching of national and continental initiatives in the BRAIN and Human Brain Projects, respectively, not to mention Asian and Latin American initiatives. These projects intend not only to elucidate disease mechanisms, but also to create wholly new technological approaches for exploring higher order function.

Core ethical concerns, in consequence, now touch on such significant and nervous system specific issues as the global regulation of organismal performance, an evolution in intervention that is breaching therapeutic boundaries, supraphysical notions of systemic and organizational reality, and the ontological and anthropological ground for human nature, among others. A frequent ethical theme raised by ever-greater knowledge and technical prowess over organismal regulation, for instance, is the manipulation by and interaction with technological devices, not just in regard to the potential harm that may be incurred by such devices, but also with respect to the very nature of technology and its relation to the human being. New interventional modes, accordingly, need to consider not only traditional ethical principles of medical practice, but also what is meant by health and normality. In this environment, ethical questions related to the nervous system have assumed an immediacy and significance matching the centrality of neural function in biological behavior.

Contributing to this immediacy is the fundamental value of the human being, which lends normative weight to questions, interventions, and practices influencing him or her. Additionally, the value of human well-being—or eudomaia—is of increasing normative significance. In recognition of these twin normative concerns, parallel metaethical principles invoked in such advanced technical fields as artificial intelligence, for example, place primacy on the human being and prioritize the increase of human flourishing.

On the other hand, despite a recognition of the relevance of fundamental human value, the derivation of metaethical principles that underwrite this value is by no means uniformly agreed to and reflects a turbulence in broader metaphysical notions of material reality, among other factors. This dissonance is singularly and uniquely acute in ethical issues related to the nervous system, seen, for example, in the normatively charged issue of death determinations. On the one hand, the human being is regarded as individuated and holistic, with invested value contingent to the human being in his entire corporality. Such a view is adopted in Karol Wojtyla's ethical perspective, and ascribed to in a number of religious traditions. Here the ground for value contingency emerges from the capacity for the performance of the "good," which thereby establishes the personal agent as a value locus, validating the wholly referential status of the person:

"The reality of the person inheres in morality, that morality is a thoroughly specific and connatural reality with respect to the person—with respect precisely to the person and only to the person [...] man as a man, becomes good or evil through the act."

This capacity extends, crucially, to the whole individual by virtue of an integral metaphysical unity that grounds the corporal reality of the personalist subject. Death determinations in this view, for example, reference the whole individual; hence, medical criteria need to encompass the individual as a biological whole. In other perspectives, value contingent properties emerge reductively, where they relate to the function of discrete brain operations. This latter view broadly privileges the value of the brain over that of the body, thereby creating an intrinsic dichotomy within the individual. Death determinations here thus resort to criteria that philosophically equate the human being with the organ of the brain.

Why and how the human being is normatively privileged, accordingly, emerge as core questions that ground questions of ethical praxis related to the nervous system. At its extremes this foundation is characterized by a diametric polarity, where value, on the one hand, is seen to intrinsically emerge from an integral global order that is normatively endowed from above, and, on the other hand, where human value is invested by consensus discourse in the absence of recognition of a unified corporal reality that can anchor metanorms. The introductory chapter explains the philosophical origin of the current dissonance between these extremes. Chapter 2 reflects on the former approach, in which the global order is constituted by a metaphysical principle of unity, which is grounded in a norm-oriented teleology. By adopting postmetaphysical presuppositions in Chapter 3, by contrast, value investment emerges externally from collective accession.

The challenge for developing normative praxis given this philosophical polarity is evidenced by the adjustment in weight given to traditional medical principles, e.g., non-malfeasance and beneficence vs. autonomy, and expressed in documents like Advanced Directives (ADs) that alter the balance among these principles by placing greater emphasis on the right to individual autonomy. Chapter 4 illustrates such a shift in current legislative initiatives for ADs now undertaken in Brazil. Chapter 5 returns this emphasis somewhat to value primacy in the individual by advancing a case for values-based medical care of cognitive disease, in opposition to the functionalist objectives often characterizing evidence-based medicine. Finally, Chapter 6 considers the implication for ethical praxis that occurs when subdomains of the body, e.g., nervous system vs. body, are treated as distinct ethical spheres, rather than mutually and functionally integrated systems.

It is hoped that these chapters will spur greater recognition of the relationship between the philosophical foundations of value contingency in the human body and the neuroethical praxis that flows from this relationship.

Denis Larrivee
Loyola University Chicago,
Chicago, USA,
University of Navarra Medical School,
Pamplona, Spain

Section 1

Introduction and Origins of Neuroethical Tension

Chapter 1

Introductory Chapter: Reconciling Neurobioethics through Nature's Lens - Metaphysical Determinants of Subjectivity

Denis Larrivee

1. Forerunners of neuroethical debate

No more than 5 decades ago, bioethics formally took the stage as an independent discipline. Intended to normatively frame the rapidly growing knowledge of biological function, the appearance of the discipline constituted a normative response to what was viewed as a morally agnostic and scientifically aseptic attitude to the investigative and utilitarian ends of biological research [1]. Inspired by a broader recognition of a science isolated from its "ought to do" dimension, highlighted in contemporaneous debates on nuclear power by such literary elites as Huxley [2], the biological emphasis sought to address a spectrum of concerns, from ecological destruction to biological weaponry and genetic engineering, among others. In coining the term bioethics, accordingly, Van Rensselaer Potter emphasized its scope as the "science of survival" that required the bridging of two cultures, one scientific and the other humanistic and moral. Given the historical context of the Cold War era, Van Rensselaer's proposal resonated broadly in its public recognition, launching bioethics as a widely motivated and widely disciplined undertaking [3].

Nonetheless, and despite the persistent public engagement with issues of ecological misuse and military use of biological capabilities, bioethics has since and relatively quickly come to be viewed as a normative extension of clinical practice. In the evolution introduced by the Dutch obstetrician Andre Hellegers, the object of bioethics was conceived as forging an ethical structure that would give intellectual scope to the ethical dimension already implicit in medical practice. In Hellegers' scheme [4], the science of bioethics was to discover and compile values in a dialog that encircled medicine, philosophy, and ethics, which would take into account the ongoing stream of information emerging from biological discovery and medical technology.

As an intellectual stepchild of ethical practices surrounding the health care of the human being, bioethics is heir to a normative tradition extending to antiquity. Premised on the recognition of the unique value within each individual, medical care has traditionally been guided by principles meant to ensure the preservation of this recognition even in circumstances of significant health risk. While this historical legacy has clearly influenced the modern understanding of bioethics, its recent emergence as an independent discipline underscores its distinction from the former and raises questions regarding underlying factors that have driven the need for its emergence. Beyond issues of the rapidity and magnitude of information acquired at ever-grander scales—which must be adequately assimilated before any therapeutic intervention—emerging core ethical concerns have been especially influenced

IntechOpen

by their contingency to philosophical conceptions that have become increasingly pluralistic. Among these are included an increasing power over the regulation of organismal performance; an evolving conception of intervention as a therapeutic undertaking; supraphysical notions of organismal, organizational reality; and ontological and anthropological conceptions of the physical basis of human nature. A recurring theme raised by ever-greater knowledge and technical prowess over organismal regulation, for example, is the manipulation by and interaction with technological devices that bear not only on limiting their use but also on the very nature of technology and its relation to the human being. New interventional notions thus not only need to include the traditional principles of malfeasance, beneficence, autonomy, and justice but must also incorporate what is meant by health and disease, normality and deviance. Crucially, across a wide swath of the physical sciences, fundamental questions on the nature of physical reality are assuming greater prominence as the recognition of the insufficiency of compositional approaches, which have dominated scientific exploration since Descartes and Newton, impels the consideration of a more synthetic understanding of material reality, like that of entities and their relation to properties. Finally, and critically for the ethics of applied neuroscience, are ontological and anthropological concerns related to human subjectivity and its relation to the objective reality of his corporal presence in the world, concerns that have become especially acute since Heideggerian revisions of metaphysical understanding [5].

Accordingly, bioethics and medical ethics remain the scholarly objects of a philosophical tension introduced and exacerbated by the restless expansion of biological knowledge. This tension originates in the need to appropriate a philosophical conception of physical reality that can then be normatively evaluated. However, with the assimilation of pluralistic notions on the physical reality of the body—which is the direct object of medical or biological intervention—normative principles and ethical praxis themselves remain varied. That is, while ethical praxis is contingent on some action taken toward the corpus, such praxis acquires normative significance only within a conceptual framework of the contingent material reality.

The effect on ethical praxis of assimilating the current conceptual ambiguity is most acute in issues concerned with neural intervention. Indeed, ontological and anthropological tensions uniquely characterize neuro(bio)ethics as a normative discipline, which must confront concerns over the impact of intervention on global and organismal regulations, conceptually addressed in philosophy of science accounts. The uncertainty between how the individual is understood and the physical features inherent in the neural activity of the brain that enable the expression of these human features has marked the field, particularly in its development of meta-ethical principles that correspondingly evolve neuroethical praxis [6, 7]. This text, especially, proposes just such an illustration of the current ambiguity. Accordingly, the following discussion will seek to address this ambiguity by grounding the philosophical accounts in fundamental features of natural reality, articulated through the metaphysical understanding of the ontological subject. This grounding then engages a dialectic with the issues of praxis presented in subsequent chapters.

2. Appropriating a philosophical conception of disease for neurobioethics

2.1 Functionalism

The absence of a reconciliation between philosophical conceptions of physical reality and the neural activity of the brain suggest that interventional praxis may best be related to medical notions of normality and disease that entail empirically accessible parameters. Neurological impairment, especially, is a significant domain of research, with an expanding fund of knowledge on the etiology of various cognitive diseases. Accordingly, in the absence of philosophical reconciliation, viewing neural intervention by the yardstick of disease replication offers a pragmatic means of arriving at normative conclusions.

Implicit in the appropriation of a disease model, nonetheless, is a conceptual interpretation of the disease state, with its understanding of normality and deviation. According to this conception, attributions about disease etiology frequently view disease as malfunction [8] and well being as a commonly observed biological order. Such functionalist notions derive their sense from what is understood of the role of a component system in "normal" operation, where disease etiologies reflect the component system's incapacity to function according to biologically ascertained standards. Normality and variance are therefore set in the context of the malfunctioning of a component's operation, for example, a cardiovascular or retinal lesion where affected anatomical and physiological zones are clearly demarcated.

According to this epistemological approach, a disease is conceived as having a causal origin affecting a specific anatomical or functional domain and generating one or more symptomatic features indicative of the disease state. Hepatitis, for example, is "caused" by the hepatitis virus, which localizes to the liver, where it displays symptoms of fibrosis. Disease states are understood to bridge two domains, one involving empirical judgments about human physiology and another concerned with normative judgments about human well-being [9]. Stated otherwise, notions of normality are articulated through the window of empirical assessment, which is used to delimit functional adequacy. Such judgments thus evoke definitions of normality and deviation that are locally applied to the affected zone. Normative judgments, on the other hand, must be elicited on the empirical judgments to ascertain whether these constitute circumstances that are undesirable or that diminish the capacity for flourishing. Normative conclusions, accordingly, constitute value judgments that are meted out with respect to an objectively accepted value standard for an empirically circumscribed zone. In adopting an analogous approach to the neurobioethics of interventions, there is thus appropriated an empirical methodology used to delimit the range of processes for which normative conclusions may be drawn.

In a Boorsian [8] conception of disease as malfunction, notably, disease features are highly territorialized in their causal structure and zone of influence. Value judgments that are contingent to such narrowly defined empirical assessments, therefore, are restricted to normative judgments on physiological normality, that is, they are primarily conditioned by the normative valuation given to attributions of functional adequacy. In bodily domains outside the nervous system, such as the liver, and even in some brain-based regions such as stroke-related lesions, this value attribution is essentially valid. However, its invocation for many other cognitive diseases, perhaps most, must confront an intrinsic, global regulatory role of the nervous system that is required to regulate organismal properties that define the individual's ontological features.

Accordingly, normative judgments that are narrowly defined by a functionalist interpretation of the disease state, and the ethical praxis that devolves from this understanding, are insufficient for evolving metaethical principles suited to cognitive intervention. Functionalist approaches to cognitive diseases thus lend themselves with difficulty to the elaboration of a comprehensive, neurobioethical praxis, due to the broader organismal role with which the nervous system is associated.

2.2 Cognitive disease and organismal unity

This broader role pertains, minimally, to capacities for unifying organismal operation and goal orientation, that is, integral and teleological features intrinsic to the ontological status of the organisms as a whole. Indeed the widespread recognition of the unique and irreplaceable role of the nervous system in mediating organismal unity has constituted an empirical pillar for philosophical conceptions of bodily integration that underwrite clinical ethics in death determinations [10]. As a fundamental capacity for goal seeking, integration is crucial to human flourishing. Hence, impairing these mechanisms can be expected to diminish this capacity and so evoke normative concern. Cognitive diseases, as mentioned, are especially prone to impairments of these mechanisms, and interventions reproducing effects of the cognitive disease states, either whole or in part, are likely to deleteriously influence them. Accordingly, they are likely to be physical conditions that would be ethically probative.

This is manifestly evident in the limiting case of bodily death, life being predicated on the body's organismal integration. With death, mechanisms of integration are no longer operative, and organismal unity is thereby destroyed. As a conceptual position universally recognized across religious, cultural, and secular scholarship [11], the loss of all organismal unity constitutes a probative, ethical imperative of ultimate and universal significance. This is also to say that while the events of death and the organismal mechanisms that work to unify the organism are physically instantiated, it is in view of the conceptual validity of organismal unity that the normative imperative is validated. By extension, factors that diminish but do not wholly void bodily integration also lessen individual well-being. A reduced capacity for intentional self-action, that is, a hallmark of several widely prevalent cognitive diseases, for example, diminishes autonomy and the satisfaction of individual need. Disturbances of self, for instance, traditionally mark the diagnostic evaluation of the schizophrenia patient [12], seen in an abnormal sense of ownership of the body, loss of ego boundary, and confused sense of self-agency. Such reduced phenomenological capacities have been shown to have their counterpart in physical features of cognition. Imaging modalities reveal, for example, a consistently high correspondence between fMRI modules and those of diffusion imaging in normal individuals, whereas those from schizophrenia patients exhibit both decreases in overall modularity and in correspondence of networks [13]. These diseases illustrate that not only the absence but also the partial impairment of physical processes for organismal integration significantly impact individual flourishing.

Taken together, meta-principles premised on disease and notions of malfunction have a practical but restricted role for evolving neuroethical praxis in the absence of philosophical judgments on global, physical attributes of the individual, of which the integrative and unitive dimension is paramount.

3. The organismal dimension of neurobioethics

3.1 Metaphysical contingency of the neural architecture

Normative conclusions that relate to a global organizational order, on the other hand, resemble ethical approaches that generalize to the individual as a whole, that is, not as an epistemological abstraction only but as a metaphysical conclusion on the natural reality of the individual, who is epistemically evident. These approaches thus distinguish themselves from those that define the human being functionally and that emphasize properties to the exclusion of their source, like that premised on the "stream of consciousness" [7] or that of delocalized essence, like extended mind theory [6]. They are thus also distinguished from an ethical pragmatism that is contingent to notions of disease as malfunction.

Such holistic routes to metaethics typically value the individual as a normative locus that is operative in the world. By virtue of an intrinsic metaphysical unity, they then extend value contingency to the whole of the individual. Neo-Thomistic developments in the twentieth century, like that of Etienne Gilson [14], for example, draw normative value from metaphysical conclusions, prioritizing the notion of presence as action in philosophies of being. Karol Wojtyla's metaphysical approach to ethics [15], for instance, anchors the personalist dimension of intentionalized action in the unitary reality of the whole individual. As a metaethical principle, this dimension appeals to a dual normative contingency present within the individual. The personalist subject is considered, first, as an agent of ethical activity and, second, as an end for the pursuit of the good, that is, as a value contingent locus. Here the appeal is chiefly theoretical and conditioned by the analysis, since bridging these contingencies is the experience of morality in action. Consequently, as a metaethical "object" for ethical praxis, the individual capacity for moral behavior validates the acquisition of a wholly unique, value-laden referential status for the person. Kant, significantly, adopts a strikingly similar perspective, identifying the individual exclusively as an end and not as a means.

In Wojtyla's theoretical exploration, the specific focus entails the phenomenal experience of subjectivity, that is, a cognitive and conscious dimension unique to each individual. His ethical analysis, accordingly, experientially and superficially, resembles ethical approaches that are phenomenologically and functionally driven. Unlike these approaches, however, Wojtyla explicitly views these as epistemological features only and so merely outward indicators of an inner and integral unity that he terms the "human suppositum," that is, a metaphysical essence that is subjectively constituted and phenomenologically manifested.

For ethical praxis this is significant for linking all dimensions of the individual to an integral reality that is phenomenologically expressed. In fact, the absence of such a unifying dynamic leaves ethical praxis inchoate, without either a contingent locus for value or a medium for its execution. Accordingly, the identification of the subject as a metaethical principle thereby extends value to the cognitive dynamics and physical organization of the neural architecture also. Indeed, it is on the basis of the integral unity of the individual that he later cautions in *Veritatis Splendor* [16] "against a manipulation of corporeity that would alter its human meaning." For neuroethics, the utility of this metaphysical conclusion thus relates directly to the contribution of the nervous system to the unity of the person, that is, as a corporal manifestation that is enabling to a human ontological, subjective, and integrative order. In other words, by invoking the unity of the uniquely human subject, the metaphysical subject identifies in the neural operation a normative terrain.

3.2 The metaphysical subject as an ordering principle for the neural architecture

3.2.1 Integration and systemic operation

The reality of the metaphysical subject is evident through the objective manifestation of the phenomenal subject; that is, it is a reality apparent through epistemological inference. Importantly, the absence of direct empirical confirmation does not imply the absence of the subject's reality, which can be seen in the variety of human functions that are nonetheless united in each individual. The subject's epistemic appearance thus reveals the role of the metaphysical subject to be the physical realization of the integral and uniquely human subject.

This role is apparent first in a unified organizational order that is operationally confined, which is to say that the metaphysical subject is seen through the reality of organismal integration. Its dynamic unity, for instance, is a fundamental feature shaped by evolutionary forces [17]. As one entity in an adaptive space, the organism constitutes a "unit of interaction" [18] where the whole organism is molded by evolutionary pressures to acquire a suite of behavioral features maximizing its fitness.

The subject's neural "manifestation," accordingly, is not autonomously determined but is shaped by an extrinsic metaphysical order that is determinative for its expression. Indeed, it is generally recognized that material reality is subject to immaterial priors, for example, organizational principles. Recognition of these externally imposed orders can be seen in the need to invoke non-causal explananda in natural design, like the accounts used to explain the design of flagellar motors [19]. These immaterial determinants are even more apparent in the case of neural operation, where dynamic brain activity is necessarily linked to a system-wide network that subsumes regional activity to global performance [20].

Because such metaphysical determinants are only epistemically evident, however, empirically elucidating the physical mechanisms of integration becomes key to a principled neuroethical praxis. In consequence, praxis remains subject to both empirical and philosophy of science accounts for its evolution. For integration, the reconciliation of these accounts has been the subject of much debate. Although the reality of integration is evident in the natural world, its conceptual articulation through philosophy of science accounts has restricted the choice of hypothetical presuppositions used to define empirical resources. This has exposed current accounts of integration to factual inconsistencies and delayed the evolution of more realistic and comprehensive frameworks.

The somatic integrity thesis, for example, which has served as the conceptual platform for clinical determinations of death, invokes a causal, brain-directed model of integration, through which the functioning of the body's varied physiological systems is coordinated [21]. According to this understanding of integration, ethical practice is contingent on the empirical demonstration of an irreversible loss of the capacity to maintain cohesive and coordinative function, the causal origin of which is identified with the brain. Loss of brain function is therefore equated with loss of the capacity. This conception now constitutes the philosophical linchpin for what has become a global clinical praxis. Probative actions, in consequence, such as the removal of vital organs, are defined in reference to the loss of a single organ, the brain.

Its validity, however, is challenged by a number of empirical observations following a diagnosis of brain failure, including continued heart and whole body circulation [22], wound healing, temperature regulation, and even pregnancies [23]. These apparent contraindications, claims of technological artifacts notwithstanding, thus raise the issue of the nature of the brain's relation to bodily processes and so how this relation impacts the physical conception of the death event.

The challenge to the somatic integrity thesis, in fact, retrieves a systemic notion of integration, where the source of integration is understood to be delocalized and distributed within and throughout the body rather than being confined to a single anatomical region. Such a conception of unity substantially differs from the strict causal notion of imposed control used to achieve an aggregate coordinative order. By siting its origin to a single organ within the individual, the latter notion has the conceptual and diagnostic effect of segregating the brain from the body's remainder, physically, hierarchically, and functionally. Normatively, this division has created a chasm between the brain and body where the brain has acquired a valued status and the body's remainder has been relegated to a dependency on the brain's vital operation. The empirical contraindications thus evidence a form of integration that more closely resembles an integral unity shared equally by all material components and processes of the body, *that is, a form of integration more closely corresponding with the metaphysical notion of unity invoked by Wojtyla. This altered conception has the important normative consequence of valuing the individual as a whole*. Importantly, it reveals how the understanding of normative value is itself influenced by the epistemic order of the material body.

Considerable neuroscientific evidence favoring a systemic model of bodily integration has in fact now been gathered, particularly with regard to motor dynamics. Existing studies reveal, for instance, that peripheral and central nervous system activities mutually and reciprocally contribute to integration at multiple levels. These largely plastic influences have been shown to be progressively and hierarchically scaled within the nervous system to (1) shape inward and outward flow between the brain and body, (2) generate stable representations of bodily interaction with the world, and (3) yield a dynamic, bodily integrated performance unit.

These studies underscore the unity of the body by showing that bodily sensory input molds connectivity patterns in the brain to shape the brain's responses to afferent input, that is, the body is responsible for configuring the brain's reaction to sensory information; the functional outcome of this molding is to modulate the brain's "perception" of the world as a function of the body [24], that is, to unify bodily responses to external events with respect to the whole individual.

The generation of the bodily percept appears to unify the body for performance [25]; that is, the percept is generated to unify action as originating from a single source. Accordingly, the dynamic nature of this process precludes the functional segregation of the events of the body from those of the brain. The need to achieve unity in performance, accordingly, implies that the perception of the world through the body requires the integration that is effected by the dynamical and reciprocal relations between the body and brain, *that is, a delocalized source of unity*, which relates the body to the world and which is fundamental to its interaction with it.

3.3 The metaphysical subject and higher-order properties

Nonetheless, the delocalization that distinctively characterizes systemic forms leaves unexplained the presence of goal-directed behavior that is essential to autonomous living and the relation of such behavior to the mediation of systemic unity. Notions of integration premised on a systemic model, notably, fail to account for higher order (i.e., organismal and not merely cellular and organic, organizational, and behavioral) properties constitutive of multicellular organisms generally and of humans with highly evolved nervous systems, in particular. This is also to say that while systemic models are consonant with the holistic character of living organisms [19], they do not account for autonomous behavior [26] and so are unable to account for a material realization of ontology. Such an explanation is crucial for neurobioethics in order to identify an empirically salient source of material processes undergirding ontology and structuring a systemic model of integration. The account for the "emergence" of ontology in fact is likely to conciliate with intrinsic metaphysical features of natural reality, like the relational and communicative features described by Etienne Gilson [15], *that is, these intrinsic features are fundamental determinants for the ontological form that is generated. In particular, they yield the most advanced expression of physical reality, the subjective entity, which, accordingly, is constituted as a metaphysical reality, as noted by Wojtyla*. Indeed, neuroscientific evidence on the phenomenal subject is consonant with a role for their metaphysical evocation.

Critically, empirical studies indicate that higher-order properties emerge from the corpus as a whole and that these properties implement organismal integration, here understood as an outcome of intentional, goal-oriented behavior. Accordingly, the integral unity of the individual is directly attributed to the autonomy of the intentional subject. Drawing from Mossio and Moreno's theoretical account of organismal autonomy, notably, human ontological faculties share a profound intimacy with the body [27] both mediating bodily integration [28, 29] and sustaining life. As predicable properties of the whole, that is, emerging for the "good of the whole organism" [17], such properties are intimately linked to processes both influencing and influenced by its extended organizational form, and so are manifest in the mutually constraining influences of the peripheral and central nervous system. In other words, higher-order properties emerge from the body as a whole where they unify the body through intended global actions, including self-identity, agency, and consciousness, and so mediate a delocalized, systemic mode of integration.

The need for the emergence of these properties from the body can be seen in the case of self-identity and understood as an ability to differentiate the physical breadth that is subsumed by processes belonging to itself from those of the contiguous environment. An organism like *Caenorhabditis elegans*, for example, must identify this range through the dynamical operation of its neural architecture [30], which regulates individual motor movements in reference to this global activity. In humans this perception of self has also been shown to be a process arising from afferent, somatotopic input of the whole body [27]; indeed, in the body's absence, there would be no percept.

Similarly, the ability to initiate actions by oneself requires that these be stably linked to the self-percept [25] now known to entail a neural dynamic termed the motor image [31]. As currently understood the motor image constitutes a covert action undertaken only mentally and as a simulation of a non-executed action. That is, the motor image contains the feature elements of a motor trajectory and so contains the projected series of motions that are prospective for execution. Insights drawn from the motor image reveal that bodily representation is a key feature that frames the elements of the plan as teleologically oriented, that is, one that inscribes actions linking an agent with an objective destination. So inscribed, actions are thereby executed as a coherent and coordinated dynamical ensemble, which have a causal origin linked to the whole individual. Accordingly, features of the motor plan entail mutual though distinct contributions from peripheral as well as central origins, underscoring the essential unity of dynamic performance even in its covert formulation, and directing it toward a unique goal.

Consciousness, likewise situates as a global property enable both responsible action and the execution of higher faculties. Current insights suggest a decentralized physical origin [32], where the body contributes to the emergence of consciousness in at least two ways, by (1) creating a generalized platform that sustains a phenomenological background of mental awareness and (2) stimulating its focal emergence. Together these results argue for a complex but nonetheless shared participation of brain and body in eliciting and sustaining all higher order properties, that is, *a unified and delocalized source of bodily emergence*.

4. The advancing future: prospects for neurobioethics from a metaphysics of subjectivity

As noted, for Wojtyła, it is the dimension of metaphysics that situates the ethics of the personalist subject, where the person "constitutes a privileged locus for the encounter with being, and hence with metaphysical inquiry." In the Wojtyłan formulation, the normative value of the personalist subject thus emerges from its metaphysical and immaterial mooring, constituting the ground for its physical instantiation and the essential metaethical dimension for neuroethical praxis.

Accordingly, it grounds his claim against "dehumanizing" corporal intervention. In doing so it has a direct bearing on the construction of ethical standards that are probative, that is, the construction of normative statements that pertain to actionable standards that would or would not infringe on a specifically human meaning.

By contrast, prevailing models of the subject that are a legacy of Cartesian metaphysics, challenge, the specifically human meaning of the personalist subject that flows from his ontological primacy in the order of being. It is a challenge, moreover, also directed to the understanding of material reality. As Gillett has pointed out [33], what is evident in current debates over the nature of material reality is the extent to which the Cartesian segregation of immaterial and material dimensions and the invocation of a strictly causal model of relations suffice for ontic adequacy, that is, whether materialism alone or dualism offer adequate explananda to account for the material order. The debate on physical reality has significant repercussions in the ethical sphere, with normative consequences that impact neuroethical praxis and leads, increasingly, to dehumanizing tendencies.

How metaphysics grounds ethical praxis, accordingly, is a critical dimension often ignored in debates about human nature and its modification that are exacerbated by the advent of neuro and genetic technologies. The culmination of a multistaged metaphysical divorce has transpired since Descartes; however, its current understanding has left efficient causal and mechanistic commitments to drive the prevailing materialism of modern neuroscience, leaving a decompositional and reductive philosophy to determine how brain operation is interpreted for the foreseeable future. *Presuppositions invoked by these efforts belie the consilience with neuroscience that is more evident in Wojtyła's proposal.* Crucially, the need to account for the emergence of subjectivity from the material order, that is, the hallmark of the neural architecture, is left unexplained by the Cartesian metaphysical segregation. The ferment in current efforts to explain the reality of the brain and mind, however, indicates that modern metaphysical presuppositions that undergird neuroethics are in a process of flux. The current uncertainty surrounding the metaphysical status of subjectivity, therefore, suggests that the Wojtyłan metaphysical subject may open a new window on the objective reality of the subjective mind that will offer surer philosophical ground for neurobioethics.

Author details

Denis Larrivee
University of Navarra, Spain

*Address all correspondence to: sallar1@aol.com

References

[1] Potter VR. Global Bioethics: Building on the Leopold Legacy. East Lansing: Michigan University Press; 1988

[2] Huxley A. Science, Liberty, and Peace. New York: Harper and Brothers Publishers; 1947

[3] Reich WT. The word 'bioethics': The struggle over its earliest meanings. Kennedy Institute of Ethics Journal. 1995;**5**(**1**):19-34

[4] Sgreccia E. Personalist Bioethics: Foundations and Applications. Milan: Vita e Pensiero; 2007

[5] Rae G. Heidegger's influence on posthumanism: The destruction of metaphysics, technology, and the overcoming of anthropocentrism. History of Human Sciences. 2014;**27**(1):51-69

[6] Levy N. Neuroethics and the extended mind. In: Iles J, Sahakian B, editors. The Oxford Handbook of Neuroethics. Oxford; 2011

[7] Parfit D. Another defense of the priority view. Utilitas. 2012;**24**(3):399-440

[8] Boorse C. On the distinction between disease and illness. Philosophy and Public Affairs. 1975;**5**:49-68

[9] Thagard P. How Scientists Explain Disease. Princeton: Princeton University Press; 1999

[10] Bernat JL. The biophilosophical basis of whole-brain death. Social Philosophy and Policy. 2002;**19**(2):324-342

[11] Jones DA. Loss of faith in brain death: Catholic controversy over the determination of death by neurological criteria. Clinical Ethics. 2012;7(3):133-141

[12] Hur JW, Kwon JS, Lee TY, Park S. The crisis of minimal self-awareness in schizophrenia: A meta-analytic review. Schizophrenia Research. 2014;**152**: 58-64

[13] Alexander-Bloch A et al. The discovery of population differences in network community structure: New methods and applications to brain functional networks in schizophrenia. NeuroImage. 2012;**59**:3889-3900

[14] Clarke WN. Person and Being. Vol. 8. Milwaukee: Marquette University Press; 1993

[15] Wojtyła K. Man in the Field of Responsibility. Vatican City Press; 1991

[16] John Paul II. Veritatis Splendor. Vatican City: Vatican City Press; 1993

[17] Hooker CA. Interaction and bio-cognitive order. Synthese. 2008;**166**:513-546

[18] Maturana HR, Varela FJ. Autopoiesis and Cognition. Boston: Reidel Publishing; 1979

[19] Braillard PA. Systems biology and the mechanistic framework. History Philosophy of Life. Science. 2010;**32**(1):43-62

[20] Friston K. Free energy and global dynamics. In: Rabinovich M, Friston KJ, Varona P, editors. Principles of Brain Dynamics. London: MIT Press; 2013. pp. 261-292

[21] Swedish committee death Swedish Committee on Defining Death. The Concept of Death. Summary. Stockholm: Swedish Ministry of Health and Social Affairs; 1984

[22] Verheijde JL, Rady MY, McGregor JL. Brain death, states of impaired consciousness, and physician-assisted

death for end-of-life organ donation and transplantation. Medicine, Health Care, and Philosophy. 2009;**12**:409-421

[23] Shewmon DA. The brain and somatic integration: Insights into the standard biological rationale for equating "brain death" with death. The Journal of Medicine and Philosophy. 2001;**26**(5):457-478

[24] Moya P. Habit and embodiment in Merleau-Ponty. Frontiers in Human Neuroscience. 2014. DOI: 10.3389/fnhum.2014.00542

[25] Smith L. Stability and flexibility in development. In: Spencer J, Thomas MSC, McClelland JL, editors. Toward a Unified Theory of Development. Oxford: Oxford University Press; 2009

[26] Moreno A, Mossio M. Biological Autonomy: A Philosophical and Theoretical Inquiry. Dordrecht: Springer Publishing; 2015

[27] Damasio A. Self Comes to Mind: Constructing the Conscious Brain. San Francisco: Pantheon Books; 2012

[28] Corbetta D. Brain, body, and mind: Lessons from infant motor development. In: Spencer J, Thomas MSC, McClelland JL, editors. Toward a Unified Theory of Development. Oxford: Oxford University Press; 2009. pp. 51-56

[29] Sandamirskaya Y, Zibner SKU, Schneegan S, Schoner G. Using dynamic field theory to extend the embodiment stance toward higher cognition. New Ideas in Psychology. 2013;**31**:322-339

[30] Kato S, Kaplan HS, Schrodel T, et al. Global brain dynamics embed the motor command sequence of *Caenorhabditis elegans*. Cell. 2015;**163**:656-669

[31] Jeannerod M. Levels of representation of goal directed action. In: Freund HJ, Jeannerod M, Hallett M, Leiguarda R, editors. Higher Order Motor Disorders. Oxford: Oxford University Press; 2005

[32] Dehaene S. Consciousness and the Brain: Deciphering How the Brain Codes Our Thoughts. New York: Penguin Group; 2015

[33] Gillett C. Reduction and Emergence in Science and Philosophy. Cambridge: Cambridge University Press; 2016. p. 2016

Section 2

Metaphysical Sources of Value Uncertainty

Chapter 2

Doing and Being: A Metaphysic of Persons from an Ontology of Action

Simon Smith

Abstract

A significant and worrying lacuna lies at the heart of neuroethics: viz., a coherent conception of personal identity. Philosophically, the consequences are serious; morally, they are disastrous. The entire discourse is constrained by a narrow empiricism, oblivious to its own metaphysical and epistemological presuppositions; worse still, it remains hostage to a latent Cartesianism, which logically and ontologically isolates neuroethicists from their subjects. Little wonder neuroethics lacks an anchor for its normative judgements. This chapter aims to supply that anchor. The key lies in action: action as essentially personal; acts owned; acts intended; and acts that embody those intentions that embody *meaning*. Such acts are the primary manifestation of 'personhood'; they are also socially oriented, therefore morally interesting. Action locates persons in a world of objects and, most importantly, others. Crucially, relocating neuroethics within this context of personal activity supplies the logical and ontological foundations for both its judgements and its participants.

Keywords: action, agency, anti-metaphysical, applied metaphysics, Austin Farrer, intending, intentionality, interaction, interpersonal, Ludwig Feuerbach, neuroethics, personal identity, personalism, personalist metaphysics, persons

1. Introduction

A significant and worrying lacuna lies at the heart of neuroethical debate. What it lacks is the anchor of a *desideratum*: namely, a full and proper understanding of persons. Given that persons and personal relations are the neuroethicist's primary subjects, both of observation and judgement, this is no minor omission. Philosophically, its consequences are serious; morally, they are disastrous. They leave neuroethics caught on the prongs of a fork quite as uncomfortable as any David Hume might proffer. On one side, the entire discourse is constrained by a kind of empiricism, narrowly reductive and oblivious to its own metaphysical and epistemological presuppositions; an empiricism constituted not by controlled experiment but by the products of an outdated and radically abstract rationalism-cum-realism. On the other, and pointing uncomfortably in the opposite direction, is a latent Cartesianism that logically and ontologically isolates the neuroethicist from her subjects. Ultimately, both sides can only end by eliminating the moral subject, so drive the discourse into literal non-sense. Little wonder, then, that neuroethics lacks an anchor for its normative judgements.

This chapter aims to supply that anchor, to articulate a conception of persons that will overcome this piercingly divisive dichotomy. It does so, not by privileging one side over the other; a pointless exercise in any event, since neither one is coherent and, besides, they terminate in the coinciding of reductive and flattened abstractions with inflationary, transcendentalised ones. Rather, the dichotomy is overcome by a conception of consciousness grounded in action: action as essentially personal; actions owned, intended; actions that embody those intentions, embody *meaning*. Such actions are the most fundamental manifestation of 'personhood.' They are also socially oriented, therefore morally interesting. Action locates persons in a world of objects and, most importantly, others. Crucially, locating neuroethics within this context of personal activity supplies the logical and ontological foundations for both its judgements and its participants.

It is in this empirical sense—the philosophically well-brought-up reader may be reassured to learn—that our conception of persons is to be understood as metaphysical. Our aim, in short, is not to critique the neurosciences or rebut their discoveries. It is no part of our case to deny the role played by understanding the brain and brain-function in understanding consciousness and 'personhood.' We wish, rather, simply to demonstrate that—if we may be forgiven—there is more to persons than meets the fMRI.

Personal action is ontologically primitive; it is also empirically, which is to say experientially, irrefragable. I cannot deny the reality of my actions without self-stultification, let alone self-contradiction; no more can I deny the actions of others, actions in which my own are but one ingredient. Action is the foundation, the condition, of experience, so meets Ockham's razor, edge to edge. As such, action is also *anti*-metaphysical. It refutes absolutely those classical abstractions that claim existence beyond or apart from our experience, the being or essence, secure in its ontological priority, which, having no effect upon us, makes no claim on our knowledge.

Put simply, personal action is an anti-metaphysical metaphysics. As such, it is also an *applied* metaphysics. It supplies the clue to real existence, such as the ephemera of mere appearance and classical being-concepts cannot do. In the words of the Oxford philosopher and theologian, Austin Farrer, *esse est operari*: to be is to act, better still, to *inter*act [1, p. 21].

There is one further point before embarking on the discussion proper. What follows operates solely from a philosophical perspective; for it is this perspective, we are reliably informed, that neuro*ethics* most sorely needs. As such, we hope to introduce to current neuroethical debates several thinkers with whom the reader may be unfamiliar but who may, nevertheless, have a valuable contribution to make.

2. Empiricism, realism, and absence

Let us begin with an account, in general terms, of the philosophical problem circumscribed by this lacuna in the discourse.

It is tempting, at first, to state the obvious and assert that the dichotomy threatening to tear neuroethics asunder is a product of reductive physicalism or philosophical materialism. Such reductivism is, after all, characteristic of the scientific method that determines the course of neuroscience and so must inform the neuroethicist's outlook. In consequence, said neuroethicist will inevitably identify consciousness with the neurological, i.e. physical, processes mapped by fMRI scans and, therefore, persons with brains. All this may be true. And yet, we would do well to remember that the obvious does not always stand on solid philosophical ground; besides which, the assertion is easily countered.

During the last century, the physical sciences have seen such extraordinary—one might even say *miraculous*—advances in almost every area of human knowledge that their efficacy is not seriously to be gainsaid. The origins and nature of our species, of the universe, of life itself, have been brought within the purview of human understanding, thanks in no small part to the rigorous and systematic application of scientific method. That method's powers of description and prediction have repeatedly and with remarkable consistency proved their worth; that the exercise of such powers stands firmly upon evidence which can, by and large, be replicated and validated surely settles the matter. Under the circumstances, it is difficult to imagine what more scientific method and its practitioners could reasonably do to demonstrate their epistemic credentials.

So much for tilting at windmills. In reality, we surrender to that first temptation and point our superior philosophical finger at the neuroscientist, only to commit the very mistake we accuse her of, thereby reinforcing an already apparently intractable conflict between two different modes of thinking. Fortunately, it is an important principle of our anti-metaphysical metaphysics that pointing fingers point in two directions at once: acts unfold in consequences, so identify the objects on which they bear; simultaneously, however, they reveal intentions and, crucially, the agent of intentions. The root of the problem, that is, lies not in a faulty science, but in bad philosophy; our obvious assertion is itself symptomatic of the very confused and erroneous thinking that gives rise to the problem. We have, in short, transformed method into metaphysic, and a wholly incompatible metaphysic at that.

The results are incompatible because the transformation issues in some form of realism. It is not, perhaps, that naïve realism which supposes, in Russell's pithy phrase, 'things are what they seem.' Nevertheless, it is close cousin to that self-same 'plebeian illusion' which Einstein described, 'according to which things "are" as they are perceived by us through our senses;' excepting that, in this instance, experiment and observation substitute for sensory perceptions [2, p. 20]. In fact, this substitution means that our method-cum-metaphysic mirrors most closely Peter Byrne's 'innocent realism' [3]. This, we are told, 'merely reflects on the content of our empirical claims, notes that most of them do not speak about how the world looks from a human perspective and concludes that the world, its things and properties, is for the most part independent of us and our representations' [3, p. 40]. That we do not articulate our presuppositions, it does not, of course, follow that there are none to articulate. However, the point is clear: no matter what the epistemic medium may be, we are still claiming to identify, to know about, a world that lies, logically and ontologically, beyond the reach of any actual or possible experience.

Any such claim must prove deeply problematic for the empirically minded, not least because it marks an attempt to found scientific knowledge on that which is *a priori* unknowable.[1] The realist claim to know the world as it is *in itself* is one for which no evidence, for or against, can be found. We do not have the epistemic tools needed to "get behind" our experiences even to establish *that* such a world exists, let alone what it might be like. Logically speaking, therefore, the claim is evidently not false as such, but meaningless. To gloss over such implications, as Byrne does, with an airy expression such as 'minimally dualist' cannot help us [3, p. 35]. Minimal or maximal, it makes no difference; the breech is opened between our experience of the world and the world as it *really* is.

Per contra, empirical investigation deals in the products of experience; scientific method, in those of experiment. Those products are, in effect, maps of the physical

---

[1] The realist is faced with, in Farrer's words, 'an X absolutely undefined;' and so must answer the question, 'How do I know that it is not the snort of a hippopotamus or the left great toe of an archangel or the taste of asparagus?' [4, p. 88].

universe, diagrams, not of the world as it is *in se*, but as it is diagrammatisable: known and knowable by those who explore and explain it. This may seem clearest in those fields, such as quantum physics and speculative cosmology, where mathematics is the *lingua franca*. It should, perhaps, be clearer still in those where computer modelling has become a vital tool, as in the cognitive and, specifically, neurosciences themselves.

Those maps, models, and diagrams are endowed with objectivity by the formulation and application of rules for their construction, rules that constitute the theoretical framework within which any scientific enquiry must be pursued. The more completely and systematically those rules can be defined, the more likely it is they will supply objective facts; but they are not and cannot be 'independent of us and our representations' as the realist imagines. They are objective insofar as they overcome the limitations of the individual enquirer's perspective by abstracting from the subjective immediacy of ordinary sense experience. As the philosopher and physical chemist, Michael Polanyi explained, rules disregard the individual's 'normal approach to experience,' so remain 'unaffected by the state of the person accepting... [them].' They come 'between our senses and the things of which our senses otherwise would have gained a more immediate impression,' so regulate the organisation and interpretation of those impressions. What is more, and in some ways more important, those rules are open to evaluation by all those qualified and equipped to do so: viz., the community of enquirers. Hence, their objectivity is underwritten by universal acceptance: the acceptance of all those participating in scientific research, whatever their field [5, pp. 3–4].

To suggest, as we have done, that empiricism and metaphysical realism are incompatible may be strictly true, but it is also, in one rather limited sense, somewhat misleading. In fact, there comes a point within the rationalist's abstract conceptualising when the opportunity arises for, not merely for compatibility, but for full-blown coincidence. This is the precise point at which realism becomes idealism and vice versa.

For realism, the point arrives when it finally acknowledges the implications of its supposedly 'minimal dualism': 'how we say things are is one thing, how things *really* are is another' [3, p. 115]. Empiricism, by contrast, reaches this point when it conceives itself as a kind of phenomenalism or sense datum theory. In search of absolute objectivity, it adopts the pose of the passive observer, there only to discover that its 'only contact with objects, and with the world of physical things, is through perception, in which objects are presented to...[the] passive mind' [6, p. 50].[2] Stuart Hampshire called this the 'deepest mistake in empiricist theories descending from Berkeley and Hume;' that is, the 'representation of human beings as passive observers receiving impressions from "outside" of the mind, where the "outside" includes their own bodies' [6, p. 47]. Faced, not with real things, but only appearances, phenomena, the products of our sensory apparatus, the empiricist, like the realist, is forced to admit that 'we know nothing about that part of the world existing independently of us' [3, p. 44].

The root cause of this metaphysical mistake lies in the assumption that the neuroscientist's models and diagrams obtain a precise correspondence with the objects modelled and diagrammatised. In representing the biochemical processes of the brain, it is supposed, the fMRI scanner supplies a literal image of, not the corollary of consciousness, but of consciousness itself. Persons, then, are at most a product of, and at least equivalent to, those biochemical processes.

2 See also Farrer: 'Abuse of the analogy between sight and understanding is one of the great philosophical delusions' [7, p. 29].

The difficulties that beset such reductive conceptualising are both numerous and notorious; not least, is the tendency to eliminate the moral subject, thereby rendering the whole neuroethical debate redundant. There is little profit to be had from arguing about the moral properties and capabilities of physical processes which are incapable of choice and therefore of responsibility. Any attempt to do so can be no more than anthropomorphic projection: the imaginative conception of impersonal forces as personal ones, which are themselves, we must remember, reducible to the very forces being imaginatively conceived. The rank confusion and, indeed, circularity, entailed by such a move is, we trust, entirely obvious.

A more serious problem, however, may be that equating persons to sheer physical process threatens to eliminate the possibility of meaningful discourse. It does so because, in and of themselves, physical processes do not possess logical properties. The firing of neurones may occur or it may not, but such an event cannot be *true* or *false*. There is, as Farrer points out, 'no physical act... which consists in [affirming or] negating,' [8, p. 41] only the actualising of one particular process or another, the impact of one force or another. Determine conscious, personal actions, such as the forming of hypotheses or the performing of experiments, as nothing but physical processes functioning according to causal regularities, however, and we refute the 'whole assumption of logical study. In effect, we deny that 'meaning governs the formation of discourse' [8, p. 79]. Not only does this put paid to all forms of systematic enquiry, such as the sciences and philosophy, it leaves us, as P.F. Strawson pointed out, unable to explain the meaning or function of personal pronouns such as 'I' and 'my', 'you' and 'your' [9, p. 98]. The realist, in short, lacks the means to identify herself or anyone else.

It is worth repeating, for clarity's sake, that it is not the reductive materialism, so called, of the neuroscientist or her *methodology* at fault here; it is the realism of the philosopher. The moral and metaphysical consequences of that are quite serious enough to be going on with, not least because they tempt us into that latent Cartesianism alluded to at the beginning of this chapter.

Put simply, the neuroscientist may, if she chooses, conceive of the subjects of her research in purely physical terms, but she cannot conceive herself in the same way. Deny this, and she must concede that her own descriptions of neurological phenomena and all the activities that give rise to them are themselves purely physical phenomena. As such, they must be governed by the same laws of cause and effect that govern all other physical phenomena. There can be no exceptions: the formulation of hypotheses, the devising and performing of experiments to test them, the analysing of results; the sharing of ideas: none of these events can be governed by meaning.

But that is absurd. The neuroscientist's experiments do not occur, either by accident, or as a function of causal impacts; no more than do the institutions in which neuroscientists work. They are intended activities that some*one*—as opposed to some*thing*—*meant* to do.[3] Their enactment is governed, as all personal actions are governed, by the ideas being expressed and explored; specifically, they are governed by the meaning of the terms in which they and the methodology used for exploring them are expressed. Ultimately, they are governed by the rules, the conventions and traditions, of the scholarly community to which the neuroscientist belongs. That is the social and intellectual framework in which her work is undertaken and without which would not be possible, let alone meaningful. Logically speaking, then, what is true of persons and brains in general cannot be true of the neuroscientist herself in

[3] See Robert Spaemann: '[t]o be 'someone' is not a property of a thing, whether animate or inanimate; it is not a predicate of some previously identified subject. Whatever we identify, is identified either as someone or as something from the word go' [10, p. 237].

particular. To avoid self-contradiction, she must, as Farrer put it, take herself 'clean out of the system of nature' [8, p. 79].[4] She cannot be physical as the subjects of her research are physical because physicality reduces to causal uniformity. *Ontologically* speaking, therefore, she must conceive of herself as utterly unlike the persons and brains found in her neuroscientific descriptions. She is, by necessity, a different order of being.

Having styled herself, no doubt unwittingly, after Descartes' *res cogitans*, the neuroscientist-cum-neuroethicist finds herself without a physical *modus operandi*: i.e. a body. She has logically and ontologically disconnected from her sensory apparatus and, consequently, all conceivable objects of experience. Her thoughts, then, whatever they may be about, have no experiential content; what remains but thought thinking itself in isolation? Most poignantly, perhaps, her thoughts can have no moral content either, for she has neither means nor opportunity to encounter moral selves. She cannot, in fact, even be sure that any others *like herself* exist, as Descartes himself memorably observed [11, p. 85]. Finally, and perhaps worst of all, along with her physicality, she has surrendered even the most basic forms of *self*-reference and *self*-knowledge. In abstraction from its *modus operandi*, thought thinking itself lacks the 'directedness' or 'aboutness', which makes it what it is. In abstraction, consciousness cannot act deliberately or intentionally. The attempt to preserve some notion of meaningful activity from physical reduction has backfired. Real relations have been surrendered to arbitrary connections, the random collisions and mutual modifications of impersonal forces: no consciousness required. Echoing Hampshire, the neuroscientist is forced to admit that 'I do not know how I would identify myself as a disembodied being and I do not know what this hypothesis means' ([6], p. 50; see also [9], p. 102).

The bridge between consciousness and the world is broken. We no longer have the means to identify other persons or even ourselves, let alone effect any kind of moral impact. The question we must face, then, is this: under such circumstances of Cartesian ego-isolation, what, in the end, is neuroethics actually *about*?

3. Empiricism, action, and presence

To answer that question, we need only return to our empirical starting point. Consciousness must be reconnected with the world; an easy task since we have, the sciences remind us, the very tools to hand. As Ludwig Feuerbach put it, 'the necessity of this connection is only sensation' [12, p. 52]. So saying, Feuerbach admonishes us to reject the demand for mind-independent reality and turn instead to those engaged in exploring and explaining the world, those for whom '[t]ruth, reality and sensation are identical' [12, p. 51]. Only there we shall find the conditions of real knowledge. In their activities, he argued, we may plainly see that '[o]nly a sensuous being is a true and real being. Only through the senses and not through thought for [or in] itself is an object given in a true sense.' Crucially, we must be as rigorous as Feuerbach in the application of this principle, so insist that 'not only the external

[4] This, as Farrer observed, gives rise to a whole host of curious questions, not the least of which concerns the place of the neuroscientist herself in evolutionary history. How, that is, did the neuroscientist's own mind evolve? Since it is no longer a feature of the natural universe, neither is it subject to the requirements of 'natural utility' or 'survival value' as these terms are currently understood. According to Farrer, it seems that the neuroscientist can only consider the existence of her own mind as being some kind of 'treat' or gift bestowed upon her by nature. Such a supposition, however, evidently requires the kind and degree of personification of the natural world that is hardly tenable [8, p. 78].

but also the internal, not only the flesh but also the mind, not only the object but also the ego are objects of the senses' [12, p. 58].

That 'sensuousness' lays the foundations for a more cogent and, ultimately, altogether practical epistemology. At the same time, it provides the terms for constructing—or perhaps more accurately, *construing*—an empirically sound metaphysics. According to Marx Wartofsky, the key to both epistemology and metaphysics may be found in a 'much-inflated yet workaday German expression' [13, p. 18]. With it, he argues, Feuerbach could unlock the significance of sensuousness and sensory experience while resisting the Cartesian lure to transform empiricism into phenomenalism and physical reduction into realism. In Feuerbach's hands, that is, sensory experience is not 'to be understood...on the "observer" or "perceiving subject" or "spectator" model of [traditional or simple] empiricist epistemology.' By extension, consciousness is neither 'a conglomerate of physical atoms, nor...a bundle of sense impressions' [13, p. 5]. Rather, Feuerbach's empiricism, his sense and sensibility, points to a conception or 'model of a being that is already involved in the world by its very nature. The context of *sensation* is therefore this primary involvement, this *Dasein*' [13, p. 377].

While it is perfectly true that, for Feuerbach as for Heidegger, '[t]o-be-here [*Dasein*] is the primary being, the primary determination,' [12, p. 61] this *Dasein* is not, *nota bene*, that later and better known manifestation: Heidegger's neutral substrate, which apparently lacks the virtue of being any particular being, any particular where; in David's Jasper's words, 'not...my being or any specific "being"... [but] simply "being there" in the universe' [14, p. 104]. Contrariwise, Feuerbach's *Dasein* is a philosophical baseline, for *Dasein* or 'being *here*' is active existence. Wartofsky explains: it denotes 'the original locus of being itself, as *a spatio-temporal here and now*, a concrete *being here and now*' [13, p. 376; emphasis added].

Metaphysically speaking, it follows from this that consciousness and the world are ontologically co-terminus: the two cannot be separated, are not 'abstractable in isolation as a subject that has then to be put in relation to an object' [13, p. 377]. Instead, Hampshire agreed, we are all of us *only* aware of ourselves as 'one item of furniture in the world,' 'one physical fact among others' [6, pp. 45, 46]. It is, moreover, *only* by identifying those other physical facts that we are able to fix our own situation *in* the world. In such identifications lie the most basic existential conditions for both subject and object. This is because 'here' and 'there' are not absolute positions in space, but relative locations; more, they are concrete stages of interaction.

Otherwise put, the very possibility of self-identification depends logically on being one 'self-moving body among other bodies' [6, p. 46]. The 'being' that is *here* must, if it is to identify itself *as a self* at all, be able to change its position in relation to those other physical facts: move from *here* to *there*. The coherent conception of 'subject' and 'object' demand it, for only by being able to change its position in relation to other objects can it control its access to the world, its point of view. Further, only by controlling that point of view can it claim ownership of it, of, that is, its perceptions; and only by controlling and claiming ownership of its point of view, can it direct its attention to particular features of its environment. Last, but by no means least, only by doing all of that can any 'being' distinguish itself from the other physical features which constitute its environment. At its simplest, perhaps, '[o]nly by the exclusion of others from the space it occupies does personality prove itself to be real' [15, p. 91]. In this, it differs absolutely from the 'abstract, vague, empty personalities' of Cartesian realism.

All of which means that our Feuerbachian *Dasein*, 'being *here*', is necessarily 'being' in the operative mode, fully expressed or actualised in 'doing *that*', whatever 'that' may be. In short, consciousness is a mode of activity: not *a* being, but a *way* of being.

What we have on our hands, philosophically speaking, is a logically and ontologically primitive conception of human being as physically (and, ultimately therefore, socially) embodied. Embodiment delimits the worldly physical fact that consciousness, personality, is, so determines the self, locating it in one place *rather* than any other. It supplies what Feuerbach would call the essential 'property of impenetrability,' which distinguishes the self as one *object* rather than any other.

> *The body alone is that negativing, limiting, concentrating, circumscribing force, without which no personality is conceivable. Take away from your personality its body and you take away that which holds it together. The body is the basis, the subject of personality. Only by the body is a real personality distinguished from the imaginary one of a spectre* [15, p. 91].

No inert substance, then, but the locus of a self-moving, self-directing agency; bodily existence is the focal point from which the impacts and interactions wherein consciousness elaborates and extemporises itself are expressed. Hence, Feuerbach's avowal: 'I am a real, sensuous being, and, indeed, the body in its totality is my ego, my essence itself.' Otherwise put, the body supplies consciousness with that much-needed *modus operandi* whereby experience is granted and thought filled with experiential content. It is for this very reason that Feuerbach would so vehemently repudiate 'those philosophers who pluck out their eyes that they may see'—or as Wartofsky tellingly translates it, '*think*'—'better'. '[F]or my thought,' he insisted, 'I require the senses, especially sight; I found my ideas on materials that can be appropriated only through the activity of the senses' [13, p. 368, 15, p. xxxiv].

If consciousness is to be sufficiently determinate to know anything or do anything, then it must, in Farrer's phrase, be 'perfectly embodied;' at once, both subject and object of experience, consciousness is a feature of the world and so 'does nothing here without the body' [8, p. 60]. Crucially, it is this capacity for doing that supplies the ontological and epistemological foundations of a concrete— i.e. combinatorial—ego-profile. That is the ground upon which we shall build our anti-metaphysical metaphysics. Put simply, the physical extensions of consciousness supply our criterion of real being. They do so, because our first and most fundamental experiences are, as the empiricist knows full well, objects 'of the senses, perception and feeling' [12, p. 55]. So saying, Feuerbach would use action, more properly *inter*action, to elevate empirical principle. Real beings are known, he argued, only 'where my self-activity finds its boundary or resistance in the activity of another being' [12, p. 51]. That is why, first Farrer would identify 'the primitive sense [as] "touch"' [1, p. 232] and then Hampshire would do likewise, describing '[t]ouch, and not sight, [as]... primitively the most authoritative of the senses, the natural criterion of physical reality' [6, p. 48]. For both men, the reasoning was the same: 'because acting upon objects necessarily involves touching, the contact of my body with the resisting body that is not my own' [6, p. 48]. Thus, our very conception of 'real' is conditioned by contact, designating the boundaries laid by 'resisting bodies' as they impact on our activities.

In accessing our environment, so to speak, we are not simply pushing on an open door. We are not, as Farrer put it, 'swimming in a perfectly featureless medium;' there is no action *in vacuo* [1, p. 233]. We are, of course, 'walking the earth among all sorts of obstacles,' obstacles which evoke or elicit our actions, either by resisting our efforts to achieve some goal or by providing the means to overcome resistance. Those obstacles, those resistances, thereby determine the boundary conditions for conscious activity; without them, we could do nothing at all. Indeed, we can only walk because the ground beneath our feet provides friction and talk because other objects reflect the sounds we make. This is not to say, however, that, in setting the boundaries of our actions, those obstacles also determine their limits. They may exhort us in the strongest possible terms not to attempt to imitate the birds; but properly managed and controlled, they enable us to build the apparatus which does just that. Their resistance, then, is the force against which intentional consciousness, 'self-activity', actively defines itself.

It follows from this that the resistance activity by which our environment is known cannot be random or arbitrary as such; otherwise our attempts to understand and ultimately control it would be fruitless. Without regularity and predictability, consciousness would have no purchase on the world. Hence, as Farrer pointed out, '[o]ur conscious experiences find themselves from the start framed by this system' this regularity and predictability [1, p. 67]. Consequently, experience of resistance, and our engagement with it, take the form of systematic intercourse or controlled interference; that, in turn, supplies consciousness with 'shape' or 'form'. In other words, the interplay between self-activity and resistance activity supplies what Farrer described as the 'natural unit of thought' [16, p. 210]. Apart, that is, 'from my experience of impinging upon, and being impinged upon by, other things or forces, I have no conceivable clue to physical existence, or physical force, or physical interaction' [16, p. 210]. This is Farrer's 'causal solution' to the problems of realism, 'minimal dualism'. The world, he reminds us, 'is not known but as the playground of human thews and human thoughts; were there no free play, there would be no knowledge' [8, p. 171]. Subject and object are therefore disclosed to one another only as agents of 'free play'; the features or furniture that occupy our field of action alongside us 'only become features and so perceptible in so far as they disturb and diversify the field' [1, p. 234]. In short, the world is (recognisable as) a field of conscious activity and real knowledge is a product of our encounters in and with this field: one may come to know an object 'only in so far as it varies the disturbances of... [one's] field—[one] knows it as a class of disturbances.' We encounter 'real being' as it exercises resistance activity; we recognise it by the 'imprint' it leaves on our exploratory activities.

To speak 'objectively,' then, the world is no more or less than the combination of forces that are continuous with our active explorations. This means that the resistance activities by which the world is known to us and the controlled interference that constitutes our knowing acts are necessarily coeval: consciousness-and-the-world—if we may reiterate a central point—are co-constructed, actualised *in pari materia*. 'The bond to nature, to an objective world,' as Wartofsky puts it, 'lies in the very form of consciousness as requiring an other, that is, in the subject-object relation that is the essential form of human consciousness' [13, pp. 337–338]. This is important; it means that 'real being' is no more a corollary of physical effects than it is a by-product of conscious projection (as realist philosophers will no doubt suppose). 'Real being' is the constitutive activity of conscious physical agency, of human being.

This takes us to the ground level of a coherent epistemology. It is also the foundation stone of our metaphysics. To explain: from all that has gone before, it follows that reality as it is known, both by ordinary agents and the most scientifically well-equipped investigators, is to be found, not in inert stuff or substance, but in dynamic process. In Farrer's Latin phrase, *esse est operari*: 'real being' is full-bodied being-in-action [1, p. 21]. Being fully operational, 'being' is also fully interactive, for 'an *operatio*, *energia*, has a plurality of elements to it.' The universe and its furniture are not made of 'solid and stupid lumps of physical matter,' but of relatively stable patterns of energy, 'infinitely complicated, minute rhythms of active process, without which process, nothing would exist at all' [17, p. 40]. Pressing the point, Farrer explicitly aligned his metaphysics with the great Einsteinian advance of the twentieth century, designating '[e]nergy, rather than stuff... our ultimate' [8, p. 52].[5] Such sentiments cannot fail to resonate with the astrophysicist and speculative cosmologist, indeed, with every scientifically enlightened thinker of the modern age. They resonate, too, with that other great metaphysician of the time, Alfred North Whitehead, for whom 'the actual world is a process, and that process is the becoming of actual occasions' [18, p. 22]. In essence, process and *energia* mean the same thing: reciprocal interference, actualities disturbing a field of activity comprised of other actualities. Real things, then, are *in and as* the mutual interplay of resistance activity or, as Farrer dubbed it, 'disturbance-effect' [1, p. 235].

Action, disturbance-effect, is our metaphysical ultimate; *esse est operari*: to be is to act, better, to interact. If this is true of the physical universe, which frames our every thought and deed—and the sciences attest that it most assuredly is—then it is no less true of the conscious, physical agents who explore and explain that universe. In Feuerbachian terms, 'the mind of man is nothing but the essential mode of his activity' [15, p. 171]. Disturbance-effect is the key to consciousness: 'that to which the personal act corresponds is not, indeed, any system of stuff, however fine-drawn, but a sequence of activity' [8, p. 26].

Thus, to identify what philosophers of mind used to call the 'seat of consciousness,' Farrer averred, we need only allow consciousness to pick its own seat by sitting in it [8, p. 24]. Do so, and we shall find that the physical 'seat', or more dynamically, 'vehicle', of consciousness is located, not in any one phase or feature of the bodily process *per se*, but in the action-pattern as a whole, the full-scale sweep of bodily movement personally executed. Consciousness is actualised or enacted in what the agent actually does: the reading of a book, the writing of an essay, the meeting or missing of a deadline. Simultaneously, of course, the action-pattern *is* the operation of all the physical processes involved, including the microscopic motions constituting the entire neurological system. That system, in each and every phase of its activity, supplies the building blocks of conscious agency. Consciousness itself, however, does not bear directly upon those building blocks; no more, of course than it bears on the large-scale extensions of the physical organism. Consciousness, as we understand and experience it concerns what we *intend to do*. Otherwise put, we do not consciously or intentionally operate the system of electrochemical processes running from brain to fingertips any more that we consciously or intentionally operate the muscles in our arms and hands. What we *do* is write an essay: our consciousness concentrates upon and is concentrated *in* those large-scale intentions, trusting the system to discharge the neurological patterns that will embody it.

This is not, if we may repeat ourselves for a second time, in anyway intended to deny or even diminish the role of the brain in conscious, personal agency. Rather, it is to bestow upon the brain its rightful role and place within the larger, bodily process, which *is* conscious agency. To illustrate, Farrer offered an analogy: 'an immensely tenuous, elongated plant, rooted in several different regions of the brain, passing its stem through the spinal column, and flowering into performance in the hand' [8, p. 26]. Consciousness, then, is not to be restricted to any particular phase of the process: it is not *in* the firing nerves, the flexing muscles, or the moving hand. Consciousness 'flowers' or comes into focus in what agents *do*, but what they *do* is embodied by the *entire* 'action plant' from root to tip. Thus, the 'whole nerve-plant from brain to hand is the vehicle or instrument of the behaviour' [8, p. 26].

This is true even when that vehicle does not appear to be moving very much at all. Thinking, for example, about how to frame this sentence is an action and so

[5] See also, Farrer: 'The notion of energies in a pure or simple state, prior to mutual engagement is physical nonsense. All activity is mutual, as between energies, and all activity thus mutually engaged changes and redistributes itself' [7, p. 82].

requires a 'nerve-plant' to embody it, however foreshortened the 'plant' may be. For thinking, Farrer, reminds us, is the 'shadow of doing' and so 'must be interpreted by a full-blooded doing' [8, p. 39]. (One suspects that this is the point where many a neuroscientist and neuroethicist commits their fatal error, mistaking this act of interpretation by means of the clue or model of bodily action for ostensive indication or direct denotative reference; and that way, as we have seen, lies metaphysical realism.) For thought apart from overt behaviour, Farrer found an interpretive key right under our noses, so to speak. 'The best sort of characterisation of thinking is that it is a sort of talking to ourselves' [7, 29]. The 'shadow-patterns' of thought follow same route as speaking, from brain to mouth, taking in lips, jaws, tongue, vocal chords and so on. But they do not get so far: the action-pattern is not fully enacted and the 'nerve-plant' fails to flower in 'full-blooded doing.' In this way, the act of thinking 'ghosts' the act of speaking, stops short of engaging the full physical apparatus of bone and muscle.

The risk of physical reduction here is palpable. As we trace out the route of our action plant, it ill behoves us to ignore the ontological dangers that lie in wait: the abstractions and disjunctions, the dissolution of consciousness into confusion and self-contradiction. Forewarned is forearmed, however; almost literally in this case for, as Farrer pithily put it, we 'still have mind on our hands just as much as matter' [8, p. 7].

In fact we have already hinted at the answer more than a little. It lies in the fundamental requirement to make sense of human action as meaningful; to recognise and understand it as governed, not by the diagrammatic laws of cause and effect, but by the rules of discourse and the conventions of the community in which we act. It lies, in short, in the logic of intending. Such logic is essentially presuppositional. It means that the very concept of action in the full and personal sense—the sense, that is, in which we experience it directly in ourselves and the other persons with whom we interact—is only complete when coupled to an intending agent: the owner of the act. In acting, the agent instantiates both the intentional and consequential motifs that make agency what it is: the 'before' and 'after' of an *esse* that actualises itself purposively, that is, teleologically, by means of some *operari*. Therein lies meaning: both theme and content of the process, without which any act is reduced to mere physical event. Stripped of this purposive structure, this 'before' and 'after', the very concept of 'action' is unintelligible. Hence Farrer reminds us, the intending that arises only in those circumstances to which the physical, bodily pattern 'reacts and only in reacting to them... has neither sense nor function.' Contain consciousness within the bounds of flattened naturalism, that is, and the 'reaction which consciousness should direct takes place in the occurrence of consciousness;' and that is no consciousness at all [1, p. 235].

Evidently, we have no wish to re-open a logical and ontological chasm so recently closed; equally, no simple reduction will do. Instead, Farrer held out for an agency 'overplus' or 'prior actuality', insisting that '[t]he *intending* is ahead of the *intended*, though it be but a hairsbreadth' [8, p. 48].[6] Note the repetition; it is as important as the differentiation it represents, for it refutes absolutely the separatist tendencies of metaphysical realism, demanding instead continuity between *intending* agent and acts *intended*. Put simply, actions, in the full and personal sense, *are* intentional; they require an agent of *sufficient* priority to intend them. Like 'a hairsbreadth', 'sufficient' denotes the briefest logical pause between becoming aware of one's circumstances and responding to them: sufficient, that is, to displace merely reflex action while the owner-*esse* of intending consciousness takes her seat, putting the intended pattern of physical action in gear and driving it off.

[6] I am indebted to Charles Conti for pointing out the significance of the double reference here.

We are not, as all of us are no doubt aware, acting and intending in a vacuum. Action and, indeed, everything we have said about it, locates us in a physical *and* a social situation. For, as we have already observed, action is always and necessarily interaction, so involves a 'plurality of elements.' All of those elements are, in a sense, physical objects; many of them are also personal others, intending agents like ourselves. The logic of intending reminds us of this, while also circumscribing the minimal requirements of prior actuality: the demands placed upon us by the presence of other persons. So much can be clearly seen, J.L. Austin has demonstrated, from the language of apology and excuses [19]. That we need and, fortunately, are able to apologise for our actions, not only reveals the personal nature of the context in which we act, but also throws the logical emphasis back upon the intending by allowing us to express what we *meant* to do.

Put simply, acting persons aspire to a lively moral perspicuity by adopting what Charles Conti describes as a 'metaphysical [i.e. ethically informed] vantage point' [20, p. 185]. We seek thereby to oversee the means towards realising consequences we actually intend and so avoid colliding with other agents. We view our proceedings, then, not as a 'Cartesian cogitator but as actor-self and monitor-self simultaneously;' and so 'perform our being as we experience it' [20, p. 185]. In such performances the Cartesian *cogito* is revised and returned, chastened by experience and recruited by agency metaphysics to do its duty *metaphorically*. Physical extension coupled with social orientation symbolically transform the realist's non-perspectival perspective [3, p. 40] into a concrete analogue for self-transcendence *in and as* 'the "owner-occupier" of deeds done; the "performer-director" of the drama of its life' [20, p. 184]. This is the 'I' of the act, the self that listens to itself, hopefully *before* speaking, but often as not through an in-built 'moral "playback" function' [20, p. 187]. Registering the reaction on the face of the other, the self seeks to make amends by resubmitting its acts for review, reinterpreting them with a view to qualifying intentions and mitigating unintended effects. Such are the lessons we all learn to invest in our proceedings, gathering 'the rosebuds of experience in daily reflection so as to remove the thorns of further disgrace' [20, p. 187].

The social orientation of action coincides—and does occasionally collide—with the 'internal' world of conscious deliberation: 'We sense our compresence with others, so intuit the obligation to act' [20, p. 186]. Alive to that 'compresence', conscious agency is quickened by the possibilities of physical interaction, personal intercourse. That defines the obligation *in* action: simultaneously enacted—obligations undertaken – and intrinsic to the logic of action—the 'ought' of my intending. Therein, Conti concludes, lies the teleology of action: being 'retrospective and reflective all at once,' [20, p. 184] end-oriented acts factor means, motive, and opportunity into intended execution.

Unearthing the roots of thought and action, we find that the logic of intending underwrites the concept 'person' as a social reality. Logic is not, however, always the most reliable guide to what does and does not exist.[7] In view of our much-vaunted empiricism, something a little more concrete would, no doubt, be appreciated. After all, as Farrer reminds us, '[i]t is not as though we believed in our neighbour's personality *because* logical philosophers are able to exhibit the self-contradiction involved in denying it' [7, p. 128; emphasis added]. No more, of course, than we should expect logical proof of our parents personhood; do so and we surely add the insult of unnecessary demonstration to the injury of inexcusable doubt. Neighbours and parents, friends, lovers, even teachers: they do not constitute a logical puzzle for us to solve. Their presence, their reality, is a matter of practical urgency; incon-

[7] This, as J.N. Findlay reminds us, is because logic provides a guide to the use (and abuse) of language, not what does or does not exist [21]. Cf. Waismann: [22, 23].

trovertibly so, since our first encounter with other persons finds us supremely helpless. John Macmurray put the point with paradoxical perspicuity when he pointed out how well 'adapted... to being unadapted' we are, 'adapted,' that is, 'to a complete dependence' on others [24, p. 48]. In short, we are 'made to be cared for'; and cared for we must be if we are to survive. Being so 'adapted', how fortuitous then that we are born into a manifold of personal agencies or, to warm the face of such schematics, a world of families and friends, of intrinsically personal love-relationships. Farrer concurred: '[f]rom first infancy,' he said, 'our elders loved us, played us, served us and talked us into knowing them' [25, p. 74]. Had they failed us, we would not be here to question their reality or cast aspersions on the meaning of their being. Indeed, we only learned to talk 'because they talked to us;' and in that talk, consciousness took its first stuttering, stumbling steps: '[b]ecause we could first talk, we can now think; that is, we can talk silently to the images of the absent, or... pretend to be our own twin, and talk to ourself' [25, p. 74].

Consciousness, then, is awakened, better still *invested*, in us by those who supply the mental and physical resources with which we explore our world, shape our place and part in it. Otherwise put, our parents and teachers—among many, many others—supply the primary conditions of our conduct, both mode and circumstance of developing personality. We can think, that is, talk to ourselves, because they first talked to us and taught us to reply. Sometimes, we can even think objectively, that is, abstract from the immediacy of experience because they taught us rules for consistently organising and interpreting it. Those rules, as we have seen, they called theories: scientific, philosophical, psychological, etc.; they mitigate the particularity of my perspective by co-opting me into a community of explorers, so make *me* one of *them*.

In this way, others supply the terms and conditions of our actions and transactions, thereby staking their claim to the very self they helped create, instilling it with what Feuerbach called 'the inner life of man': our social self, our 'species being' [15, p. 2]. Like her talk, the other is internalised, metaphysically and morally incorporated into the structure of the self. This process displaces the subjectivity of the subject: its needs, activities, perspective—all felt as intrinsically, immediately present and real, *as* its *self*—these are *first* 'filtered' by a more basic presence in the shape of the 'otherness' 'inside'. Being 'filtered', the self evaluates and re-evaluates itself, conceiving and constructing, re-conceiving and re-constructing, itself *in and as* relation. The self learns to double itself, so play the part of the other within it. In the vernacular, we might say I become a self by learning to put myself in the place of another: I become *a* self, an *I*, by re-enacting that place, that primary otherness; I become a self by being appropriated by others and learning to appropriate them in turn. In this way, the transactional structure of social conscience and conscious action are built-into the mode and manifestations of self-construction *by the other*. This overrules any ontological privilege or priority the 'I' might seek to claim over deeper interpersonal connections. Prior actuality cannot belong *essentially* to the self, for, as Farrer avers, 'mentality *always* was a social, not a solitary, thing' [25, p. 74]. Both metaphysically and psychologically, priority resides *in* the other for that is where the self is born.

Taking this one step further, it is, perhaps, sufficiently well known that the derivation of the word 'person' lies in the Latin *persona*, meaning 'an actor's mask.' A vital metaphor, this: agent and alter-ego in one. The metaphysical hint is unmistakable. Give someone a mask, as Oscar Wilde quipped, and they reveal their true selves; and in revealing, we add, so they become. As consciousness is bodied forth by the other (inside) so it is embodied *in* the self. Theirs is the mask we wear, the *persona* we appropriate and transform into a self, a conscious, personal reality, commissioned by the other. Thus does '[m]ind... everywhere flow into mind' [26, p. 143] and I learn to play my part in the exchange of perspectives on my self-enactment.

Our first performance, then, is no monologue but a dialogue with the other. In such transactions, are we made to be self-making.

The essence of consciousness, of 'personhood', is fragmentary, consolidated by these exchanged perspectives. This is a commonplace of postmodern identity theories as well as the 'metaphysical personalism' (as Conti's titled his exegesis of Farrer) that we have been mapping here. The 'unity' we call a self is actually a function of that primary dialectic of perspectives, the love-relationships into which we are born. In this way, those who had and held us have inexorably bound themselves, their image, into our *every* experience of consciousness. We are who we are by their gift; wherein, St. Paul reminds us, works the grace of God [27].[8] Others give us the tools with which to make or 'mend' ourselves (as Eugene O'Neill suggests) using that grace as 'glue' [28, p. 101].[9] They give us the language, the symbols, in which we think our thoughts and live our lives.

4. Conclusion

It seems we have, at last, reached the philosophical bottom-line. These first and most fertile encounters shape the development of conscious thought and action; they are the grounds which supply form and purpose, sometimes even content, to our explorations and explanations. This is the well-spring of human being, in Martin Buber's poignant phrase, the 'cradle of real life' [22, 29].

Here, then, is an opportune moment to take stock. Let us make the point of moral application plain. Immediately obvious is the absence of any ethical theory, our conception of persons as active agents offers no system or set of rules for the formulation of normative judgements. Being rooted in the personal relations wherein we all, quite literally, find ourselves, our anti-metaphysical, *applied* metaphysics is profoundly averse, even hostile, to such things. Indeed, as the history of Western philosophy—and any decent textbook—will show, such theorising and systematising is always inherently flawed, unable as it is to accommodate the messy and complicated cases that moral practice inevitably throws up. Real life is never black and white; for every rule there is an exception; although even the best system-builders frequently forget this, preferring as they do to exalt their abstract conceptual constructs such as reason and utility.

Applied metaphysics may leave us without a moral theory, but it does not leave us empty-handed. Instead, it supplies the very anchor that our normative judgements demanded from the start: concrete personal connection, the embodiment of moral agency. This rebuts absolutely that Cartesian ghost in—or rather *out of*—the machine, that 'being-beyond,' which remains forever quarantined from physical experience, physical knowledge, physical reality. And so the transcending ego, which passes judgement on a reality it can neither experience nor, consequently, understand, is exorcised at last. Along with it, goes the flattened naturalism which reduces personal reality to causal mechanism. In their place stands, not a concept, but a person, a conscious physical agent. This is the other with whom I am intimately and intrinsically interconnected, the living, breathing reality at the very heart of my own existence: co-constituent of my becoming, whose rightful claim upon me demands that I reciprocate, respond in kind and participate in his or her becoming. We demur at our own risk, for that way lies self-stultification; worse still, perhaps annihilation. Deny the presence of the other and coherence is corrupted:

[8] 'But by the grace of God I am what I am: and his grace which was bestowed upon me was not in vain; but I laboured more abundantly than they all: yet not I, but the grace of God which was with me.'

[9] 'Man is born broken. He lives by mending. The grace of God is glue!'

our entire moral discourse will rot. Reject their claims upon us and our very existence may be in dire peril. Regard them as mere objects, as a function of physical process or even interpenetrating forces, and we transform ourselves likewise. Action is reflexive: it reveals the nature of the agent and in revealing, actualises. Bluntly, that is, I am who and what I am through the grace (and glue) of others; without them, I am not. Therein lies the moral imperative of our anti-metaphysical metaphysics.

Philosophically speaking, of course, we have found more than a moral anchor; we also have a coherent logical and ontological framework for our discourse. Personal action supplies the context in which we may clearly see both the particular and the general: first, the analyses and judgements of neuroethics; second, the discipline as a whole and all its participants. Within this framework we may recognise, then understand, and finally overcome the 'self-sufficing speculation,' [15, p. xxxiv] which threatens to undermine our efforts. On the one hand, we recall the personal presuppositions of our empiricism: the epistemological requirements of exploring agents that reconnect experience with action, real knowledge with the controlled interference which is the neuroscientist's stock in trade. On the other, it reveals and resists the temptation to align methodology too closely with metaphysics. This, in turn, allows us to reconcile those binary oppositions—mind and body, intending and intended, subject and object—which do so much to incapacitate every branch of moral philosophy. Reconciliation comes, not by over-inflating empiricism with the transcendental pretensions of metaphysical realism, but by returning us to the only place where those abstract notions can possibly make sense. Mind is a mode of bodily action, body the physical manifestation of mind. Intending and intended are phases of that manifestation, conceptually separable but in reality, i.e. in action, continuous. Subjectivity is essentially other-oriented by virtue of being a reflection of the other who invokes and evokes it in us. Ethically, it denotes obligations owned: my responsibilities as presupposed and, moreover, delimited by my capacity to act in response to a physical and social or personal environment. Being a communal act, objectivity is coeval with this environment: it represents the truth-conditions and epistemic norms laid down by the community of knowing persons. Thus, subject and object are not independent as such, but theoretical perspectives, ways of seeing, of thinking about and understanding the world, the use of which is sanctioned by that community. This does not detract from their truth-value but merely reminds us of the context in which they are first negotiated and defined; that is, transacted with the world by the community of thinkers. Both ethically and epistemologically, then, these theoretical perspectives represent, in their contrasting but congruent ways, the very 'claimingness' of others that is our anchor.

Ultimately, then, being firmly anchored by our concept of persons to the solid, social, and inherently ethical ground that entails it, uncouples neuroethical analyses from the arbitrary dictates and philosophical fiats of classical rationalism-cum-realism. Diverted from the rabbit hole of incoherence and irrelevance, which awaits so much philosophical discourse, and possessed of a renewed social conscience, our thoughts and actions are oriented back towards the communities in which even neuroethicists must live and work. Most immediately, perhaps, is the scholarly community whose job it is to map out and delineate our discipline. Beyond that, is the academy itself, whose traditions, standards, and requirements we have imbibed, deploying them rigorously in our own practice. And if we care to look still further, beyond the halls of academe, we may even see the society whose various institutions—from the logico-linguistic to the socio-political—make our investigations possible and before which our contributions will no doubt be held to account.

Author details

Simon Smith
British Personalist Forum, University of Surrey, Haslemere, United Kingdom

*Address all correspondence to: simon.smith@surrey.ac.uk

References

[1] Farrer A. Finite and Infinite. 2nd ed. Westminster: Dacre Press; 1959

[2] Einstein A. In: Seelig C, et al., editors. Ideas and Opinions, Based on Mein Weltbild. New Translations by Sonja Bergmann. New York: Crown Publishers, Inc.; 1960

[3] Byrne P. God and Realism. Aldershot: Ashgate; 2003

[4] Farrer A. Metaphysics and analogy. In: Conti C, editor. Reflective Faith. London: SPCK; 1972. pp. 82-90

[5] Michael P. Personal Knowledge, Towards a Post-Critical Philosophy. Chicago: University of Chicago Press; 1962

[6] Hampshire S. Thought and Action. Notre Dame: University of Notre Dame Press; 1983

[7] Farrer A. Faith and Speculation. London: Adam & Charles Black; 1967

[8] Farrer A. The Freedom of the Will (The Gifford Lectures for 1956-1957). New York: Charles Scribner's Sons; 1960

[9] Strawson PF. Individuals. London: Methuen & Co.; 1959

[10] Spaemann R. Persons: The Difference between 'Someone' and 'Something'. Translated by Oliver O'Donovan. Oxford: Oxford University Press; 2006

[11] Cottingham J, Stoothoff R, Murdoch D, translators. Descartes Selected Philosophical Writings. Cambridge: Cambridge University Press; 1993

[12] Feuerbach L. The Principles of the Philosophy of the Future. Translated by M.H. Vogel. Cambridge: Hackett Publishing Co.; 1986

[13] Wartofsky MW. Feuerbach, Cambridge: CUP; 1982

[14] Jasper D. A Short Introduction to Hermeneutics. Kentucky: Westminster John Knox Press; 2004

[15] Feuerbach L. The Essence of Christianity. Translated by George Eliot. New York: Harper & Row; 1957

[16] Farrer A. In: Conti C, editor. Causes' in Reflective Faith. London: SPCK; 1972. pp. 200-218

[17] Farrer A. Does god exist? In: Conti C, editor. Reflective Faith. London: SPCK; 1972. pp. 39-47

[18] Whitehead AN. In: Griffin DR, Sherburne DW, editors. Process and Reality, Corrected Edition. New York: Free Press; 1978

[19] Austin JL. A Plea for excuses. In: Urmson JO, Warnock GJ, editors. Philosophical Papers. Oxford: Clarendon; 1961. pp. 123-152

[20] Conti C. Metaphysical Personalism. Oxford: Clarendon; 1995

[21] Findlay JN. Can God's existence be disproved? In: Flew AGN, MacIntyre AC, editors. New Essays in Philosophical Theology. London: SCM Press; 1955. pp. 47-56

[22] Waismann F. Verifiability. In: Parkinson GHR, editor. The Theory of Meaning. Oxford: OUP; 1968. pp. 35-60

[23] Waismann F. The resources of language. In: Black M, editor. The Importance of Language. Englewood Cliffs, N. J: Prentice-Hall; 1962. pp. 107-120

[24] Macmurray J. Persons in Relation. New Jersey: Humanities Press International; 1991

[25] Farrer A. Thinking the trinity. In: Houlden L, editor. A Celebration of

Faith. London: Hodder & Stoughton; 1970. pp. 72-77

[26] Farrer A. You want to pray? In: Houlden L, editor. A Celebration of Faith. London: Hodder & Stoughton; 1970. pp. 141-144

[27] James K. Bible. 1 Corinthians. 1611;**15**:10

[28] O'Neill E. The Great God Brown and Lazarus Laughed. London: Jonathan Cape; 1960

[29] Buber M. I and Thou. Translated by Ronald Gregor Smith. Edinburgh: T&T Clark; 1996

Chapter 3

Naturalizing Neuroethics? A Syncretic Approach

John R. Shook and James Giordano

Abstract

Neuroethics is uniquely situated to socially interpret what brain sciences are learning about social and moral cognition while helping society hold neuroscientific research and neurotechnological applications to firm moral standards. Both tasks, if they are to be pursued successfully, must find ways to closely relate the "neuro" with the "ethical." Keeping them apart has been the objective of nonnaturalist worldviews worried about scientism and reductionism, and now they complain about "neuroessentialism" and similar labels for dissolutions of agency and responsibility into mere brain activity. A nonnaturalistic neuroethics, on whatever metaphysical basis, insists that the biology of brains could not explain moral decisions or ground moral norms. We agree on that much, since the methodology of brain sciences presumes, and cannot replace, behavioral and psychological attributions of moral capacity and conduct. But the social and the neurological are always related through the anthropological; and that common basis is, not coincidentally, also where the ethical is grounded, as humanity upholds persons as bearers of moral worth and moral capacity. Neuroethics, by focusing on persons, need never resort to nonnaturalism to uphold what ultimately matters for ethics, and "naturalizing" neuroethics is also unnecessary for a humanity-centered neurobioethics.

Keywords: neuroethics, neurobioethics, naturalism, nonnaturalism, neuroscience, psychology, ethics

1. Introduction

In this chapter we present a syncretic approach to neuroethics, opening a conciliatory and convergent path forward for this interdisciplinary area. This approach can (1) align neuroethics with cognitive and social neuroscience as well as neurology and (2) situate neuroscience within a capacious philosophical naturalism. Keeping "neuro" primary to neuroethics for its perspective on humanity and keeping "ethics" for humanity central to neuroethics and its mission are paramount goals. Yet, those goals anticipate that neuroethics will have sufficient generality and applicability for all humanity. If the "neuro" and the "ethical" cannot be somehow harmonized, any such universality for neuroethics is unattainable. To that end, we argue here that relationships and continuities connecting (neuro)science and (neuro)ethics should be traced through domains of (natural) philosophy.

IntechOpen

2. Metaethics and philosophy

Elsewhere, we have labeled the higher goal of universal relevance for humanity as a "cosmopolitan" aim, to solicit ethical wisdom from many cultures and elicit principles fostering ethics across societies. That aim falls under the purview of ethical theorizing, but it cannot be beholden to any particular ethical theory (such as deontology, consequentialism, virtue ethics, and so forth) or to the perennial debates among them. By setting a high methodological standard for ethical theorizing, a cosmopolitan approach enters the area of metaethics as well. However, cosmopolitan ethics, due to its attentiveness to humanity, strongly doubts that metaethics by itself is oriented toward human universality. Metaethics can easily amount to validations bestowed on one society's conventional morality over other societies or fixations with some country's linguistic habits about moral matters or a meditation upon a single culture's moral tradition.

Just as metaphysics eventually lost its credibility as an adjudicator of moral norms, skepticism toward metaethics as a lone arbiter of moral concepts and truths has also been warranted. Will further refinements to metaphysics, or metaethics, at last permit deductions of binding moral principles? That also seems dubious, as proffered derivations continue to be a plentiful source of diverse and inconsistent results. That profligacy, at least, could be reasonably expected. No narrow intellectual base could sufficiently support broad practical norms.

Looking to metaethics to adjudicate ethical theorizing and deliver a principled moral framework relevant to humanity cannot be encouraged, unless a different kind of metaethics is engaged—one that is based upon and employs a metaphysics that consults other areas of philosophy and is informed by fields across the humanities, social sciences, and life sciences. Tentative efforts and initial results on our part illustrate how such a broadly informed metaethics can yield a cosmopolitan ethical framework, which in turn suggests some principled ethical guidelines [1, 2]. We do not replicate that work here. Instead we address certain metaethical and philosophical issues of neuroethics, as it develops as an interdisciplinarity of several scientific fields. Analyses and inquiries of a philosophical nature seem inescapable, and likewise, we regard them as essential to the success of neuroethics.

But taking neuroethics to be fundamentally indebted to philosophy would not be apparent upon a survey of the many fields contributing to neuroethical concerns and inquiries [3]. The centrality of philosophical inquiry comes into view with the primary assignments given to neuroethics as an interdisciplinary enterprise (consult [4, 5]). In brief, neuroethics (i) ponders the brain's functions that are involved with personal identity, autonomy, and moral judgment/action and (ii) evaluates ways that neuroscience and technology (i.e., neuroS/T) can be developed and implemented while respecting human dignity and ethical norms. Indeed, as many have begun to acknowledge, each assignment yields information and actionable assessments that are relevant to the other assignment.

Harmony between these two assignments is hardly automatic or straightforward. Consider again the hazardous intersections of ethics and neuroscience where neuroethics has offered its supervision: first, the growing responsibility to advise or even adjust social views about psychological and neurological processes involved in moral and immoral conduct and second, the expanding ability to alter cognitive processes in ways affecting conceptions of the self and moral capacity. Unless neuroethics can coordinate the advice to society with an assessment of neuroscientific interventions, neuroethics will be unable to distinguish itself amid the cacophony of opinions about what brain science does and means.

For example, what neuroethical advice and guidance will be offered about these matters in the area of criminal justice? Imagine a defense lawyer making this argument during a trial: "Ladies and gentlemen of the jury, my client cannot be guilty because neuroscience shows that no brain is really capable of moral responsibility." And then imagine another trial, where a judge imposes this sentence: "The court requires this convicted criminal to undergo neurological treatment to restore the capacity for moral responsibility." As discourses in neurolaw are already indicating, such scenarios may not remain as fictional as they once seemed [6]. But it appears that a forced choice lies ahead: moral responsibility is either "in the brain" or it is not. Criminal law and legal theory require consistency and try to eliminate confusion. And many other civic institutions, social structures, and cultural frameworks will encounter conflicting interpretations of new neuroS/T. If and when neuroethical consultation is sought, will it be able to speak with one voice?

One might think that the aforementioned kinds of confusing scenarios would be preventable, or at least manageable, if neuroethics is steered in a less naturalistic direction. Assertions that "We are not just our brains!" have an appealing clarity. Disparaging labels for an excessive fixation upon brain functions now include "neurocentrism" and "neuroessentialism" to join the oft-heard charges of "reductionism" and "scientism" [7]. Such labels conceal more than they expose. How does a blanket rejection of scientific reductionism enlighten legal theory about utilizing empirical evidence that adjusting neurological functioning in a brain region actually makes a person less indifferent to hurting other people? How does a scornful repudiation of neuroessentializing illuminate a better definition of moral responsibility, while societies dispute different conceptions of culpability? Deeper philosophical investigations are evidently necessary.

3. Naturalistic and non-naturalistic neuroethics

The counterpart to naturalism would presumably be nonnaturalism, as a catch-all classification. Any alternative to naturalism sets up its opposition by pointing out selected matters that are (allegedly) unaccounted for and left inexplicable, by the resources of naturalism. A nonnaturalistic neuroethics therefore is a neuroethical approach taking the view that authentic moral responsibility and moral decision-making are matters requiring something unnatural about human beings. As unnatural, that feature cannot be generated or directly affected by natural causes, although natural causes may be able to interfere with human capacities (e.g., "free will" is held to be necessary for moral responsibility). In addition, a nonnaturalistic neuroethics would hold that authentic moral responsibility and moral deeds must meet normative standards that remain independent of physiological/neurological/cognitive processes, although such processes can help explain human behaviors (e.g., "ethical rules" must prevail as normatively binding).

In sum, nonnaturalistic neuroethics rejects what it takes to be the opposed position of "naturalistic neuroethics" and the neuro-reductionism and ethical naturalism which naturalistic neuroethics could foster. Such a nonnaturalistic perspective has its own distinctive stance on the two tasks assigned to neuroethics. For nonnaturalistic neuroethics, psychological matters needed for one's moral capacity and moral conduct cannot be explained by any amount of information about the structures and functions of brains; and ethical norms needed for judging someone's morality cannot be grounded by any amount of information from biology or neurology. Neuroscientific reductions or replacements of moral capacity are severely questioned (NB: for a current survey, see [8]), and attempts to ground ethics directly upon nature have long been scrutinized (a recent analysis is offered by [9]).

At this stage, we make our urgent plea for a philosophical pause, before the paired tasks of neuroethics proceed toward a contested divorce, and false dichotomies compel differing worldviews to collide. Although it is the case that "neuro" was hitched to "ethics" with the sort of haste that intellectual fads display, no such mistake was made with "neuroethics." Rather, the true mistake is to presume that each component rests upon a basis that is independent from the other. Philosophy, even naturalistic philosophy, does not so presume, which receives our elaboration in what follows. We remain convinced that the "neuro" and the "ethical" can be closely related and their grounds should be somewhat integrated. We provocatively raise the question of "Naturalizing Neuroethics?" not to advocate for that one-sided agenda, or to instigate counter-responses from naturalism's adversaries, but rather to point the way to a conciliatory philosophical setting that is broader than both sides.

Physician-philosopher Henk ten Have has recounted how the central tasks of any philosophy involve metaphysical, epistemological, anthropological, and ethical domains [10]. Naturalism is no exception. Naturalism, as a philosophical worldview, cannot avoid a metaphysical perspective about what counts as real. For naturalism, the universe, as it is empirically experienced and known, represents phenomena of nature, which are accessible for inquiry. On this view, the tools and methods of science—inclusive of those exploring and demonstrating how organisms arise, exist, and interact with each other and their ecologies—are applicable to the universe, and they are able (at least in the long run) to reveal the nature of anything accessible by inquiry.

To be sure, practicalities limit what can be investigated and understood, especially at the outer bounds of size and scale. The epistemic basis of naturalistic understanding, while ever-widening from the minute to the massive, has to respect constraints of technologies and techniques (i.e., the tools) that humans develop and employ to define what is known and can be known. From such capabilities and constraints arise hypotheses and theories. Through methods of observation, evaluation, and corroboration, hypotheses conjoin currently accepted facts and established physical laws to develop theories: well-substantiated, valid explanations of some aspect(s) of the natural world. Common definitions apply:

> *Fact: In science, an observation that has been repeatedly confirmed and for all practical purposes is accepted as "true." Truth in science, however, is never final, and what is accepted as a fact today may be modified or even discarded tomorrow.*
>
> *Hypothesis: A tentative statement about the natural world leading to deductions that can be tested. If the deductions are verified, it becomes more probable that the hypothesis is correct. If the deductions are incorrect, the original hypothesis can be abandoned or modified. Hypotheses can be used to build more complex inferences and explanations.*
>
> *Law: A descriptive generalization about how some aspect of the natural world behaves under stated circumstances.*
>
> *Theory: In science, a well-substantiated explanation of some aspect of the natural world that can incorporate facts, laws, inferences, and tested hypotheses* ([11], 2).

Humans engage in their empirical inquiries with investigational and decisional tools they implement and put acquired knowledge (information, understandings, meanings) and invented technologies to use for other human enterprises. Everything about science is thoroughly human in embodiment as well as in intellect. Science (qua *Scientia*: knowing, and epistemic means and methods at hand), no less than technology (qua *Techne-logos*: an accounting of tool development and use), falls entirely within the range, and limitations, of human activity in general. To examine what science does is to study ways that humanity lives. Humans use science and its tools for human endeavors: of comprehension, articulation, interaction with the world, survival, competition, cooperation, and flourishing. Examining, explaining, and proposing how humans enact and implement science include epistemic matters, but they all instantiate the anthropological domain.

Moreover, as Thomas Kuhn, Bruno Latour, and other philosophers and historians of science have elucidated, human ways of life and thought are able to influence and impact each other (for overviews, consult [12, 13]). Because science is a human endeavor, its conduct and employment render it amenable to interpretations and redirections based upon a worldview or philosophy, and/or on cultural tenets and traditional beliefs, which both reflect and foster particular sociocultural ideas, norms, and mores. As philosopher and cognitive scientist Daniel Dennett points out, there is no "philosophy-free" science, "only science whose philosophical baggage is taken on board without examination" ([14], 21). Furthermore, since science is part of the human drama of life, it cannot help but manifest an ethical dimension. Human enterprises pursue ends and defined "good(s)" which are taken to be valuable for something and someone, and thus the ethical domain is engaged.

For naturalism, or any other worldview, the "natural" cannot be very distant or detached from the "human" and the "ethical." That relationship works both conceptually and pragmatically. Neuroethics is no exception, and indeed, it should exemplify that kind of relationship. If and when the "nature" of moral meanings, decisions, and actions are understood in connection with "neural" matters, *and* the nature of brain operations are understood in relation with meaningfully "moral" behaviors, then we can ascertain that the "neuro" is placed securely in "neuroethics" [15].

Can so much "neuro" for neuroethics be trusted? Nonnaturalistic neuroethics lacks that confidence. However, neuroscience cannot dictate what counts as morality and moral cognition, on scientific grounds alone. The neuroscience of morality cannot be scientifically conducted without guidance from social understandings of morality. Scientists premise inquiries into "moral" brain functioning upon ethical views about what shall count as moral situations, moral thinking, moral decisions, and moral values. No amount of cognitive neuroscience and neurology, on their own, could determine what counts as a moral emotion, value, or belief had by any subject. Nor do any of those fields, by themselves, identify the occurrence of a moral decision among the innumerable brain processes happening at any moment. Any perusal of current literature from those fields will illustrate such scientific modesty, independent of conclusions that researchers themselves happen to make about moral cognition (Ample citations to that body of literature are provided by [16–18]). A fuller discussion of neural processes involved in moral cognition, decision-making, and action is beyond the scope of this chapter, but the reader is referred to references cited above.

This methodological point deserves some additional expansion. Exploratory experiments proceed as a human subject (an encultured person, to be specific), who is told what to think about, is asked for a judgment about a certain situation, or the subject is watched for some specific type of conduct, etc., so that experimenters know when morality (among numerous matters for one's attention) has some relation to ongoing cognitive processes. For example, Keith Yoder and Jean Decety survey key brain regions involved with the neuroscience of morality in this manner:

> *Converging evidence from functional neuroimaging studies and neurological observations indicates that the same regions implicated in social decision-making play*

> *important specific roles in morality. Specifically, a set of interconnected regions encompassing the vmPFC, OFC, amygdala, TPJ, ACC, aINS, PCC, and dlPFC are reliably engaged across tasks which involve explicit or implicit evaluations of morally-laden stimuli, regardless of whether the outcome of an action affects the participants directly or another individual* ([19], 285).

Neuroscientific terms predominate, yet key conditioning factors—such as "morally-laden stimuli"—are already deemed by experimenters to be *moral* prior to peering into the brain. In general, unless conditions are amenable to moral sensitivity and judgment, and a person could be mentally oriented under those conditions toward possible moral behaviors, nothing about that person's brain could be interpreted as *moral* cognition [20]. Brains are not examined for signs of moral cognition, while subjects are focused on preparing a dinner meal or operating a lawn mower, unless some distinctively moral feature were added, and that cannot be added by brain science alone. Nevertheless, neuroethics would lack vital content and credibility without consulting neuroscience, so we believe our call for "no neuroethics without neuroscience" to be a sensible demand [21].

In short, epistemic, anthropological, and ethical frameworks together transmute a neurological assessment of brain activity into a neuroethical assessment of moral competency and performance. These methodological considerations lend reassurance that our approach does not conceal a "neuro"-reductionist or essentialist agenda. The discoveries of empirical relationships, stable connections, cause-effect patterns, and conditioning factors among observable events are the very opposite of concluding that some of those matters are unreal or "really" something else entirely. As an illustration, if two observed matters are empirically correlatable, they both remain just as real. References to neural correlates of psychological events, or to neurological events preceding and preparing behaviors, are not covert concessions to reductionism (see, e.g., [22, 23]). Neuroethics pursued in light of well-confirmed neuroscientific discoveries is just well-informed neuroethics, not a neuroethics already co-opted by a metaphysical worldview.

We have also endorsed a call for "no neuroscience without neuroethics" [21, 24], to support an agenda already promoting the development and impact of neuroethics. Yet neuroethics has characteristically been equivocal at best, and at worst mute (if not blind), about the corresponding call for "no neuroethics without neuroscience." Ethical rules and principles ready-made for application to neuroethical issues relieve philosophical intercessions from the burden of incorporating cognitive and neuroscientific information about moral judgment and action. A *philosophical* neuroethics can do better than that. The dictum that "Is cannot imply an Ought" appeals to positivists, yet the converse notion that "Ought cannot supply an Is" is too simplistic and pessimistic as well. What is devoutly pursued with ethical devotion must make its material difference in human practices and psychological operations, or else it has no footing or effectiveness (anywhere) in the natural world.

To this point of our argument, we have defended our view that reflective philosophical approaches to neuroethics should acknowledge a "natural-ethical" continuity and entanglement. Due recognition of that relationship has not been naturalism's insight alone. After all, idealisms, phenomenologies, existentialisms, and theologies have perennially sought to integrate the ideal and the real. Perhaps answering the question, "Which philosophy or philosophies best undergirds neuroethics?" need not choose one front-runner, if enough shared philosophical ground could be found.

Philosophical anthropology, as the fulcrum point midway between metaphysics and ethics, is ideally situated to stimulate realistic reflections on the capacity of various cultural constructs and practices to ground a global neuroethics. The plurality displayed by ethics around the world is the key to forging an applicable ethics for humanity. Since it is naturally human for societies to develop and uphold their cultural ethos in diverse ways, all ethics is undeniably human in aspiration and service. Our search for a universally relevant neuroethics, securely grounded in humanity's capacities and endeavors, has brought us to the question of cultural diversity. How might neuroethics comport with, and best serve, the varied world-views, wisdom traditions, and philosophies exemplified in the global heterogeneity of the twenty-first century?

To begin with, neuroethics in definition and practice should not be viewed as only another subfield of applied ethics, despite certain advantages to doing so. If neuroethics were entirely subsumed under philosophical ethics, then its supervision by philosophy would bind neuroethics to the humanities, where human values can be insulated from scientific encroachment and the "naturalistic fallacy." That security might relieve anxieties about dissolving what is most "human" into the biological realm. However, neuroethics has already acquired and apprehended far too much from the behavioral and brain sciences to expect and propose that human values float freely and apart from individual and groups' plans, pursuits, and practices. We would hope that dismissing the scientific study of human beings and retreating into idealistic enclaves should not be the destiny of neuroethics.

Perhaps neuroethics is instead destined to play an ancillary role, supporting the lead taken by the brain sciences. Ethics, to be most realistic in nature, would presumably be discerned somewhere in the cognitive processes generating the actual moral judgments that humans make in the course of living (more or less) moral lives. That would allow neuroethics to appeal to ethical standards pre-approved by the embodied human brains of people trying to be moral in the first place, so neuroethics gets subsumed under the "neuroscience of morality." But that leaves moral psychology torn between two masters: shall it conform to strictures set by neuroscience (such as the eliminationist abandonment of much moral vocabulary as fictional folk psychology), or shall it remain loyal to one or another ethical theory (e.g., by taking the dualist route of awarding moral thinking an ontological status among other brain processes). Is neuroethics similarly caught between serving two masters?

Treating ethics as something that is materially instantiated in the brain, as many academic writings on neuroethics expect, is only a half-way measure that contorts both ethics and science. Crafting just-so interpretations "showing" how the brain does what this or that ethical theory requires amounts to committing the naturalistic fallacy in reverse! Far too much work on behalf of one preferred ethical theory or another has to be put into designing experiments and selectively interpreting results, from either experimental psychology or imaging neuroscience, to reasonably conclude that any ethical theory enjoys an obvious empirical advantage. Uniquely *moral* sentiments (and moral values, etc.) have no singular cerebral locale, and they are not ready-made for guiding purely *moral* judgments somewhere in the brain [8, 15, 25].

However, a third option beckons, presented by philosophical anthropology. Like neurophilosophy, and its revisions of philosophical issues with a due measure of scientific information, neuroethics could collaborate with the sciences in a pragmatic and judicious manner. Neuroethics can be suitably naturalistic with respect to advances in behavioral and brain sciences, without descending into a naturalistic submission to science. On that basis, then—and only then—will human "ethics" be fully aligned with "neuroethics."

Here, proponents of nonnaturalistic neuroethics may intercede, observing that their protection of moral values surely merits considerable anthropological validity. To reiterate, a nonnaturalistic neuroethics follows the lead of privileged nonscientific or anti-scientific ideas about why and how people are moral/immoral, and it conforms to traditional moral norms endorsed by one culture or another. What could be more human? We cannot disagree, having drawn attention to the way that humanity flourishes through many diverse cultures.

However, such laudable diversity compels nonnaturalistic neuroethics to subdivide into numerous neuroethics, each beholden to one or another ethical tradition that seems as "natural" for human beings as any. What they retain in common is their reluctance to accept neuroscientific claims about human morality without ample reinterpretation and amendment in light of their tradition(s). And in this way, each nonnaturalistic neuroethics will tend to display a contradictory stance toward brain science: while denying that neurological evidence could count against preferred moral judgments, they expect brain evidence to somehow support the naturality of those judgments. To conceal that tension, a nonnaturalistic neuroethics may appeal to two allies: moral philosophy (about what morality really is) and ethical theory (about principles grounding moral norms). A suitably parochial moral philosophy and a parochial ethical theory, sharing a sociocultural basis, can lend support a nonnaturalistic neuroethics. No admission of relativism will be forthcoming, as they purport to address what is genuinely moral for humanity.

A concern for human morality is admirable, yet nonnaturalistic neuroethics is not alone in its anthropological focus. Naturalistic neuroethics, by definition, will not follow ideas about humanity and human morality that prove incompatible with the behavioral, biological, and brain sciences. Inconsistency cannot be ruled out in advance. Naturalistic neuroethics is not silenced by claims to the effect that "What we think about morality cannot be placed in doubt by anything brains are doing." For a naturalistic neuroethics, what human brains are really doing (and not doing) can expose mistaken ideas about how people are able (or fail) to behave morally.

Human capacities to learn morality and incorporate moral norms into daily conduct are studied closely by developmental, social, and moral psychology, and cultural anthropology can be coordinated with those fields [26]. As for cognitive and social neuroscience (i.e., what could be considered "neuroscience of moral cognition and behavior"), their role here is adjunct to psychology, since they presuppose that experimental subjects are sometimes thinking about, and occasionally performing, moral behaviors. Moral philosophy should cooperate with the behavioral sciences as well: moral philosophizing that ignores anthropology and psychology lacks sufficient content, devolving instead into either rationalism or sentimentalism.

4. Integrative, realistic, and neuroethics

Naturalistic neuroethics, heeding moral anthropology and psychology, finds that only socialized and encultured brains enact moral practices. As previously explained, no answer to "What is morality?" or "Who is moral?" will arrive solely from studying neural functioning and brain processes. A "naturalistic" stance for neuroethics should affirm, as firmly as nonnaturalistic neuroethics, that ethics will not be determined by brain sciences, and narrow "neuro-reductionism" will not replace moral philosophy or dictate neuroethics. Nevertheless, what human brains are really doing (and not doing) sets factual bounds to pondering how people are able (or fail) to behave morally.

Nonnaturalistic neuroethics would be best served by heeding and upholding the realistic advice that ethical theorizing should attend to actual moral capacities and practical methods able to improve them. Naturalistic neuroethics has the same boundaries, attending to humanity as it has biologically evolved, and morality as actually practiced by humanity. Only socialized and encultured individuals (with their embodied brains) understand and enact moral practices; hence there is no such thing as a culture-free morality, unstructured by historical tradition embedded in some society or another. Any neuroethics relies on ethics and cannot create it. Ethics displays considerable variation with regard to concrete moral norms, but it never wavers from its primary devotion to moral agency and the moral subject, without which morality would be an empty gesture. It is ethics itself, a thoroughly human ethics that requires neuroethics to protect the human capacity for personal identity, dignity, and moral responsibility. And it is ethics that demands neuroethics to accordingly apply the highest ideals and principles for evaluating neuroS/T. Thus, the answer to the question, "From where does neuroethics get its ethics?", can only be an anthropological answer: from humanity itself.

In comparison, nonnatural neuroethics cannot be as faithful to humanity as a whole. Fixations upon unnatural psychology and transcendent ethics only seem to satisfy metaphysical quests for permanence and certainty. Epistemic tensions tend to render any nonnatural neuroethics apart. Neuroscience cannot be conducted or trusted without reinterpretation from unscientific stands, while allies from moral philosophy and ethical theory are culture-bound and somewhat resistant to revision. Anthropological problems will also mount: human moral capacities are misconceived or minimized in contrast with idealized moral expectations, while the effects of neuroS/T interventions on moral behavior are regarded as mysterious or tenuous. Finally, when it comes to practical ethics, nonnatural neuroethics is bereft of resources for constructive ethical theorizing about workable ways to adjust and improve moral conduct.

A nonnatural neuroethics need not exalt metaphysics to the detriment of epistemology, anthropology, and ethics. A cultural heritage or religious tradition can avoid the problems inherent to a staunchly nonnatural neuroethics. Abandoning ethical principles and embracing reductionism is not necessary; indeed, naturalistic neuroethics is admittedly metaphysical about nature yet it need not, and should not, devolve into value-free physicalism. Even if metaphysical insights distinguish the worldview of a religious tradition, scientific insights into the whole human being and the human capacity for moral agency can be accepted and implemented for worthy ethical goals. As for naturalistic neuroethics, it must never lose sight of the personal self that bears moral worth and pursues moral ends. Here, it is important to assert that neuroscience—and neuroethics—must appreciate the functions of brains that are embodied in organisms that are embedded in their ecologies, inclusive of culture and religious traditions and practices [27]. In this way, naturalistic neuroethics will be indebted to ethical wisdom conveyed by cultural and religious heritages.

From this broader vantage point, the chasm separating naturalistic and nonnaturalistic neuroethics no longer seems so wide. With anthropology and ethics leading this approach, a closer convergence is coming into view. We can now confess that the initial (and admittedly artificial) dichotomy that we erected between "naturalistic" and "nonnatural" neuroethics had to collapse. The shared humanistic basis to any ethical neuroethics, grounded in humanity and its moral ways, brings ethics and science into conceptual and practical coordination:

> *Only socialized and encultured brains understand and enact morality. No science has a basis for inquiries or judgments about morality apart from this human arena of life.*
>
> *Moral values and norms are instilled and perpetuated through one or another culturally embedded heritage. No science is inquiring into anything about morality outside of these ongoing practices.*

> *Cognitive science and neuroscience cannot independently understand human moral capacities. Alleged discoveries about moral cognition from brain science alone have, in fact, tacitly presumed psychological or philosophical frameworks.*
>
> *Developmental, social, and moral psychology is best positioned to comprehend how people participate in the moral practices of their societies. Brain sciences yield adjunct inquiries to moral capacities by presuming frameworks from the behavioral sciences.*
>
> *The behavioral and brain sciences are discovering the cognitive functions and neurological processes permitting moral behaviors. What human brains are really doing (and not doing) sets factual bounds to pondering how people are able (or fail) to behave morally.*
>
> *Ethics offers bridges between moral practices that humans promulgate and desired moral ends worthy of pursuit. Ethics should deal with actual moral capacities and practical methods of improving them.*
>
> *Effective means of understanding and improving real-world moral conduct are the practical tools in service of meeting moral standards and realizing ethical ends. Imagined threats to morality from nature and causality unwisely thwart motives to make a more moral world.*

So long as humanity as a whole is an objective of both scientific study and ethical interest, then neuroethics can be cohesive and complete. "Naturalizing" neuroethics actually names no urgently needed project. As unwarranted worries over reductionism subside, "nonnaturalistic" neuroethics only names a reactionary agenda without a real opponent.

5. Conclusion

We posit that the truly urgent project facing neuroethics today is this query: *Given the cultural heterogeneity characterizing the global stage where advanced neuroS/T is emerging, how should neuroethics wisely learn from, and lend advice to, humanity's worldviews, wisdom traditions, and philosophies?* Elsewhere we have urged that a cosmopolitan approach to ethics can elicit deliberations converging on useful principles [1, 28]. Here, we add our warning against emphasizing metaphysical differences or moral disagreements at the expense of our shared humanity, so that "neuro-bio-ethics" has a consolidated foundation and consists of more than just a hybrid term [22, 29]. A human-centered and person-oriented neuroethics will prove capable of assessing how neuroscience is exploring and affecting cognition, emotion, and behavior (inclusive of moral conduct), while upholding ethics to guide the application of neuroS/T as an endeavor seeking the good for humanity.

Acknowledgements

This work was supported in part by the European Union's Horizon 2020 Research and Innovation Programme under grant agreement 720270: HBP SGA1 (JG); by federal funds UL1TR001409 from the National Center for Advancing Translational Sciences (NCATS), National Institutes of Health, through the Clinical and Translational Science Awards Program (CTSA), a trademark of the Department of Health and Human Services, part of the Roadmap Initiative, "Re-Engineering the Clinical Research Enterprise" (JG); and by the Austin and Ann O'Malley Visiting Chair in Bioethics of Loyola Marymount University (JG).

Author details

John R. Shook[1]* and James Giordano[2,3,4]

1 University at Buffalo, Buffalo, New York, USA

2 Department of Neurology, Georgetown University Medical Center, Washington, DC, USA

3 Department of Biochemistry, Georgetown University Medical Center, Washington, DC, USA

4 Neuroethics Studies Program, Pellegrino Center for Clinical Bioethics, Georgetown University Medical Center, Washington, DC, USA

*Address all correspondence to: jshook@pragmatism.org

References

[1] Shook JR, Giordano J. A principled, cosmopolitan neuroethics: Considerations for international relevance. Philosophy, Ethics, and Humanities in Medicine. 2014;**9**(1):article 1

[2] Shook JR, Giordano J. Neuroethics beyond normal: Performance enablement and self-transformative technologies. Cambridge Quarterly of Health Care Ethics. 2016;**25**(1):121-140

[3] Shook JR, Giordano J. Neuroethical engagement on interdisciplinary and international scales. In: Racine E, Aspler J, editors. Debates About Neuroethics. Berlin: Springer; 2017. pp. 225-246

[4] Clausen J, Levy N. What is neuroethics? In: Clausen J, Levy N, editors. Handbook of Neuroethics. Vol. 1. Berlin: Springer; 2014. pp. v-vii

[5] Johnson LSM, Rommelfanger KS. Introduction. In: Johnson LSM, Rommelfanger KS, editors. The Routledge Handbook of Neuroethics. London: Routledge; 2018. pp. xviii-xvxix

[6] Koi P, Uusitalo S, Tuominen J. Self-control in responsibility enhancement and criminal rehabilitation. Criminal Law and Philosophy. 2018;**12**(2): 227-244

[7] Satel S, Lilienfeld SO. Brainwashed: The Seductive Appeal of Mindless Neuroscience. New York: Basic Books; 2013

[8] Wiseman H. The Myth of the Moral Brain: The Limits of Moral Enhancement. Cambridge, MA: MIT Press; 2016

[9] Audi R. Ethical naturalism as a challenge to theological ethics. Journal of the Society of Christian Ethics. 2014;**34**(1):21-39

[10] ten Have H. From synthesis and system to morals and procedure: The development of philosophy of medicine. In: Carson RA, Burns CR, editors. Philosophy of Medicine and Bioethics. Dordrecht: Kluwer; 1997. pp. 105-123

[11] National Academy of Sciences. Science and Creationism: A View from the National Academy of Sciences. 2nd ed. Washington, DC: National Academy Press; 1999

[12] Blok A, Jensen TE. Bruno Latour: Hybrid Thoughts in a Hybrid World. London: Routledge; 2011

[13] Richards RJ, Daston L, editors. Kuhn's 'Structure of Scientific Revolutions' at Fifty: Reflections on a Science Classic. Chicago: University of Chicago Press; 2016

[14] Dennett D. Darwin's Dangerous Idea. New York: Simon and Schuster; 1995

[15] Giordano J, Becker K, Shook JR. On the 'neuroscience of ethics': Approaching the neuroethical literature as a rational discourse on putative neural processes of moral cognition and behavior. Journal of Neurology & Neuromedicine. 2016;**1**(6):32-36

[16] Becker K, Shook JR, Darragh M, Giordano J. A four part working bibliography of neuroethics: Part 4—Ethical issues in clinical and social applications of neuroscience. Philosophy, Ethics, and Humanities in Medicine. 2017;**12**(1):1-32

[17] Darragh M, Buniak L, Giordano J. A four part working bibliography of neuroethics: Part 2—neuroscientific studies of morality and ethics. Philosophy, Ethics, and Humanities in Medicine. 2015;**10**(1):1-22

[18] Martin A, Becker K, Darragh M, Girdano J. A four part working

bibliography of neuroethics: Part 3—The ethics of neuroscience. Philosophy, Ethics, and Humanities in Medicine. 2016;**11**(2):1-55

[19] Yoder K, Decety J. The neuroscience of morality and social decision-making. Psychology, Crime & Law. 2018;**24**(3):279-295

[20] Turiel E. The relevance of moral epistemology and psychology for neuroscience. In: Zelazo P, Chandler M, Crone E, editors. Developmental Social Cognitive Neuroscience. New York: Taylor and Francis; 2009. pp. 313-331

[21] Giordano J, Shook JR. Minding brain science in medicine: On the need for neuroethical engagement for guidance of neuroscience in clinical contexts. Ethics in Biology Engineering and Medicine. 2015;**6**(1-2):37-42

[22] Avram M, Giordano J. Neuroethics: Some things old, some things new, some things borrowed...and to do. AJOB Neuroscience. 2014;**5**(4):1-3

[23] Avram M, Hennig-Fast K, Bao Y, Pöppel E, Reiser M, Blautzik J, et al. Neural correlates of moral judgments in first- and third-person perspectives: Implications for neuroethics and beyond. BMC Neuroscience. 2014;**15**:39

[24] Kushner T, Giordano J. Clinical neuroethics—From bench to bedside... and beyond. Cambridge Quarterly of Health Care Ethics. 2016;**25**(4):570-572

[25] Sinnott-Armstrong W. The disunity of morality. In: Liao SM, editor. Moral Brains: The Neuroscience of Morality. Oxford: Oxford University Press; 2016. pp. 331-353

[26] Wheatley T, Decety J, editors. The Moral Brain: A Multidisciplinary Perspective. Cambridge, MA: MIT Press; 2015

[27] Giordano J, Benedikter R. An early—and necessary—Flight of the Owl of Minerva: Neuroscience, neurotechnology, human socio-cultural boundaries, and the importance of neuroethics. Journal of Evolution and Technology. 2012;**22**(1):14-25

[28] Lanzilao E, Shook JR, Benedikter R, Giordano J. Advancing neuroscience on the 21st century world stage: The need for—and proposed structure of—An internationally relevant neuroethics. Ethics in Biology Engineering and Medicine. 2013;**4**(3):211-229

[29] Giordano J, Benedikter R, Kohls NB. Neuroscience and the importance of a neurobioethics: A reflection upon Fritz Jahr. In: Muzur A, Sass H-M, editors. Fritz Jahr and the Foundations of Integrative Bioethics. Berlin: LIT Verlag; 2012. pp. 267-280

Section 3

Neuro-Ethical Praxis Amidst Pluralistic Value Sourcing

Chapter 4

Terminality Advance Directives and Nursing Practice in Brazil: Bioethical Issues

Jacqueline Resende Boaventura, Juliana Dias Reis Pessalacia, Luciana Ferreira Da Silva, Ana Paula Da Silva, Larissa Da Silva Barcelos, Carlos Eduardo Pereira Furlani and Adriano Menis Ferreira

Abstract

Advance directives (ADs) are understood as the act of deciding what care the patient wants to receive in the period before death. Preserving the patient's autonomy by choosing his care guarantees human dignity during the process of dying. In Brazil, life expectancy and supportive technologies have increased, leading to growth of the number of terminally ill patients. However, there is still no legislation regulating ADs causing legal uncertainty in health professionals. Nursing professionals have the support of the Federal Nursing Council to respect the ADs, but, because it is an issue little explored, nursing professionals do not feel safe in the use of ADs, and changes in the curricula of the undergraduate courses in nursing are extremely needed, ensuring that patients have their wishes met during the dying process. Thus, this chapter deals with bioethical and legal issues involving ADs and nursing in the Brazilian context, proposing to deepen reflection and criticism on the issue and subsidies for decision-making.

Keywords: advance directives, right to die, palliative care, bioethics, nursing

1. Introduction

Life in the society is shaped by a set of principles, values, and concepts that determine approval or disapproval judgments in the interpersonal relationships and actions of the individuals. In this context, ethics seeks to reflect and understand the presuppositions of morality, aimed at achieving the best result for people and society [1].

However, this concept was expanded through scientific and technological advances, emerging bioethics in the 1970s, which means "ethics of life" in the literal sense. Bioethics proposes the dialog between the biological and human sciences. In 1971, the oncologist and university professor Van Rensselaer Potter published the book *Bioethics: A Bridge to the Future*, placing bioethics as necessary to ensure human survival in the accelerated civilization development. He reported that knowledge has been acquired at a speed far greater than the capacity and ability to know what to do with it [2].

Bioethics needs to be considered not only in the research and development area but also in interprofessional relationships in health, not limiting the analysis of such relationships only to deontological codes. In this sense, the North American principalist model is shown as a good ally in directing actions, reflections, and decisions of health professionals [1].

The beneficence, non-maleficence, autonomy, and justice principles can be applied prima facie in health decision-making. Beneficence suggests the need to do good, requiring professionals' knowledge and skills to distinguish which procedures and practices are beneficial and which can harm. Non-maleficence is not exposing the patient to risk situations, minimizing damages, and seeking other alternatives. Autonomy represents the patient's right to decide what is done to his body and health, based on his life purpose, principles, and creed. The principle of justice is the social duties and benefits, which are contemplated and guaranteed in the Federal Constitution of 1988 and in the Organic Law of Health (Law 8080/90) [3].

In different healthcare settings, terminality is a topic full of ethical dilemmas that require decision-making by the professional who is always trying to overcome death and interfere in different ways in this process. As death is still a "taboo" in our society, when it occurs in health services, it becomes more evident as a medical failure than the simple understanding of the natural course of life, leading to bioethical discussions and problems [3].

Facing the current conjuncture of advances in technological development for the extension of life, death previously seen naturally and as part of the process of human finitude is now tried to be avoided. At present the usefulness of life support therapies is questioned, such as: When to interrupt or maintain life without hurting the principles of bioethics? [4].

The problems revealed with end-of-life care express the importance of intensifying the debate about the imminence of death and human terminality, analyzing the progress of the social behaviors and the ethical precepts of health professionals in palliative care [5].

In this context, the theme of the advance directives (ADs) has been discussed in Brazil, which consists of deciding what care to receive in the period before death, ensuring to the patient more dignity and quality in this process. Refusing unnecessary interventions, pain and suffering relief, and home care around the family rather than hospital isolation are debatable issues that express the patient's autonomy.

Therefore, legal issues of effectiveness of the social rights and the affirmation if they contemplate the fundamental rights of the constitutional legal order expressed by the Democratic State of Law will be addressed, with due guarantees and legal safeguards of the existential minimum or the possible reserve, accessibility to justice as a common good.

Thus, this chapter addresses the bioethical and legal issues involving ADs and nursing in the Brazilian context, proposing a deepened reflection and criticism on the topic and subsidies for decision-making involving the nursing professional.

2. Advance directives and nursing

Brazil is following the world trend with a significant increase in the population over 65 years old, from 4.1% in 1991 to 7.4% in 2010. In 2020, it is assumed that Brazil will be sixth worldwide, considering the older adult population [6].

In this context, the increase in life expectancy and in the supportive technologies has led to a substantial increase of terminally ill patients. During the terminality of life, the individual is faced with unusual events and arduous decisions regarding health care, including communication of bad news, palliative care, advance directives (living will), order of not resuscitating, and dysthanasia [7].

Little is prepared for death. Even the health professionals are prepared to seek only life above all, putting death as something to be defeated [8]. In the situations where the medical behaviors are exhausted, the palliative care appears to offer better assistance to the patient and to minimize the suffering [9].

Biologically, death is a consequence of the vital functions, cardiac and respiratory end, and over the years, even feared, it has been postponed through the use of various technologies. Cardiopulmonary resuscitation (CPR) in some cases keeps the heart pumped only for a short period turning into an invasive and traumatic experience and sometimes depriving the patient of their choice of death that can lead to a loss of dignity and prolongation of suffering [10, 11]. Thus, the question is: What benefits are added to the state of human existence in which the person does not establish more relationships with other people, as in the case of the state of coma? Why increase the days of life, concomitantly, to the affliction of the patient and their relatives? [3].

Under some conditions, the decision to maintain life at any cost must be taken by the patient, because although death is relatively close, he is still alive and conscious, and his wishes must be respected as far as possible [12]. The act of deciding what care to receive in the period before his death guarantees more dignity during the process of dying [13] since the bioethical principle of autonomy can interfere, question, and choose procedures or treatments [3].

In the meantime, it is worth noting that the principle of autonomy foresees that decision-makers are rational agents with appropriate cognitive conditions for the understanding of their own interests and without any external controlling influences. Thus, the obligation to respect the autonomy of the patient can exceed the duty of beneficence of doctors and health professionals, if rationality and knowledge of the patient's situation can be confirmed [14].

Also a greater vulnerability of the patients with chronic neurological-incapacitating conditions should be considered, such as Parkinsonism or muscular dystrophy. In these cases, it is important to create a formal communication process, from the diagnosis of a serious illness. For neurology patients, the period between the diagnosis and the loss of communication capacity is frequently limited, and the opportunity of effective communication in this period should not be missed [14].

Under the view of humanization, the technical-scientific advance restricts the patient, since health care is directed to attend only biological and physiological aspects. Thus, ADs enable patients to express the subjectivities of their desires and, with dignity, to direct what they expect for their days to the end of life.

These advances have enabled some patients to survive in persistent or minimally conscious vegetative states for decades. In these cases, due to emotional issues, the caregivers opt for care continuity. However, such decisions have impacts on the patient's quality of life and ethical responsibility for the distributive justice of health systems. Doctors are encouraged to make decisions in individual cases since conflicts may be unavoidable. In cases of some conflict, doctors may ask help to nurses as they are professionals who are with patients most of the time, being potential experts of their wishes [14].

Given such conditions, advanced care planning (ACP) strategies have been discussed in India, ensuring that adults at any age or stage of health understand and share their personal values, life goals, and preferences regarding future medical care. In this context, the main responsibilities of neurologists in medical practice in end-of-life care appear in two situations: catastrophic brain injury (CBI) and life-limiting neurological illness (LLNI). Patients with CBI are hospitalized in an altered mental status, and life-sustaining treatments (LST) are often performed immediately after. Also the difficulties of decision-making for not presenting legislation on the declaration of death by neurological criteria were pointed out, recommending that the medical team makes decisions, in conflicting cases, in consensus with the relatives and other members of the health team [14].

In Brazil, as being a very recent topic, there is little research that explains the ADs and the understandings of health professionals and society on the theme [15].

Currently, the consideration for the patient autonomy is being discussed, as well as the power to express opinions, make decisions, and proceed according to their personal principles and rules [16]. This right is shown in Article 15 of the Civil Code and Articles 22, 23, and 24 of the Code of Medical Ethics (CEM).

In the world context, ADs appeared in the United States in the 1960s and were initially presented by the American Society for Euthanasia in 1967 through the document entitled "Living Will (TV)," in which the individual could register their wishes to cease the medical conceptions of continuity of life [17].

It is suggested that advance care planning initially includes information about the types of life-sustaining treatments available and decisions about the types of treatment that patients would or would not want if they were diagnosed with a life-limiting illness. Afterward, it is necessary to encourage the sharing of personal values by patients and their families, and only then the ADs should be written, expressing what kind of treatment they would like or not if they could not speak for themselves [18].

If the patient does not have the cognitive conditions to decide, it is suggested that the substitute decision-maker meets the following criteria: being able to make a decision, being available and willing to do so, and being legally established as representatives of the patient. In the absence of a legally established representative for decision-making, the next of kin may be considered a substitute [18].

In Brazil, from the juridical point of view, in the current Constitutional Order, principles are considered as guidelines, and unlike the norm that regulates an end, the principle regulates a means, and it is the foundation of any legal system. In the case of ADs, the principles seek to eliminate gaps, offering coherence and harmony to the legal order. Although widely discussed worldwide for years, the ADs were inserted in the national healthcare scenario only in 2012, through Resolution CFM 1995/2012 which guides the medical practice in end-of-life conditions, ensuring patient's self-sufficiency and the preservation of human integrity [19].

According to the CFM, the ADs are characterized as a grouping of wills, clearly expressed by the patients about their treatments and care they want to receive when they are unable to manifest their wishes [19]. This resolution considers the probability of the patient to name a representative so his demands can be met when he can no longer pronounce them [19]. The instruction to interrupt treatments that unnecessarily prolong the life of the patient with a severe or incurable illness allowed to the doctor was already provided for in Resolution CFM 1805 of 2006 [20].

When talking about ADs, it is essential to understand that this is the junction of the Durable Mandate (DM) and TV in a single document [17].

The DM is the patient's indication of one or more attorneys-in-fact to be consulted by the medical team in case of his definitive or momentary impossibility when it is necessary to make a decision on the treatment or not treatment [16]. The TV is a document in which the patient details the treatments and procedures he intend to do or not to do when he is incapacitated to manifest his will, being useful only in cases of terminality [16].

The TV is a legal instrument that enables to certify the domination of the individual in the decisions about his health, having the "good death" as his final purpose [19].

Brazilian doctors still do not have legal support in relation to the ADs. However, they must obey CFM Resolution 1995/2012 [16]. The doctor should transcribe in medical records the ADs that are formally declared by the patient. If the person in the hospital is not known and if there is no appointed attorney-in-fact, available relatives, or concordance between them, the doctor should refer to the Bioethics Committee of the institution. If there is no committee, the hospital's Ethics Committee or Regional and Federal Council of Medicine needs to document their opinion on ethical confrontations, when considering this measure as indispensable and appropriate [19].

Currently, the Bill 149 of 2018 is in process in the Brazilian Federal Senate, which regulates the advance directives on health treatments. The Article 2, paragraph I of this Bill defines ADs as a "manifestation documented by public deed, without financial content, of the will of the reporting person to receive or not certain medical care or treatment, to be respected when the person can not express his will, freely and autonomously" [21].

Also in Article 3, the Bill proposes that "every greater and capable person has the right to declare in advance, his or her will to receive or not certain medical treatments in the future when being in clinical condition" [20]. Article 5 of this same Bill reports that "advance directives must be met by health professionals and public or private health services, as well as by relatives, legal guardians, and the declarant's representative" [21].

The respect for the independence of the actions related to the ADs is an important benefit for their application, especially in the disease termination, not only for doctors but also for the nurse [22].

ADs are seen by nursing professionals as synonymous with attending to the principle of autonomy of the patient and their relatives, with undeniable character and with inevitable growth [23]. It is an instrument capable of facilitating decision-making on ethical issues related to the end of life [24].

Nursing is recognized as the professional category that plays a primary role in the exercise of the right to self-determination, helping and facilitating patient decision-making, as it is present throughout the death process [25]. When establishing effective and early communication with the hospitalized patient, the nursing team creates a bond of trust between patient and professional that allows the conscious and autonomous exercise of the right to self-determination, ensuring that the patient's wishes and choices are taken into account in situations involving decision-making in terminality [26].

The Code of Ethics of Nursing Professionals [26], in its Article 42, Sole paragraph, describes that the nursing professional must "Respect the person's advance directives regarding the decisions about care and treatment that he or she wishes or not to receive at the moment when he/she is unable to freely and autonomously express his/her wishes."

However, the lack of knowledge of regulations aimed at nursing professionals and the fear of ethical-legal implications interfere with the use of ADs. Faced with this reality and to avoid conflicts, nurses prefer to attend the wishes of family members, even if these wishes are not in accordance with the wishes expressed by the patient [27, 8].

For nursing professionals to feel effectively supported and safe in the use of ADs, it is necessary to include this subject in the curricula of the Nursing Undergraduate Courses, and the dissemination of scientific knowledge should be in agreement with the benefits brought to the patients with their wills met.

Currently, the National Curricular Guidelines of the Nursing Undergraduate Program indicate that nurses' training should cover issues related to the prevention, promotion, healing, and rehabilitation of the health of individuals and the community. Thus, higher education institutions guided by these guidelines offer technical-scientific training that favors therapeutic obstinacy, aiming only at maintaining life at any cost [28].

It is believed that curricular changes, which deepen the ethical debate around issues related to the dying process, are necessary in the training of the nurse since the proximity of the nursing team with the hospitalized patient provides emotional exhaustion, and these professionals feel they are helpless before death. It is necessary that the process of dying be debated within educational institutions, so future nursing professionals understand and respect terminality as a phase present in human existence [23].

Rethinking treatment related to terminal patient care within higher education institutions favors the reduction of difficulties in dealing with the death process and therapeutic obstinacy and providing more humanized care [29].

Thus, it is important that the future nurse be encouraged to know the ADs during the professional training process, to understand its applicability in their clinical practice and to stimulate its use by patients, terminal or not, informing the possibility of construction and the importance of the ADs and presenting the necessary explanations for the elaboration of a document of this nature [28].

3. Conclusion

In Brazil, there is still no legislation that deals with ADs, which makes this topic little debated and diffused among health professionals, more specifically among the professionals of the nursing team.

Guaranteeing the individuals the right to carry out their wills in terminality through the ADs is still not enough since collective work is indispensable and necessary to respect their autonomy and reflections on the cultural actions of professionals' health and family members that determine the paradigm of sustaining life at any cost.

The main challenge found during the dying process is to ensure that in practice, the patient's wishes are met. It is noticeable that the implications and obstacles resulting from the ceaseless transformations of the right to health as a whole are far from over, especially the relationships inherent to the principle of human dignity, individual freedom, and the practices of health professionals.

There is a need to disseminate among nursing professionals the importance of encouraging the free and informed autonomy of patients and of the Federal Nursing Council regulation that supports professionals who respect the ADs of the individuals under their care. The knowledge of the Code of Ethics of Nursing Professionals and the inclusion of ADs in the curricula of Nursing Undergraduate Courses are essential for Brazil to make a positive contribution to this issue.

In view of the current Brazilian health scene, the ADs are characterized as a new subject, and its applicability involves cultural change, family and health professionals' agreement, and an early approach in both undergraduate and care education.

Conflict of interest

We declare there is no conflict of interest in this research.

Author details

Jacqueline Resende Boaventura, Juliana Dias Reis Pessalacia*, Luciana Ferreira Da Silva, Ana Paula Da Silva, Larissa Da Silva Barcelos, Carlos Eduardo Pereira Furlani and Adriano Menis Ferreira
Federal University of Mato Grosso do Sul, Três Lagoas, Mato Grosso do Sul, Brazil

*Address all correspondence to: juliana@pessalacia.com.br

References

[1] Koerich MS, Machado RR, Costa E. Ética e bioética: Para dar início à reflexão. Texto & Contexto – Enfermagem. 2005;**14**(1):106-110. DOI: 10.1590/S0104-07072005000100014

[2] Zoboli ELCP. Bioética e atenção básica: Um estudo de ética descritiva com enfermeiros e médicos do Programa de Saúde da Família [thesis]. São Paulo: Faculdade de Saúde Pública, Universidade de São Paulo; 2003

[3] Xavier M, Miziara C, Miziara I. Terminalidade da vida: Questões éticas e religiosas sobre a ortotanásia. Saúde, Ética & Justiça. 2014;**19**(1):26-34. DOI: 10.11606/issn.2317-2770.v19i1p26-34

[4] Marengo M, Flávio D, Silva R. Terminalidade de vida: Bioética e humanização em saúde. Medicina (Ribeirao Preto. Online). 2009;**42**(3):350-357. DOI: 10.11606/issn.2176-7262.v42i3p350-357

[5] de Paiva FCL, de Almeida Júnior JJ, Damásio AC. Ética em cuidados paliativos: Concepções sobre o fim da vida. Revista Bioética. 2014;**22**(3):550-560. DOI: 10.1590/1983-80422014223038

[6] Kovács MJ. A caminho da morte com dignidade no século XXI. Revista Bioética. 2014;**22**(1):94-104. DOI: 10.1590/S1983-80422014000100011

[7] Comin LT, Panka M, Beltrame V, Steffani JA, Bonamigo EL. Percepção de pacientes oncológicos sobre terminalidade de vida. Revista Bioética. 2017;**25**(2):392-401. DOI: 10.1590/1983-80422017252199

[8] Vancini-Campanharo CR, Vancini RL, Machado Netto MC, Lopes MCBT, Okuno MFP, Batista REA, et al. Do not attempt resuscitation orders at the emergency department of a teaching hospital. Einstein. 2017;**15**(4):409-414. DOI: 10.1590/s1679-45082017ao3999

[9] Poletto S, Bettinelli LA, Santin JR. Vivencias en torno a la muerte de pacientes de edad avanzada en la práctica médica y dignidad humana. Revista Bioética. 2016;**24**(3):590-595. DOI: 10.1590/1983-80422016243158

[10] Campbell R. Do not attempt cardiopulmonary resuscitation decisions: Joint guidance. The Journal of the Royal College of Physicians of Edinburgh. 2017;**47**(1):47-51. DOI: 10.4997/JRCPE.2017.110

[11] Field RA, Fritz Z, Baker A, Grove A, Perkins GD. Systematic review of interventions to improve appropriate use and outcomes associated with do-not-attempt-cardiopulmonary-resuscitation decisions. Resuscitation. 2014;**85**(11):1418-1431. DOI: 10.1016/j.resuscitation.2014.08.024

[12] Santana JCB, Caldeira CLG, Martins Andrade JD, Silva CCD. Experiences of caring for patients of life in terminal: Perception of a group of students of nursing. Rev. Enfermagem Revista. 2015;**18**(2):29-41

[13] Lima MLF, Rego STA, Siqueira-Batista R. Proceso de toma de decisión en los cuidados de fin de vida. Revista Bioética. 2015;**23**(1):31-39. DOI: 10.1590/1983-80422015231043

[14] Gursahani R, Mani RK, Simha SN. End of life and palliative care in neurology: Does autonomy matter? Annals of Indian Academy of Neurology. 2018;**21**(4):239-241. DOI: 10.4103/aian.AIAN_138_18

[15] Gomes BMM, Salomão LA, Simões AC, Rebouças BO, Dadalto L, Barbosa MT. Diretivas antecipadas de vontade em geriatria. Revista Bioética. 2018;**26**(3):429-439. DOI: 10.1590/1983-80422018263263

[16] Kulicz MJ, Amarante DF, Nakatani HTI, Arai Filho C, Okamoto

CT. Terminalidade e testamento vital: O conhecimento de estudantes de medicina. Revista Bioética. 2018;**26**(3):420-428. DOI: 10.1590/1983-80422018263262

[17] Dadalto L, Tupinambás U, Greco DB. Diretivas antecipadas de vontade: Um modelo brasileiro. Revista Bioética. 2013;**21**(3):463-476. DOI: 10.1590/S1983-80422013000300011

[18] Salins N, Gursahani R, Mathur R, Iyer S, Macaden S, Simha N, et al. Definition of terms used in limitation of treatment and providing palliative care at the end of life: The Indian council of medical research commission report. Indian Journal of Critical Care Medicine. 2018;**22**(4):249-262. DOI: 10.4103/ijccm.IJCCM_165_18

[19] Cogo SB, Lunardi VL. Diretivas antecipadas: Uma análise documental no contexto mundial. Texto & Contexto - Enfermagem. 2018;**27**(3):e1880014. DOI: 10.1590/0104-070720180001880014

[20] Scottini MA, de Siqueira JE, Moritz RD. Direito dos pacientes às diretivas antecipadas de vontade. Revista Bioética. 2018;**26**(3):440-450. DOI: 10.1590/1983-80422018263264

[21] BRAZIL. Federal Senate. Bill No. 149 of 2018. Provides for the advance directives of will on health treatments. Brasília, DF; Apr 03 2018. Available from: https: //www25.senado. leg.br/web/atividade/materias/-/ material / 132773. [Accessed on: 24 April, 2019]

[22] Cogo SB, Lunardi VL, Quintana AM, Girardon-Perlini NMO, da SRS. Assistência ao doente terminal: Vantagens na aplicabilidade das diretivas antecipadas de vontade no contexto hospitalar. Revista Gaúcha de Enfermagem. 2017;**38**(4):e65617. DOI: 10.1590/1983-1447.2017.04.65617

[23] Saioron I, Ramos FRS, Schneider DG, da Silveira RS, Silveira LR. Diretivas antecipadas de vontade: Percepções de enfermeiros sobre os benefícios e novas demandas. Escola Anna Nery. 2017;**21**(4):e20170100. DOI: 10.1590/2177-9465-ean-2017-0100

[24] Vieira TGF. Diretivas antecipadas de vontade: Um estudo de revisão de literatura à luz da Bioética [dissertation]. Brasília-DF: Universidade de Brasília; 2018

[25] Cogo SB, Lunardi VL, Nietsche EA. Considerações acerca da atuação do enfermeiro das diretivas antecipadas de vontade. Enfermagem em Foco. 2018;**8**(2):26-30. DOI: 10.21675/2357-707X.2017.v8.n2.1061

[26] Ramos V. Equipa de emergência médica intra-hospitalar: Processo de decisão de não reanimar [dissertation]. Castelo Branco, Portugal: Instituto Politécnico de Castelo Branco, Escola Superior de saúde; 2017

[27] Conselho Federal de Enfermagem. Novo Código de Ética dos Profissionais de Enfermagem [Internet]. 2017. Available from: http://www.corengo.org.br/wp-content/uploads/2017/12/RESOLU%C3%87%C3%83O-COFEN-N%C2%BA-564-2017.pdf

[28] Cogo SB, Lunardi VL, Quintana AM, Girardon-Perlini NMO, da Silveira RS. Challenges to implementation of advance directives of will in hospital practice. Revista Brasileira de Enfermagem. 2016;**69**(6):1031-1038. DOI: 10.1590/0034-7167-2016-0085

[29] Cassol PB, Quintana AM, Velho MTAC. Diretiva antecipada de vontade: Percepção de uma equipe de enfermagem da hemato-oncologia. Journal of Nursing and Health. 2015;**5**(1):04-13. DOI: 10.15210/JONAH.V5I1.5497

Chapter 5

Values-Based Medicine (VsBM) and Evidence-Based Medicine (EBM)

Ahmed Ammar

Abstract

Medical care is a dynamic process to implement and use the most recent technologies, skills, and knowledge to either maintain the good health of people or to treat sick patients. Patients have the right to receive the best possible available treatment. During the course of treatment, the patient's dignity and rights should be respected and never be compromised. A patient's right to be properly treated is one of the fundamental human rights. The healthcare system is responsible for providing efficient and sufficient healthcare facilities and training and continuously educating able medical and paramedical teams. Evidence-based medicine has been popularized in the last 40–50 years in order to raise the standard of medical practice. Medical ethics and values have been associated with medical practice for thousands of years since patients felt the need for treatment. There is no conflict between evidence-based medicine and values-based medicine, as the medical practice should be always preformed within a frame of ethics and respect of patient's values. Observing the principles of values-based medicine became very relevant as multicultural societies are dominant in some countries and hospitals in different corners of the world.

Keywords: values-based medicine, bioethics, patient's rights, education, dignity, history of medical ethics

1. Introduction

Conventional clinical relationships are centered on a triad, consisting of the physician, the patient, and his/her family. Nowadays, individuals in need or seeking medical care, as well as their intimate circle, interact with a great variety of stakeholders and clustered interests. Three important factors contribute to this more complex situation.

The progress of life sciences and technological innovations as well as the development of the health system and the medical-industrial complex create new medical situations and redefine the role of both family members and health professionals.

The potential of modern healthcare, including resuscitation and life-sustaining technologies, their impact on the quality of life, as well as problems of costs and resource allocation in the context of market economies, also redefine the role of family members. This opens a myriad of ethical questions, from coping with frail, sick, or disabled relatives, over socialization and commercialization of traditional household tasks, to substitute decision-making for minors and patients with diminished autonomy, as well as dealing with end-of-life situations.

The nature of neurosurgical problems forces neurosurgeons to face their patients' families in different emotional situations, frustrated to see good results, disappointed with the outcome, confused, denying, or angry. Neurosurgeons should learn the skill to absorb the first reaction of the patients' family and work with them as one team to help their loved one. The patient's family can play a very positive part in the caregiving team for the patient and may have a great and unreplaceable input for their patient care.

2. Definition and the concept of values-based medicine

Values-based medicine (VsBM) is the concept to ensure that the principles of medical ethics are strictly implemented and observed in every step of a patient's management.

> *Values-based medicine can be defined as "medical practice that aims at maximizing value, specifically desirable or positive value in every step of a patient's medical management".*

The concept of values-based medicine (VsBM) stresses on the fact that patient, patient care, and well-being are the center of care in modern medicine. The treating neurosurgeons, physicians, or healthcare givers should spare no effort to improve their skills, update their knowledge, and learn to use the latest technology in order to provide the best care for the patient. The treating team should have a vision and build up a strategy of management and follow-up of their patients. All these necessary steps should be performed within a frame of values and medical ethics. The treating teams should respect and observe the patient and value and respect the culture of the society. Evidence-based medicine should be considered an important component of values-based medicine [1].The key elements of values-based medicine which, like evidence-based medicine, influence any clinical decisions may be taken for patients' management (**Figure 1**).

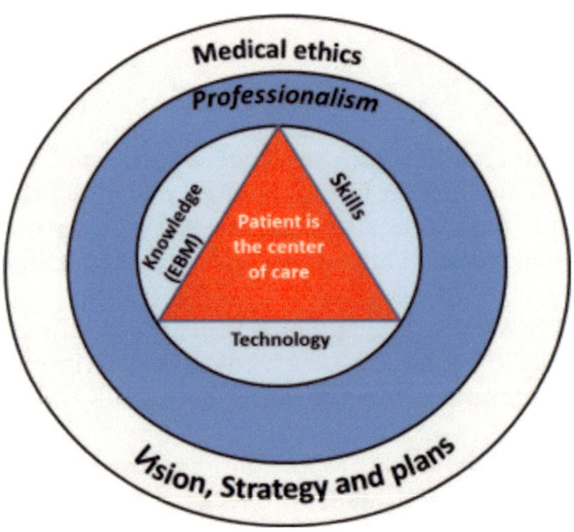

Figure 1.
The concept of values-based medicine (VsBM): patient is the center of care.

3. The principles of medical ethics

Based on the Hippocratic Oath, the main ethical principles were beneficence (do the best for patients) and non-maleficence (do no harm). These two principles were considered to be the fundamental principles of medical ethics for hundreds of years. The principles of medical ethics/bioethics were expanded to include autonomy (patient's right to accept or refuse the method of treatment) and justice. Justice in medicine considers the distribution of healthcare facilities and the access of all patients to these facilities. One of the positive characters of the last and this century is the respect and observation of human rights. Therefore the human rights were manifested clearly in the medical ethics, as the medical ethics expanded again to (a) autonomy, (b) beneficence, (c) non-maleficence, (d) justice, (e) dignity, and (f) truthfulness and honesty. **Figure 2** demonstrates these principles.

3.1 Patients' rights

The respect of patients' rights is one of the main foundations of the concept of values-based medicine. Patients should be considered as partners and share in the process of management. Patients should agree and consent to every step of treatment. Patients have the right to be fairly and properly treated; follow-up should be guaranteed. A patient's privacy, dignity, and confidentiality should be respected. Dignity encompasses a feeling of self-worth and equality. It is paramount that the patient be treated as a person with a disease, rather than a disease that a person has. The patient should also feel he is an equal partner in decision-making, and not just a bystander or subordinate. Patients should be educated and learn about their medical problems, treatment options, and the prognosis. Patients must know who the treating team is, their experiences and qualifications. Patients should have the right to complain in the cases of dissatisfaction about the treatment or lack of communication. Most of these rights are illustrated in **Figure 3**. These fundamental human rights are listed in the WHO recommendation [2] and the World Federation of Neurological Societies as good practice guideline [3].

3.2 The duties and task of the treating teams

The concept of values-based medicine draws the outlines of the duties and tasks of the treating team as illustrated in **Figure 4**. These duties include respecting the

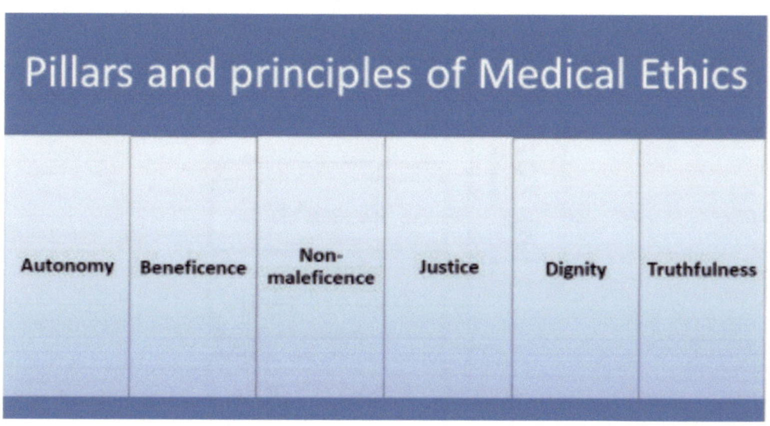

Figure 2.
The principles of medical ethics.

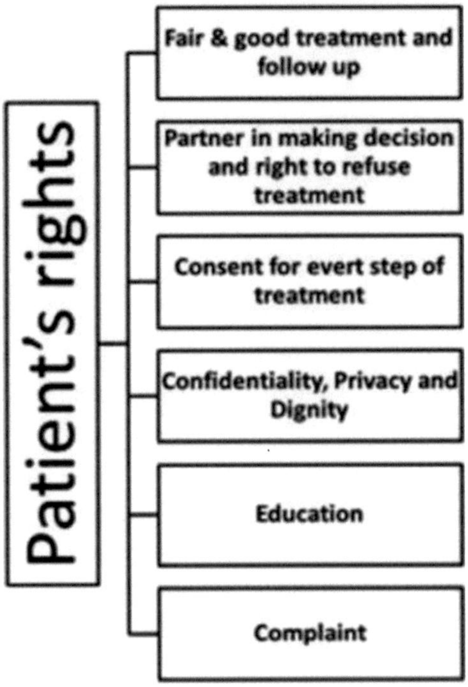

Figure 3.
The Patient's rights.

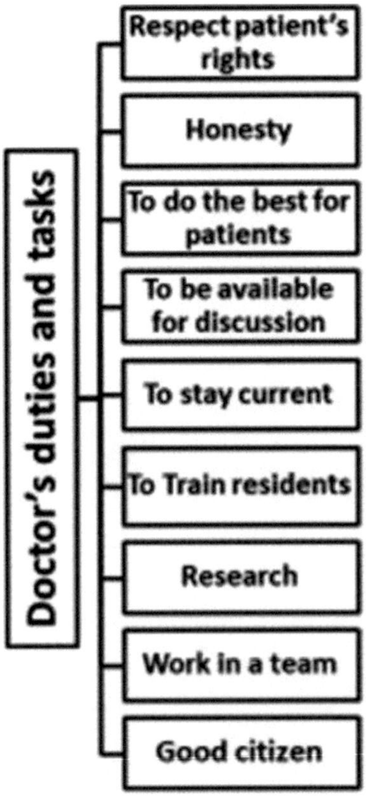

Figure 4.
The tasks and duties of a medical team.

patient and preserving their dignity. It is the duty of every doctor to improve skills and update the knowledge. Doctors should research answers to previously unanswered medical questions. Doctors should be good citizens and advocate for good health. They should maintain a high level of professionalism at all times.

4. Ethical relativism

Healthcare is considered as a universal human right. Culture, faith, socioeconomic factors, and the perception of the value of the education, work, and status of doctors in differing societies are some of the causes of the variance of healthcare in those societies. That variance cannot be deemed as right or wrong, which led to the study and introduction of ethical relativism. Ethical relativism is the view that there are no ethical standards that are absolutely true and must be applied to the societies, without variance. According to the Relativism Theory, a certain event, attitude, or practice may be considered right, if it is accepted as morally correct by the people of the involved society. The same event or attitude may be considered wrong by a society that does not accept it as morally correct.

Throughout the world, most neurosurgical training programs are designed to produce safe, effective neurosurgeons trained to find evidence for the treatment of different neurosurgical problems [4].

Neurosurgeons are obliged to establish ethical and professional relationships with their patients and to that end, should listen to and be guided by both the patient's medical complaint and their perception of the possible outcomes. It is the duty of neurosurgeons to explain to their patients all the steps of investigation, treatment, operation, and possible outcome.

The neurosurgeon can gain valuable knowledge of the patient's culture and beliefs while discussing the benefits and risks of a particular method of management during the course of obtaining informed consent. This knowledge and exchange of information assist in gaining the patient's respect and trust and compliance for both the agreed-upon treatment and its follow-up. Ethical informed consent requires that autonomy and beneficence are applied in equal measure. In applying beneficence, at the expense of autonomy, neurosurgeons may cause irreparable psychological damage [5–7] . Pressure or influence for a particular course of treatment can never be considered ethical, because, although it may be applying the principle of beneficence, it is at the expense of autonomy.

5. Evidence-based medicine (EBM) and values-based medicine (VsBM)/ EBM and VsBM

5.1 What is medical evidence?

An "evidence" is considered as evidence according to data of a particular cohort study under particular condition of some patient group somewhere. Several scholars and ethicists have raised concern about using the stereotype of evidence to promote a chosen type of therapy or surgery [8]. This attitude may cause bias in selecting evidence to justify certain methods of treatment.

Ross defined the clinical evidence as "In essence, evidence—narrowly defined or not—is a provisional departure point in the consideration of whether or not a particular course of action is to be taken in any clinical context." [9] This definition directly links the evidence to its application but not to the strength, validity, and reliability of the source of that evidence.

5.2 Evidence-based medicine: definitions and impact on medical practice

The introduction of evidence-based medicine 40–50 years ago had a great impact on medical practice almost everywhere. That concept became very popular in a very short time. The main reason being that it offers a strong foundation for the justification of decision-making in the course of management of clinical cases. The evidence-based medicine was defined by El Kayaly et al. as "Evidence-based clinical medicine can be seen as the conscious incorporation of the best evidence that is currently available into daily clinical practice covering prevention, diagnostics, clinical assessments, treatments and patient-centered care" [10]. The implementation of the concept of EBM is significantly helpful and challenging for many practitioners for several reasons such as:

a. EBM aims to manage uncertainty regarding the short- and long-term outcome of management of certain cases. However, this aim cannot be always achieved.

b. From the physicians' perspective, the conscious belief of the treating team that the best evidence and recommended method of a case management is followed has a definitely positive impact on the treating team and increases their confidence about the line of treatment they decided to choose.

c. In the cases when good and suitable evidence are not found or not agreed about, the integration of the principles of values-based medicine is a must.

d. From the patients' perspective, knowing that the course of management offered to them is supported by good evidence helps the patient and his family to accept that method of treatment. The patient's perception of receiving treatment according to EBM has good psychological impact.

e. In the cases of medical litigation or argument, the documents of the best evidence have an important value to balance the argument. EBM documents should have an important value in a court of law.

f. EBM has also important educational values as it challenges all the practitioners to continuously update their knowledge in the course of their striving to find the best evidence. It definitely promotes the practitioners' professional development. EBM seeks to inculcate lifelong learning process.

6. Clinical application of EBM: considerations

In daily clinical practice, the application and implementation of EBM simply means that choosing a treatment for a patient is based on the strongest available evidence. However, the concept of EBM does not consider as much, but should consider patient's values and beliefs or other factors such as experiences of the treating team and facilities available at that hospital. Sackett et al. defined EBM as "Evidence-based medicine is the integration of best research evidence with clinical expertise and patient values" [11]. In that definition "Patient values" is not clearly explained in that definition which may refer to what does the patient want? In fact, the implementation of EBM does not generally seek patients sharing in decision-making. The science, practice, and application of EBM do not consider that patient's values, faith, and culture are factors for grading or leveling evidence (hierarchy of evidence). Several studies showed the importance of the patient being a partner in decision-making [12, 13].

7. How evidence is ethically evidence?

Evidence-based medicine has been popularized in the last 30 years and to a certain extent has been considered a good measure of medical practice. However, the use of EBM shows these limitations:

I. Patient preferences and values were not always considered during the decision-making process [7].

II. Limitations in incorporating health-related quality of life (HRQoL) [14] .

III. EBM is based on finding and following the highest-quality evidence. However, in the absence of randomized clinical trials, the veracity of the evidence comes into question.

8. Collecting evidence

Ethically there are a few serious questions regarding presumed evidence collection. Those queries are legitimate as most of the evidence is obtained from the analysis of large data (meta-analysis) which has subsequently inherited all the problems of analyzing the large data of multiple sources. This problem has been discussed by several authors including Dagi [15]. He mentioned "The ethical question is what to do about the data once it has been collected and analyzed. It is ethically important to separate the results of statistical analysis from, for example, [1] statistically significant but clinically irrelevant outcomes, [2] judgments about how data about the set should be applied to specific individuals within the set, [3] the protection of the prerogatives of individual patients in the face of population-based protocols, and [4] the protection of the surgeon's prerogatives in personalizing the treatment of individual patients. The question of what should be done with probabilities and statistics is not statistical in the least: it is entirely a value judgment." Both scientifically and ethically, there is a clear line between what is considered fact and what should be or ought to be. The philosophical debate about is/ought (fact/value) has continued for hundreds of years and remains unsettled. Hume produced what is called Hume's law "From causes which appear similar we expect similar effects. This is the sum of all our experimental conclusions." He recognized as well the "is-ought" controversy. The idea of linking what ought to be to what is, is seriously ethically and clinically challenged.

Randomized controlled studies are the main factors that were used to level validity and strength of evidence. The value of evidence from randomized controlled studies is considered the strongest or best evidence and top leveled and graded as "Grade I Evidence." Evidence obtained from nonrandomized studies is considered as "Grade II Evidence." However, evidence based on valid experiences and thoughts and opinions of distinguished medical and surgical authorities are considered as "Grade III Evidence."

Ethical concerns have been raised about double-blind randomized controlled studies. It has been debated that denying a group of patients (control group), the experimental treatment or method of management believed to be beneficial, is ethically challenged. There is also an ethical issue concerning the validity of evidence which is a result of double-blind randomized controlled studies which were carried out in certain circumstances, homogenous or not subjects, variable controls, and particular role to be used as the base for making decision for treating patients in different circumstances. Therefore, the integration of the best research evidence with clinical expertise and patient values should be carefully and cautiously considered.

There is a very important and distinct difference between the methods and approaches of clinical randomized controlled studies and the methods and approaches to established treatment. In the cases of clinical research, the physician (researcher in that case) and the patient are not standing on the same platform and may not have the same motivation and goals of the treatment. Therefore ideal clinical equipoise may not be achieved in such cases. Clinical equipoise should be carefully observed in any clinical research. The patient-physician relationship is a complex relationship regardless of the circumstances or the status of the patient. The patient has rights which should be and must be respected fully. The treating physician or surgeon should be a partner who has the main task to provide the best available treatment to the patient and share the very same goals with patient to cure the medical illness.

Respecting and observing patient values and quality of life are core to the implementation of VsBM. These principles and values somehow are overlooked by evidence-based medicine [12, 13].

The obtained and presented clinical evidence should not be out of the ethics frame (values-based medicine). The evidence should be valid and applicable in that particular condition, scientifically proven and adherent to the ethical principles and rules. VsBM and EBM should be integrated in daily medical practice and medical research. Ross [9] wrote "attention to evidence, however conceived, is linked to commitment to care. Rather than being seen as distinct spheres, ethics and evidence become part of an integrated whole."

9. Theories of ethics

The core of the concept of values-based medicine is to value the human being's dignity and respect patient's rights and lay a foundation for ethical and meaningful good medical practice. Values-based medicine is an expression of medical ethics, considering patient as the center of care. So the frequent question of the clinician is "what is the best management for that particular patient?" If the uncertainty is the answer, the question should be brought as "which method of management ought to be better for that particular patient?" The answer to this question should be based on both clinical evidence and ethical values. Medical ethics should guide decisions in the daily medical practice. There are several branches of ethics which are normative ethics, applied ethics, descriptive ethics, and metaethics.

9.1 Normative ethics

Normative ethics are ethical theories which highlight what is morally right or wrong in order to lead to proper decision. Normative ethics constitutes/includes/is explained by several ethical theories, including:

a. **Deontological theory**—which suggests that means may justify the ends. Deontological theory considers the moral rights according to observing laws and authorities.

b. **Consequentialist theory**—which suggests the ends justify the means. It is an outcome-based ethic that says the moral right depends on the positive results.

c. **Virtue theory**—this theory's roots go back to Aristotle's which focused on the inherent person more than an analysis of the person's deeds. According to this theory, the characters of individuals or groups prevail.

d. **Ethic of caring theory**—which considers the subjective values is the determining factor to identify what is right and what is wrong. This theory suggests that relationships should be a deciding factor in deciding what is right and wrong.

e. **Ethical intuitionism theory**—which suggests that intuitions may be distorted by not accurate or complete information, prejudice, and bias.

9.2 Applied ethics

Applied ethics may be described as it mandates the professional code of ethics or ethical guidelines for a certain profession such as medical profession or counseling.

9.3 Descriptive ethics

Comparative ethics focus on the beliefs of individuals, what people believe. Descriptive ethics is concerned with what is believed, not what should be believed.

9.4 Meta ethics

This type of ethics is mainly concerned with the ethics itself. Metaethics studies the nature of values.

10. VsBM: professionalism and professional ethics (separatists)

Medical professionalism in this context encompasses all qualities obtained and expressed to conduct or perform tasks and medical duties as described by the governing organization and hospital and as expected by the society.

11. Professional ethics

Professional ethics is the use of knowledge and skills to providing patient care governed by the ethical code of the workplace [16]. It is akin to moving from abstract values to daily behavior of individuals in their workplaces or societies.

Professional ethics (as it is one of the elements of values-based medicine) should observe values and standards of medical professionals and their medical societies, along with the expected behavior of the organizations and hospitals [17]. Medical professionals have to continuously gain and update their knowledge and skills in order to improve their career and consequently the patient's care. Medical researchers strive to find facts either in deductive or inductive ways. That effort should be governed by values and ethics of the patients and patients' culture and beliefs, not purely the eagerness to obtain knowledge or achieve professional goals [9, 18, 19].

12. Code of ethics

The code of medical ethics is general ethical guidelines adopted by medical societies, organizations, and hospitals. The code is mandatory for all medical and paramedical professionals in that organization to strictly observe. The code of ethics is not only for the benefit of patients but also for benefit for the medical and paramedical professionals.

13. Decision-making

Professional decision-making cannot be overemphasized in medicine in general and neurosurgery in particular. The medical professional should be able to balance the principles of values-based medicine within the roles of the governing organization and hospital. This balance is very important to avoid conflicts of patient's values or hospital policies.

The most critical step in patient management is the decision made by the treating team. The correct decision for a particular patient at the right time is the most determinative factor for the outcome of management. Medical decision-making depends on empirical knowledge and rational and analytical thinking. Evidence-based medicine depends on knowledge and accumulated information over rational thinking and individual experiences and to a certain extent ignores the patient's own values. In brief, there are in general two ways of logical thinking in order to make medical decisions, deductive and inductive methods. However, the rapid development of science, discoveries, medical technology, understanding the roots of pathophysiological disorders, and introduction of new treatments should allow for a less tightly constructed and rigid clinical decision. With uncertainty, the increased probability of causing risk, unsure outcome, and treatment of specific problems in a field like neurosurgery, the patient's autonomy and values should be paramount. The concept of values-based medicine which focuses on patient's best care allows more flexibility to adapt any scientific method which may help the patient. Patient and patient values should be part of any management equation.

The patient's family rights should be observed. The engagement of the patient and patient's family in making decisions created what is called "Patient-patient's family-doctor complex relationship." Such relationship is needed not only for the patient's comfort and well-being but also for the treating team to prevent any misconduct and future unnecessary troubles.

14. Ascertain the immediate outcome and long-term prognosis

The nature and pathophysiology of variable types of neurosurgical disorders may not help the neurosurgeons to ascertain an accurate predication of the prognostic outcome for a specific patient. Sometimes predictable answers can be hard to attain. This unfortunately is not rare which complicates the discussion, communication, and the relationship between a medical team and the patient and patient's family. Agonized and apprehensive extremely worried families are eager to hear answers to their painful questions. It is vital to reach the right diagnosis. Right diagnosis is always the fundamental base for management of the patient, however, in pediatric group may not give an accurate predication for long outcome. Usually the families regardless of their age, culture, religion, or race have many very similar nagging and worrying questions regarding the survival and well-being of their loved one.

Effective communication with patients and their families to discuss every step of the management and the prognostic information to the family is very important to create a good relationship and trust between the treating teams and patients and patients' families. The effective communication has profound influence on decisions regarding goals of care and clinical management of the patient, especially when prognostic information is clouded with a confusion of uncertainties [18].

15. Conclusion

Modern medicine may be based on EBM, which is a positive aspect of modern medicine; however, medicine since its inception, thousands of years ago, is based on values. The core of values-based medicine (VsBM) is creating a status to provide the patients the best possible available treatment within a frame of ethics and values which appreciate their culture and keep their dignity. Evidence-based medicine is, and should be, based on ethical and clinical principles which permit the best proven method of management. Values-based medicine and evidence-based medicine are and should be integrated, complementary to each other, not conflicting. The holistic approach to a human who has a disease needs to be treated, not just the disease should be treated. Humanity comes first, always.

Author details

Ahmed Ammar
Department of Neurosurgery, King Fahd University Hospital, Immam Abdukrahman Bin Faisal University, Al Khobar, Saudi Arabia

*Address all correspondence to: ahmed@ahmedammar.com

References

[1] Ammar A. Value based medicine. In: Ammar A, Bernstein M, editors. Neurosurgical Ethics in Practice: Value Based Medicine. Berlin, Germany/New York, USA: Springer; 2014. pp. 7-9

[2] World Health Organization (WHO). Patient's Rights. 2013

[3] World Federation of Neurological Societies; European Association of Neurological Societies. Good practice: A guide for neurosurgeons. Acta Neurochirurgica. 1999;**141**:791-799. (Final Version: August 1998)

[4] Royal Institute of British Architects. Code of Professional Conduct. Archived: 2013-06-18 at the Wayback Machine

[5] Ammar A. Influence of different culture on neurosurgical practice. Child's Nervous System. 1997;**13**:91-94

[6] Engebretson J, Mahoney J, Carlson ED. Cultural competence in the era of evidence-based practice. Journal of Professional Nursing. 2008;**24**(3):172-178

[7] Brown MM, Brown GC, Sharma S. Evidence-Based to Value-Based Medicine. Chicago: AMA Press; 2005. pp. 5-7. 125-149, 151-181, 193-217, 267-279, 319-324

[8] Kerridge I, Lowe M, Henry D. Ethics and evidence based medicine. BMJ. 1998;**316**:1152

[9] Ross EG. A call to integrate ethics and evidence-based medicine. American Medical Association Journal of Ethics. 2013;**15**(1):86-89

[10] El Kayaly D, Essene I, Ammar A. Evidence based medicine—Hydrocephalus guideline for systemic reviews. In: Meta-Analysis and Evidence Based Medicine. Hydrocephalus—What We Know and What We Still Don't Know. Springer International Publishing AG; 2017. pp. 31-31

[11] Sackett D, Rosenberg W, Gray M, Haynes B, Richardson S. Evidence based medicine: What it is and what it isn't. BMJ. January 1996;**13**

[12] Hoffmann TC, Montori VM, Del Mar C. The connection between evidence-based medicine and shared decision making. Journal of the American Medical Association. 2014;**312**(13):1295-1296. DOI: 10.1001/jama.2014.10186

[13] Ammar A. Patients' rights. In: Ammar A, Bernstein M, editors. Neurosurgical Ethics in Practice: Value Based Medicine. Berlin, Germany and New York, USA: Springer; 2014. pp. 37-52

[14] Stein JD, Brown MM, Brwon GC, Irwin B, Brwon KS. The comparative effectiveness and cost-effectiveness of vitreoretinal intervention. Current Opinion in Ophthalmology. 2008;**19**:202-207

[15] Dagi TF. Seven ethics affecting neurosurgeons in the context of health care system. Neurosurgery;**80**(4S):S83-S91

[16] Black M. The gap between "is" and "should". The PReview. 1964;**73**(2):165-181

[17] Hume D. A Treatise of Human Nature. Oxford: Clarendon Press; 1739; 244ff. Available at: https://people.rit.edu/wlrgsh/HumeTreatise.pdf. [Accessed: January 15, 2016]. Reprinted from the original edition in three volumes and edited with an analytical index by L.A. Selby-Bigge. 1896

[18] Loewy EH. Ethics and evidence-based medicine: Is there a conflict?

MedGenMed. 2007;**9**(3):30. Published online 2007 Aug 6

[19] Petrova M, Dale J, Fulford BK. Values-based practice in primary care: Easing the tensions between individual values, ethical principles and best evidence. The British Journal of General Practice. Sep 2006;**56**(530):703-709

Chapter 6

Dynamic and Static Models of Body-Mind Approaches from Neurobiological Perspectives

Practical Ethics for Researchers and Practitioners in the Medical and Educational Fields

Shoichi Shiota and Michio Nomura

Abstract

Body-mind approaches (e.g., yoga, mindfulness meditation, Pilates method, and cognitive behavior therapy) are commonly used by the public today. However, the comprehensive neurobiological framework of effects of body-mind approaches is unknown. To begin, we discuss the dynamic and static models of each body-mind approaches from neurobiological perspectives, as well as from the standpoint of practical issues. By the dynamic components of body-mind approaches, people enhances meta-cognitive function, and it lead to decreases in avoidance behavior in social aversive context are suggested. On the other hand, it is assumed that static components of body-mind approaches enhance non-reactive monitoring function for baseline of self. Therefore, we discuss the implications of these findings for practitioners and for future research on body-mind researchers. Additionally, this chapter covers the essential ethical guidelines of body-mind approaches within the domain of medical or educational fields.

Keywords: body-mind approaches, psychiatric disorder, dynamic components, static components, resonance effect, meta-cognitive function

1. Introduction

No doctor or medical treatment can be comparable in efficacy to the human feelings of joy and happiness [1]. The variety of feelings we have as humans and our process of recognition make our lives interesting and meaningful. The inter-individual differences in subjective feelings and the processes of recognition are affected by individual differences in our physical function [2]. The human mind comprises both a bottom-up peripheral nervous system and a top-down central nervous system interaction that controls it. For example, playing football or baseball, which are moderate whole-body exercises, creates feelings of happiness. It is thought that this is due to an increase in body temperature, which is the result of an increase in momentum. This rise in temperature leads to an improvement in autonomic nervous system control through exercising the muscles of the torso and other parts of the body, which we then recognize as positive emotions. Also, when people hear of painful experiences of those close to them (e.g., friends, significant others, family), this affects emotions in a way that makes the listener want to help. Altruistic behavior arises when we perceive changes in own body sensations in social interactions and when we guess the feelings of others. On the other hand, before people speak in public, individuals often have shortened breath and a rapid heartbeat, feelings we understand as being nervous. Subsequently we attempt to relax. Stress in both the workplace and academic situations increases our sympathetic nervous system, long-term stress which is difficult to control is harmful for physical and mental health. According to the World Health Organization, one in three people suffer from some type of psychiatric disorder, a statistic that holds true in many countries around the world. In Japan, the economic loss related to mental illness exceeds seven trillion yen yearly, a number that combines direct and indirect expenses. Psychiatric disorders can be interpreted as abnormalities in bodily functions due to external factors, and a breakdown in basic mental functions. For example, depression and anxiety disorder result in abnormalities in the control of cardiac autonomic nervous system. Also, persons with depression and anxiety disorder have abnormal functional connectivity between the prefrontal cortex and insula when compared to healthy subjects. Recently, there is increased attention to body-mind approaches as effective treatment for psychiatric disorders. However, as in terms of the treatment mechanisms of these body-mind approaches, there has been little discussion of a comprehensive framework from neurobiological perspectives. Therefore, the current paper explores two basic frameworks: (1) a dynamic and static model of body-mind approaches from neurobiological perspectives and (2) basic ethical guidelines of the body-mind approach when practicing in the fields of medical care and education.

2. Body-mind approach

Body-mind approaches (e.g., yoga, mindfulness meditation, Pilates method, and cognitive behavior therapy) are commonly used by the public today [3]. A body-mind approach focuses on the relationships between the brain, mind, body, and behavior, and their effects on health and disease [4]. To begin, we discuss the dynamic and static models of each body-mind approach from neurobiological perspectives, as well as from the standpoint of practical issues (**Figure 1**).

2.1 Theoretical framework and practical evidence of yoga

Yoga is constructed by practices of postures, breathing techniques, and meditation. Many of the elements of yoga that have been adjusted to Western cultures and became more popular in recent years focus on weight reduction through vigorous physical exercise. However, yoga in general not only aims to help people lose weight but also seeks to modulate an individual's physical or mental condition during practice. Previous meta-analysis studies indicated that yoga is an effective intervention for psychiatric disorders [5–7]. Previous studies have demonstrated that yoga improves one's brain functions and cortical thickness, resulting in improvements in attention control, emotional regulation, and meta-cognitive function. Interestingly, it also seems to improve telomere length and autonomic nervous control in both healthy individuals and those with physical ailments [8–16]. These results are interpreted as demonstrating that asana, breathing techniques, and meditation work interactively. Here, we explain the treatment mechanisms of asana, breathing technique, and meditation. We also illustrate the dynamic and static components that work in concert with asana, breathing techniques, and meditation.

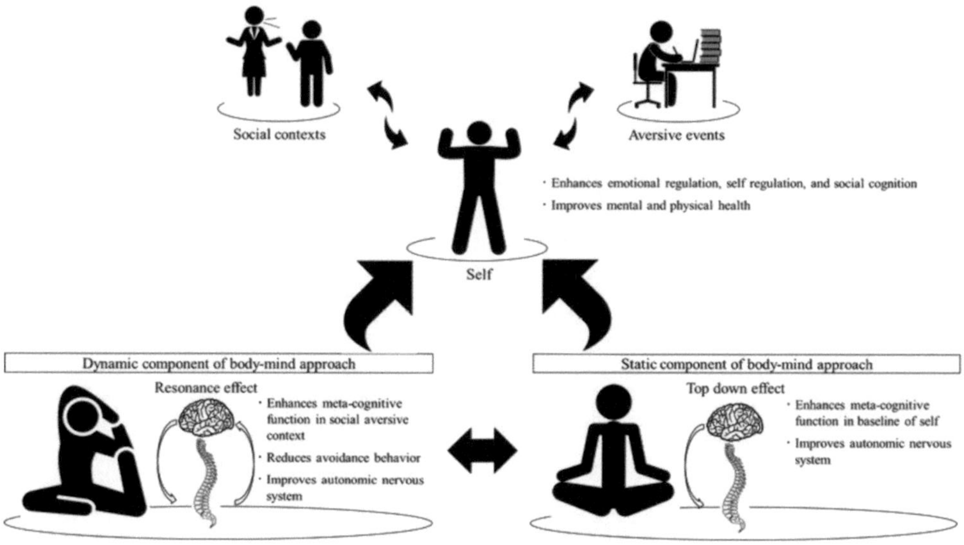

Figure 1.
The dynamic and static model of body-mind approaches.

2.2 The bottom up effect of asana

Asana points to specific physical postures that involve using one's whole body during yoga practice. These physical postures are categorized as standing, seated, and supine postures; they also include forward folds, adopted forward bend, back bends, hip-openers, twists, and inversions [17]. Some practices, such as Ashtanga Yoga, are characterized by quite intense and continuous physical motion with a focus on creating a "flow" of movement by linking one posture to the next. In other practices, such as Hatha Yoga, the movement is less dynamic and the focus is on holding individual postures for a longer period of time. The effect of asana during yoga practice is briefly explained in the following. First, we examine the effects of asana on autonomic nervous system as a result of exercise for the dorsal vertebrae, musculus erector spinae, musculus trapezius, latissimus dorsi muscle, and adductor longus muscle. Previous review articles have indicated that yoga intervention improved autonomic nervous system control for people with psychiatric disorders and individuals with cardiovascular disease [9, 15]. Iyengar yoga, which is characterized by improving toughness and stamina and correct body distortion, has been shown to reduce anxiety, depressive symptoms, anger, neurotic symptoms, and low frequency heart rate variability for people with depression [18]. According to Lakkireddy et al. [19], structured Iyengar yoga decreased anxiety, and depressive symptoms, while improving quality of life, heart rate, and systolic and diastolic blood pressure for individuals with arrhythmia burden. Streeter et al. [20] reported asana practice significantly increased brain GABA levels. Common asana, which includes exercise for the dorsal vertebrae, musculus erector spinae, musculus trapezius, latissimus dorsi muscle, and adductor longus muscle, is included in these studies. For example, the Sun Salutation, the most popular asana, was studied by Steer et al. [20]. It includes exercises for dorsal vertebrae, musculus erector spinae, musculus trapezius, latissimus dorsi muscle, and adductor longus muscle during flow movements. Adhomukhavirasana (modified child posture), which was used Lakkireddy et al. [19], expands the latissimus dorsi muscle and lower back. The latissimus dorsi muscle is related to extension of shoulder joint, and extending this muscle eases deep breathing (abdominal breathing). During Salamba

Sarvangasana, which was used in Shapiro et al. [18], the focus in on individual exercise of the dorsal vertebrae and several muscles (e.g., musculus erector spinae, musculus trapezius, latissimus dorsi muscle, and adductor longus several muscle). We must not disregard the interaction between asana and abdominal breathing; however, from the evidence above, we speculate asana exercise improves autonomic nerve system control which should then lead to the improvement in the symptoms of psychiatric disorders. However, possible side effects of asana exercise should be carefully investigated. Asana is regarded as having bottom up treatment effects during yoga practice.

2.3 Top down effect of breathing techniques

The conscious practice of altering breathing patterns may have a number of different effects depending on the characteristic of the practice [21]. For instance, slow and rhythmic breathing is said to promote a shift to parasympathetic dominance via vagal afferent stimulation with consequent stress reduction [22], whereas more forceful breathing practices may promote sympathetic activation [23]. Voluntary change of breathing patterns can alter emotional states and influence well-being [21, 24, 25]. In fact, a typical autonomic reaction to stressful situations is rapid thoracic breathing, which in turn leads to hyperventilation, altered tidal volume, and hypocapnia [26]. Yoga is a practice that emphasizes linking breath and movement. For example, in Ashtanga Yoga each asana is coupled to a specific breathing rhythm so that the specific breathing technique helps enhance movement. Sudarshan Kriya Yoga is a yoga practice that incorporates powerful breathing, Ujjiay—slow and forced breathing, 3 cycles per minute; Bhastrika—rapid exhalation at 20–30 cycles per minute; Sudarshan Kriya—rhythmic, cyclical breathing of slow, medium, fast cycles [21]. In the practice of yoga, various breathing methods such as chest respiration, which increases the sympathetic nervous system, and abdominal breathing, which increases the parasympathetic nervous system are used. Previous studies have demonstrated that yoga breathing techniques when used alone improved symptoms in patients with psychiatric disorders and healthy elderly individuals [27–29]. Santaella et al. [28] reported that the Sudarshan Kriya Yoga breathing technique significantly improves maximum expiratory and inspiratory pressures of pulmonary function, and significantly decreases low component and low frequency/high frequency ratio (marker of sympathovagal balance) of heart rate variability in healthy older individuals. Toschi-Dias et al. [29] demonstrated that the Sudarshan Kriya Yoga breathing technique improved subjective symptoms while decreasing sympathetic modulation and cardiac autonomic control; specifically, it was shown to increase parasympathetic modulation and cardiorespiratory coupling in in patients with anxiety-depression disorders. Intentional change for respiratory rhythms translates into changes in the neural activity of brainstem [30]. Both cardiorespiratory coupling and the cardiac autonomic nervous system are controlled by a network of neurons located within the lower brainstem [31, 32]. Based on this evidence, we hypothesize that yoga breathing techniques change brain stem activation in patients with psychiatric disorders and lead to improvements in the cardiac autonomic nervous system (mainly associated with parasympathetic nervous system) and cardiopulmonary coupling through the vagus nerve. These breathing techniques represent a top down treatment mechanism of yoga. Therefore, during yoga practice, participants experience both bottom up and top down effects of yoga, and these effects can improve cognitive functions. In the next section, we discuss a third treatment mechanism in yoga, a physical technique that improves cognitive function.

2.4 Neurobiological resonance effects in dynamic components of yoga

Resonance effects between bottom up and top down effects within individuals produced by yoga practice generate a third type of treatment effect. During an asana sequence, the range of motion in a person's joints expands and joint load will largely be maintained at submaximal levels. As a result, physical stress increases over time, manifesting in the muscles, joints, and connective tissue. Therefore, by stimulating the autonomic nervous system, individual arousal is accelerated. As a result, subjective emotional reaction increases, which prompts avoidance behavior. These negative emotional reactions are similar to emotional reactions in negative situations individuals face in social contexts. This is a bottom up effect of yoga. On other hand, the yoga breathing technique used during asana sequence enhances parasympathetic nervous control and cardiopulmonary coupling. This top-down relax effect reduces the subjectively negative emotional reaction that occurs in the asana sequence. This is the top down effect of yoga. The bottom up and top down effects are functionally resonant within an individual during the asana sequence. These resonance effects reduce one's subjectively negative emotional reaction and promote awareness of bodily sensations that produce them. Through this increase in body awareness, an individual can monitor (meta-cognition) perceived emotional events that may occur from moment to moment that arise in the context of yoga practice. Therefore, by enhancing meta-cognitive function, an individual's emotion regulation and self-regulation in practical an aversive context are improved. Previous meta-analysis studies indicated that yoga intervention improved cognitive function for both people with psychiatric disorders and healthy individuals [33, 34]. Eyre et al. [12] reported that patients with mild cognitive impairment who participated in yoga classes had statistically significant improvements in alleviating depression and enhancing visuospatial memory. Jensen and Kenny [13] demonstrated that children with attention deficit hyperactivity disorder who participated in yoga intervention had significantly improved emotional lability at post intervention compared to pre intervention. Furthermore, some studies indicated that yoga intervention significantly enhanced body awareness in individuals with eating disorders [10, 11]. A previous neuroimaging study also demonstrated that gray matter volume of bilateral insula was positive correlated with pain tolerance, and also had positive correlation with yogic experience in yoga practitioners [16]. Additionally, another fMRI study reported healthy elderly yoga practitioners significantly increased gray matter volume in the left lateral prefrontal cortex compared to an age matched healthy control group [8]. The resonance effect of yoga promotes cognitive reappraisal of individuals in terms of negative emotional reactions faced in practical contexts. Cognitive reappraisal gained by the resonance effect of yoga may give new meaning to an individual's emotional reactions, which in turn lead to improved emotional regulation and self-regulation. Thus, interoceptive awareness and monitoring are essential for most affective, cognitive, and interpersonal processes [35]. These observations suggest that the experience of yoga practice decreases avoidance behavior, and this experience may be generalized to other behaviors in social contexts. These are the dynamic components of yoga. Next we focus on meditation, which is a static component of yoga.

2.5 Meditation and breathing technique in static components of yoga

As a static component of yoga, meditation aims to develop mental silence and non-reactive consciousness. Before yoga meditation, participants are instructed to maintain focus on abdominal breathing and observe their interoceptive and physical sensations while keeping their minds blank. During yoga meditation, individuals develop awareness of both their inner experience, and how this experience functions on a meta-cognitive level. Here, the top-down control of using abdominal breathing reduces the emotional response occurring in an individual during meditation. One's awareness of both their emotional reactions and body are enhanced due to the resonance effect generated by the dynamic component of yoga. Through these effects, individuals can observe emotions and thoughts objectively (non-reactive) without being caught up in them. Static components of yoga promote cognitive reappraisal of one's self as a baseline. Therefore, static components are also found for mindfulness meditation.

3. Theoretical framework and practical evidence of mindfulness meditation

Mindfulness can be defined as the ability to observe thoughts, and bodily sensations or feelings in the present moment with an open and accepting orientation toward one's experiences [36]. Mindfulness meditation that develops mindfulness uses abdominal breathing in a way similar to yoga, and it is seen as a body-mind approach with static components. Mindfulness meditation has been employed for centuries within Buddhist traditions, yet it is has only been since the 1970s that mindfulness has become a target of intervention for several psychological problems [37]. Through facilitating awareness and non-judgmental acceptance of moment-to-moment experiences, these mindfulness-based meditation techniques alleviate intense emotional states [37, 38]. As evidenced by previous meta-analyses, mindfulness meditation based intervention has proven effective in reducing psychological distress, anxiety, depression, and improving well-being and quality of life in individuals with mental disorders [39–41]. In this section, we explain the interaction between three types of meditation (focused attention meditation, open monitoring meditation, and compassion meditation) and breathing technique; these are basic techniques that employ several types of mindfulness meditation.

3.1 Focused attention meditation, open monitoring meditation, and compassion meditation: mindfulness meditation involving a static component

Meditation that develops mindfulness consists of three types of meditation: focused attention meditation, which improves concentration abilities, open monitoring meditation, which improves the ability to monitor our experiences without reactions or judgments, and compassion meditation, which integrates focused attention meditation and open monitoring meditation [42, 43]. Focused attention meditation is a type of systematic training aimed at directing and sustaining attention on a chosen neutral object (e.g., the breath), noticing when the mind wanders from the object, and disengaging from distractions, negative emotions, rumination, or worry by redirecting or shifting one's attention back to the chosen neutral object [42]. Focused attention meditation cultivates both calmness and stability of mind and reduces attention on negative thoughts and emotions [42]. Open monitoring meditation does not involve any specific object of focus, nor does it focus on disengagement from negative thoughts or emotions or expecting them to diminish [42]. Open monitoring meditation entails cultivating non-reactive awareness of automatic cognitive and emotional interpretations of sensory, perceptual, and endogenous stimuli, regardless of valence [42]. During compassion meditation, meditators focus on developing love and compassion first for themselves and then gradually extend this love to evermore "unlikeable" others, and various other creatures [44]. Compassion meditation is often entails that helps practitioners develop cognitive schemas which cultivate a sense of equanimity and hopefulness. According to a previous review article [45], mindfulness meditation, which consists of focused attention meditation, open monitoring meditation, and compassion meditation, enhances attention control, emotional regulation, and self-awareness in both healthy subjects and individuals with psychosis. Goldin and Gross [46] reported that mindfulness meditation intervention improved self-esteem, and lessened anxiety and depressive symptoms. They additionally reported reduced amygdala activity that corresponded to emotional reactivity during reacting to negative self-beliefs in people with social anxiety disorder. Tomasino and Fabbro [47] demonstrated that focused attention meditation increased activation in the right dorsolateral prefrontal cortex and in the left insula, and that it decreased activation in the rostral prefrontal cortex and in right parietal area. According to Fujino et al. [48], both focused attention meditation and open monitoring meditation specifically reduced functional connectivity between the striatum and posterior cingulate cortex, which is a core hub region of the default mode network. Additionally, open monitoring meditation reduced functional connectivity of the ventral striatum in both the visual cortex related to intentional focused attention in the attentional network and the retrosplenial cortex related to memory function in the default mode network. In contrast, focused attention meditation increased functional connectivity in these regions. Furthermore, other previous studies revealed stronger neural responses to emotional sounds in the anterior insula and anterior cingulate cortex during compassion meditation than when an individual was in a resting state [49, 50]. From these reports, we speculate that mindfulness meditation increases emotional regulation, attention control, and self-awareness. Additionally, we assume the abdominal breathing technique, which is a physical movement, is enormously important in this respect.

3.2 Breathing technique of mindfulness meditation

Prior to mindfulness meditation, participants are instructed to focus on breathing and to let their minds wander, not to focus attention on worries or negative thoughts [51]. Previous studies demonstrated that mindfulness breathing technique used alone alleviated subjective distress and improved meta-cognitive function, emotional non-reactivity, and autonomic nervous control in healthy individuals and those with physical ailments [51–53]. According to Ng et al. [53], 5 minutes of brief mindfulness breathing technique lessened subjective distress, and improved blood pressure, pulse rate, and breathing rate in subjects in palliative care cancer patients. Furthermore, Arch and Craske [51] indicated that 15 minutes of mindfulness breathing enhances an individual's emotional non-reactivity during presentation of negative pictures. Based on these reports, focused attention on breathing is seen to reduce the attention given to distressing experiences or thoughts, and abdominal breathing reduces the role of the sympathetic nervous system and increases that of the parasympathetic nervous system during distressing experiences or thoughts.

3.3 Meditation and breathing technique in static components of mindfulness meditation

The purposes of mindfulness meditation, which is one of the body-mind approaches including static components, alleviate intense emotional states and self-awareness for psychological problems accompanied by aversive emotions, and develop cognitive schemas, which cultivate a sense of equanimity and hopefulness. Here, the psychological problems accompanied by aversive emotions include the problem that is currently occurring and occurred in the past. Participants develop the objective monitoring function for inner emotions and thoughts without being caught up in them during focused attention meditation and open monitoring meditation. It should be also noted that participants observe psychological problems that are obstacles to cultivating love and compassion for themselves and others with objectively monitoring function during compassion meditation too. Therefore, we hypothesize that these meditations enhance individuals' metacognitive function. Furthermore, before each mindfulness meditations, participants are instructed to maintain focus on abdominal breathing. The top-down control of using abdominal breathing reduces the emotional response occurring in an individual during each meditation. There is suggested that these effects promote cognitive reappraisal of psychological problems which forming the core of the current self and as a result develop cognitive schemas which cultivate a sense of equanimity and hopefulness. This is the effect of the static component which adjusts baseline of self. Thus far, we have explained the characteristics and therapeutic effects of yoga and mindfulness respectively. Mindfulness meditation and yoga are both body-mind approaches which have static components. In addition, previous studies for patients with psychiatric disorders have demonstrated that symptom reduction via attention control, emotional control, and self-awareness are viable treatment mechanisms. On the other hand, mindfulness meditation does not have a dynamic component. Individuals must continue to focus on their own interoceptive sensations and breathing during mindfulness meditation. However, with the dynamic component of yoga, participants are able to automatically focus on their interoceptive sensations or breathing. We assume that yoga-based interventions may be more appropriate for ADHD children who have difficulty sustaining attention. Recently, in order to overcome the problems that currently exist in psychotherapy, yoga, mindfulness, and other body-mind approaches have been aggressively promoted for patients with mental disorders. For example, the aim of conventional cognitive behavioral therapies has been to modify maladaptive cognitive content affecting emotions and behavior. On the other hand, when cognitive behavioral therapy for major depressive disorder is performed, if negative self-cognitive modification is incomplete, it can lead to a return of symptoms [54]. There are also problems in the change of cognitive bias for patients with PTSD, which can increase their pain and emotional burden. These issues can lead to individuals dropping out of the treatment protocol [55–57]. Therefore, there has been more attention given to body-mind approaches that have an effect on cognitive functions through bodily functions. However, in terms of body-mind approach treatment mechanisms, there has little discussion of a comprehensive framework based on the dynamic and static component models. In the next section we examine the Pilates method, which is another body-mind approach, and behavior activation, a third generation cognitive behavior therapy.

4. Theoretical framework and practical evidence of Pilates method

Pilates method was developed in the 1920s by Joseph Pilates and consists of comprehensive body conditioning, which aims to develop better body awareness and improve posture. The Pilates method requires core stability, strength, and flexibility, as well as attention to muscle control, posture, and breathing [58]. At first, the Pilates method gained popularity in rehabilitation settings [59]; however, in recent years Pilates based exercise has become popular among the general population. In the modern Pilates method, after adjusting one's breath (a costal breathing technique), an individual performs a series of approximately 25–50 simple, low-impact flexibility and muscular endurance exercises with emphasis on muscular exertion in the abdominals, lower back, hips, thighs, and buttocks in combination with timed breathing [60, 61]. The Pilates method is one of the body-mind approaches featuring a dynamic component. According to previous meta-analysis studies, the Pilates method improves physical flexibility, dynamic balance, and muscular endurance in healthy people [62], as well as physical balance in older adults [63]. Additionally, some randomized controlled trials studies have demonstrated that the Pilates method improved subjective degree of pain, subjective degree of disability, and kinesiophobia [62, 64, 65]. However, to the best of our knowledge, few studies have investigated intervention effects of the Pilates method for symptoms of psychiatric disorders, as compared to the research in this area employing other body-mind approaches. We assume that the primary objective of the other body-mind approaches is improving mental condition, while the primary goal of Pilates method is to improve physical health. Second, we speculate that present interventions which use the Pilates method are not sufficient to be effective for psychiatric disorders. However, if the dynamic component of the Pilates method could be adjusted, it is possible this method could be an effective intervention for some psychiatric disorders. In the next section we examine the potential intervention effect of the Pilates method for individuals with psychiatric disorders.

4.1 Potential intervention effects of the Pilates method for individuals with psychiatric disorders

In the Pilates method, participants adjust their physical condition using costal breathing before exercise. This is one of the main differences from yoga. As previously mentioned, costal breathing increases the activity of the sympathetic nervous system. This boost of the sympathetic nervous system both increases the heart rate and enhances the metabolism of one's body. We speculated that if the aim of the Pilates method is dieting or physical fitness for healthy individuals, this breathing technique is appropriate. However, previous meta-analysis studies have demonstrated that patients with psychiatric disorders had reduced high frequency of heart rate variability (which is influenced by the parasympathetic nervous system) compared to healthy subjects [66, 67]. Therefore, we consider that it may be better to adopt the breathing technique which increases parasympathetic activity, such as abdominal breathing, in the Pilates method. In fact, a numerous interventions which use the modern Pilates method have adopted this breathing technique [58]. However, these techniques are used only to adjust physical condition prior to exercise and are not used during exercise. We assume if one adjusts abdominal breathing while engaging in an easy pose, such as a "cat stretch" or "mermaid stretch", the effects of the dynamic component of Pilates method may be more effective. In this case, the Pilates method may be an effective intervention for psychiatric disorders.

5. Theoretical framework and practical evidence of behavioral activation

Based on the approach of Lewinsohn et al. [68], behavioral activation is focused on enhancement of self-monitoring, increasing healthy goal-oriented behavior, and increasing environmental reward frequency. In the course of behavioral activation interventions, participants monitor and assess their daily activities and work to change their habitual behaviors in a way that aims to increase pleasant events and interactions and reduce depressive symptoms [69]. Behavioral activation is another body-mind approach including a dynamic component. Previous meta-analysis studies have demonstrated that behavioral activation is an effective treatment for depression [70, 71]. Dimidjian et al. [72] indicated that treatment effects of behavioral activation are comparable in efficacy to pharmacological therapy for individuals suffering from depression. Our previous studies reported that behavioral activation improved abilities both to access positive reinforcing activities and to engage in rewarding behaviors under adverse circumstances [73, 74]. Additionally, Jacobson et al. [69] showed behavioral activation significantly improved self-concept in people with depression. A few previous neuroimaging studies have also demonstrated that behavioral activation enhances one's cognitive function and corresponds to brain activations in people with subthreshold depression [75–77]. Specifically, our previous studies indicated that brief behavioral activation had increased activation in the dorsomedial prefrontal cortex in individuals with subthreshold depression, which is associated with metacognitive function, and that this activation is also correlated with an improvement in depressive symptoms [76, 77]. Based on these reports, we hypothesized that there should be two treatment mechanisms of behavioral activation for depression. The first is involved in reducing depressive symptoms to improve the reward system, and the second involved in improving depressive symptoms to enhance meta-cognitive function. Future research is needed to verify the above hypotheses related to these two treatment mechanisms.

6. Ethical guidelines of body-mind approach within the medical and educational domains

The primary purpose of medical research involving human subjects is to understand the causes, development, and effects of diseases and improve preventive, diagnostic, and therapeutic interventions (methods, procedures and treatments). Even the best proven interventions must be evaluated continually through research for safety, effectiveness, efficiency, accessibility, and quality [78]. In this section we review four body-mind approaches that have gained attention in recent years. Each approach has different characteristics (see **Table 1**). Here, for practitioners and researchers, we discuss the current and future issues of each approach. First, further neurobiological examination is necessary for the body-mind approach. For example, yoga and mindfulness are speculated to be very similar approaches in their emphasis on enhancing attention control, emotional regulation, and self-awareness which using one's interoceptive sensations or breathing. However, to the best of our

	Dynamic component	Static component	Subject	Degree of structuralization	Intervention effect
Yoga	Asana sequence and abdominal breathing	Meditation	Healthy -mental diseases	Medium	Medium
Mindfulness meditation	—	Meditation	Healthy -mental diseases	High	High
Pilates method	Pose sequence and costal breathing	—	Healthy	Medium	Low
Behavioral activation	Positive activities	—	Healthy -mental diseases	Low	High

Table 1.
The difference of characteristics for each body-mind approaches.

knowledge, there are few neurobiological studies that compare yoga and mindfulness. This is also true for research comparing the effects of the Pilates method to other approaches. A second important point regards the enhancement of treatment effects in each of the body-mind approaches. According to a previous meta-analysis study [79], the treatment effect of yoga is not sufficient compared to other types of active control (Hedges' g = 0.30). However, this study did not fully examine the therapeutic effect of each asana. We assume that a structured asana sequence is necessary to more greatly enhance the therapeutic effect of yoga. Third, as we noted above, there are many therapies applying the mindfulness meditation in recent years (e.g., dialectical behavior therapy, mindfulness-based cognitive therapy, and acceptance and commitment therapy). This is because the disease to be treated, the duration of the treatment effect, and the intervention duration are different for each therapy. On the other hand, it can be more conveniently implemented by someone, and versatility treatment is necessary. Thereby, it is necessary to examine the treatment model used in conventional mindfulness-based therapies from neurobiological perspectives to extract essential factors. Furthermore, new mindfulness meditation-based treatment, which integrates essential factors in conventional mindfulness-based therapies, should be developed. Forth, we speculate it is necessary to examine the treatment effects of body-mind approach for not only basic emotions (e.g., fear, anger) but also complex emotions (e.g., awe, shame) and social cognition. A few previous studies [80] indicated that mindfulness meditation alleviated subjective symptoms of anxiety and enhanced social skills for people with learning disabilities. From the evidence, it could be considered that other body-mind approaches may enhance complex emotions and social cognition. It is necessary to provide a higher-quality body-mind approach based on previous evidence that can be adjusted to fit the needs of medical institutions and school schedules. Finally, the research that uses the body-mind approach for psychiatric disorders is at an early stage at present. We speculate that it is necessary to establish more detailed ethical guidelines for each approach corresponding high-quality body-mind approach in the near future.

7. Conclusion

In this chapter, we introduced and discussed neurobiological treatment effects and mechanisms of yoga, mindfulness meditation, Pilates method, and cognitive behavior therapy. In recent years, these body-mind approaches have been actively adopted in the educational and medical fields in Western countries. In the future, it is necessary to clarify the detailed neurobiological mechanisms of each body-mind approach and provide higher quality service in both medical and educational settings. At the same time, we should also extend knowledge and technology to countries and regions where body-mind approaches are not widely available.

Source of funding

This article was supported by a Grant-in-Aid for the Japan Society for the Promotion of Science (JSPS) fellows (18J01157).

Conflict of interest

None of the authors have any conflicts of interest to declare regarding the findings of this study.

Author details

Shoichi Shiota[1,2*] and Michio Nomura[1]

1 Graduate School of Education, Kyoto University, Kyoto, Japan

2 Japan Society for the Promotion of Science, Tokyo, Japan

*Address all correspondence to: syo.shiota@gmail.com

References

[1] Nakamura T. Give You Success. Tokyo: Tenpu-kai; 2001

[2] Damasio AR. Looking for Spinoza: Joy, Sorrow, and the Feeling Brain. Boston: Houghton Mifflin Harcourt; 2003

[3] National Institutes of Health. What Is Complementary and Alternative Medicine? [Internet]. 2007. Available from: http://www.health.state.mn.us/divs/fpc/cww/CamBasics.pdf. [Accessed: 2018-07-04]

[4] Wahbeh H, Haywood A, Kaufman K, Zwickey H. Mind-body medicine and immune system outcomes: A systematic review. The Open Complementary Medicine Journal. 2009;**1**:25-34. DOI: 10.2174/1876391X00901010025

[5] Cabral P, Meyer HB, Ames D. Effectiveness of yoga therapy as a complementary treatment for major psychiatric disorders: A meta-analysis. The Primary Care Companion to CNS Disorders. 2011;**13**: PCC.10r01068. DOI: 10.4088/PCC.10r01068

[6] Meyer HB, Katsman A, Sones AC, Auerbach DE, Ames D, Rubin RT. Yoga as an ancillary treatment for neurological and psychiatric disorders: A review. The Journal of Neuropsychiatry and Clinical Neurosciences. 2012;**24**:152-164. DOI: 10.1176/appi.neuropsych.11040090

[7] Ross A, Thomas S. The health benefits of yoga and exercise: A review of comparison studies. The Journal of Alternative and Complementary Medicine. 2010;**16**:3-12. DOI: 10.1089 acm.2009.0044

[8] Afonso RF, Balardin JB, Lazar S, Sato JR, Igarashi N, Santaella DF, et al. Greater cortical thickness in elderly female yoga practitioners—A cross-sectional study. Frontiers in Aging Neuroscience. 2017;**9**:201. DOI: 10.3389/fnagi.2017.00201

[9] Chu P, Gotink RA, Yeh GY, Goldie SJ, Hunink MM. The effectiveness of yoga in modifying risk factors for cardiovascular disease and metabolic syndrome: A systematic review and meta-analysis of randomized controlled trials. European Journal of Preventive Cardiology. 2016;**23**:291-307. DOI: 10.1177/2047487314562741

[10] Dittmann KA, Freedman MR. Body awareness, eating attitudes, and spiritual beliefs of women practicing yoga. Eating Disorders. 2009;**17**: 273-292. DOI: 10.1080/10640260902991111

[11] Daubenmier JJ. The relationship of yoga, body awareness, and body responsiveness to self-objectification and disordered eating. Psychology of Women Quarterly. 2005;**29**: 207-219. DOI: 10.1111/j.1471-6402.2005.00183.x

[12] Eyre HA, Acevedo B, Yang H, Siddarth P, Van Dyk K, Ercoli L, et al. Changes in neural connectivity and memory following a yoga intervention for older adults: A pilot study. Journal of Alzheimer's Disease. 2016;**52**:673-684. DOI: 10.3233/JAD-150653

[13] Jensen PS, Kenny DT. The effects of yoga on the attention and behavior of boys with attention-deficit/hyperactivity disorder (ADHD). Journal of Attention Disorders. 2004;7:205-216. DOI: 10.1177/108705470400700403

[14] Kumar SB, Yadav R, Yadav RK, Tolahunase M, Dada R. Telomerase activity and cellular aging might be positively modified by a yoga-based lifestyle intervention. The Journal of Alternative and Complementary Medicine. 2015;**21**:370-372. DOI: 10.1089/acm.2014.0298

[15] Streeter CC, Gerbarg PL, Saper RB, Ciraulo DA, Brown RP. Effects of yoga on the autonomic nervous system, gamma-aminobutyric-acid, and allostasis in epilepsy, depression, and post-traumatic stress disorder. Medical Hypotheses. 2012;**78**:571-579. DOI: 10.1016/j.mehy.2012.01.021

[16] Villemure C, Čeko M, Cotton VA, Bushnell MC. Insular cortex mediates increased pain tolerance in yoga practitioners. Cerebral Cortex. 2013;**24**:2732-2740. DOI: 10.1093/cercor/bht124

[17] Schmalzl L, Powers C, Blom EH. Neurophysiological and neurocognitive mechanisms underlying the effects of yoga-based practices: Towards a comprehensive theoretical framework. Frontiers in Human Neuroscience. 2015;**9**:1-40. DOI: 10.3389/fnhum.2015.00235

[18] Shapiro D, Cook IA, Davydov DM, Ottaviani C, Leuchter AF, Abrams M. Yoga as a complementary treatment of depression: Effects of traits and moods on treatment outcome. Evidence-based Complementary and Alternative Medicine. 2007;**4**:493-502. DOI: 10.1093/ecam/nel114

[19] Lakkireddy D, Atkins D, Pillarisetti J, Ryschon K, Bommana S, Drisko J, et al. Effect of yoga on arrhythmia burden, anxiety, depression, and quality of life in paroxysmal atrial fibrillation: The YOGA my heart study. Journal of the American College of Cardiology. 2013;**61**:1177-1182. DOI: 10.1016/j.jacc.2012.11.060

[20] Streeter CC, Jensen JE, Perlmutter RM, Cabral HJ, Tian H, Terhune DB, et al. Yoga asana sessions increase brain GABA levels: A pilot study. The Journal of Alternative and Complementary Medicine. 2007;**13**:419-426. DOI: 10.1089/acm.2007.6338

[21] Brown RP, Gerbarg PL. Sudarshan Kriya yogic breathing in the treatment of stress, anxiety, and depression: Part I—Neurophysiologic model. Journal of Alternative & Complementary Medicine. 2005;**11**:189-201. DOI: 10.1089/acm.2005.11.18

[22] Sovik R. The science of breathing—The yogic view. Progress in Brain Research. 2000;**122**:491-505. DOI: 10.1016/s0079-6123(08)62159-7

[23] Beauchaine T. Vagal tone, development, and Gray's motivational theory: Toward an integrated model of autonomic nervous system functioning in psychopathology. Development and Psychopathology. 2001;**13**:183-214. DOI: 10.1017/s0954579401002012

[24] Boiten FA, Frijda NH, Wientjes CJ. Emotions and respiratory patterns: Review and critical analysis. International Journal of Psychophysiology. 1994;**17**:103-128. DOI: 10.1016/0167-8760(94)90027-2

[25] Blom EH, Serlachius E, Chesney MA, Olsson EM. Adolescent girls with emotional disorders have a lower end-tidal CO_2 and increased respiratory rate compared with healthy controls. Psychophysiology. 2014;**51**:412-418. DOI: 10.1111/psyp.12188

[26] Laffey JG, Kavanagh BP. Hypocapnia. New England Journal of Medicine. 2002;**347**:43-53. DOI: 10.1056/NEJMra012457

[27] Doria S, De Vuono A, Sanlorenzo R, Irtelli F, Mencacci C. Anti-anxiety efficacy of Sudarshan Kriya Yoga in general anxiety disorder: A multicomponent, yoga based, breath intervention program for patients suffering from generalized anxiety disorder with or without comorbidities. Journal of Affective Disorders. 2015;**184**:310-317. DOI: 10.1016/j.jad.2015.06.011

[28] Santaella DF, Devesa CR, Rojo MR, Amato MB, Drager LF, Casali KR, et al.

Yoga respiratory training improves respiratory function and cardiac sympathovagal balance in elderly subjects: A randomised controlled trial. BMJ Open. 2011;**1**:1-8. DOI: 10.1136/bmjopen-2011-000085

[29] Toschi-Dias E, Tobaldini E, Solbiati M, Costantino G, Sanlorenzo R, Doria S, et al. Sudarshan Kriya yoga improves cardiac autonomic control in patients with anxiety-depression disorders. Journal of Affective Disorders. 2017;**214**:74-80. DOI: 10.1016/j.jad.2017.03.017

[30] Liou CH, Hsieh CW, Hsieh CH, Wang CH, Lee SC, Chen JH. Comparison of fMRI bold effect and arterial pulsation harmonic distribution among different breathing rate. In: 27th Annual International Conference. Engineering in Medicine and Biology Society; 2005. pp. 5313-5316. DOI: 10.1109/IEMBS.2005.1615680

[31] Napadow V, Dhond R, Conti G, Makris N, Brown EN, Barbieri R. Brain correlates of autonomic modulation: Combining heart rate variability with fMRI. NeuroImage. 2008;**42**:169-177. DOI: 10.1016/j.neuroimage.2008.04.238

[32] Spyer KM, Gourine AV. Chemosensory pathways in the brainstem controlling cardiorespiratory activity. Philosophical Transactions of the Royal Society of London B: Biological Sciences. 2009;**364**: 2603-2610. DOI: 10.1098/rstb.2009.0082

[33] Balasubramaniam M, Telles S, Doraiswamy PM. Yoga on our minds: A systematic review of yoga for neuropsychiatric disorders. Frontiers in Psychiatry. 2013;**3**:1-16. DOI: 10.3389/fpsyt.2012.00117

[34] Gothe NP, McAuley E. Yoga and cognition: A meta-analysis of chronic and acute effects. Psychosomatic Medicine. 2015;**77**:784-797. DOI: 10.1097/PSY.0000000000000218

[35] Cameron OG. Interoception: The inside story—A model for psychosomatic processes. Psychosomatic Medicine. 2001;**63**:697-710. DOI: 10.1097/00006842-200109000-00001

[36] Bishop SR. What do we really know about mindfulness-based stress reduction? Psychosomatic Medicine. 2002;**64**:71-83. DOI: 0033-3174/02/6401-0071

[37] Keng SL, Smoski MJ, Robins CJ. Effects of mindfulness on psychological health: A review of empirical studies. Clinical Psychology Review. 2011;**31**:1041-1056. DOI: 10.1016/j.cpr.2011.04.006

[38] Baer RA. Mindfulness training as a clinical intervention: A conceptual and empirical review. Clinical Psychology: Science and Practice. 2003;**10**:125-143. DOI: 10.1093/clipsy/bpg015

[39] Klainin-Yobas P, Cho MA, Creedy D. Efficacy of mindfulness-based interventions on depressive symptoms among people with mental disorders: A metaanalysis. International Journal of Nursing Studies. 2012;**49**:109-121. DOI: 10.1016/j.ijnurstu.2011.08.014

[40] McCarney RW, Schulz J, Grey AR. Effectiveness of mindfulness-based therapies in reducing symptoms of depression: A meta-analysis. European Journal of Psychotherapy & Counselling. 2012;**14**:279-299. DOI: 0.1080/13642537.2012.713186

[41] Strauss C, Cavanagh K, Oliver A, Pettman D. Mindfulness-based interventions for people diagnosed with a current episode of an anxiety or depressive disorder: A meta-analysis of randomised controlled trials. PLoS One. 2014;**9**:e96110. DOI: 10.1371/journal.pone.0096110

[42] Lutz A, Slagter HA, Dunne JD, Davidson RJ. Attention regulation and monitoring in meditation. Trends in

Cognitive Sciences. 2008;**12**:163-169. DOI: 10.1016/j.tics.2008.01.005

[43] Lippelt DP, Hommel B, Colzato LS. Focused attention, open monitoring and loving kindness meditation: Effects on attention, conflict monitoring, and creativity—A review. Frontiers in Psychology. 2014;**5**:1-5. DOI: 10.3389/fpsyg.2014.01083

[44] Hofmann SG, Grossman P, Hinton DE. Loving-kindness and compassion meditation: Potential for psychological interventions. Clinical Psychology Review. 2011;**31**:1126-1132. DOI: 10.1016/j.cpr.2011.07.003

[45] Tang YY, Hölzel B, Posner MI. The neuroscience of mindfulness meditation. Nature Reviews Neuroscience. 2015;**16**:213-225. DOI: 10.1038/nrn3916

[46] Goldin PR, Gross JJ. Effects of mindfulness-based stress reduction (MBSR) on emotion regulation in social anxiety disorder. Emotion. 2010;**10**: 83-91. DOI: 10.1037/a0018441

[47] Tomasino B, Fabbro F. Increases in the right dorsolateral prefrontal cortex and decreases the rostral prefrontal cortex activation after-8 weeks of focused attention based mindfulness meditation. Brain and Cognition. 2016;**102**:46-54. DOI: 10.1016/j.bandc.2015.12.004

[48] Fujino M, Ueda Y, Mizuhara H, Saiki J, Nomura M. Open monitoring meditation reduces the involvement of brain regions related to memory function. Scientific Reports. 2018;**8**: 1-10. DOI: 10.1038/s41598-018-28274-4

[49] Lutz A, Brefczynski-Lewis J, Johnstone T, Davidson RJ. Regulation of the neural circuitry of emotion by compassion meditation: Effects of meditative expertise. PLoS One. 2008;**3**:e1897. DOI: 10.1371/journal.pone.0001897

[50] Lutz A, Greischar LL, Perlman DM, Davidson RJ. BOLD signal in insula is differentially related to cardiac function during compassion meditation in experts vs. novices. NeuroImage. 2009;**47**:1038-1046. DOI: 10.1016/j.neuroimage.2009.04.081

[51] Arch JJ, Craske MG. Mechanisms of mindfulness: Emotion regulation following a focused breathing induction. Behaviour Research and Therapy. 2006;**44**:1849-1858. DOI: 10.1016/j.brat.2005.12.007

[52] Feldman G, Greeson J, Senville J. Differential effects of mindful breathing, progressive muscle relaxation, and loving-kindness meditation on decentering and negative reactions to repetitive thoughts. Behaviour Research and Therapy. 2010;**48**:1002-1011. DOI: 10.1016/j.brat.2010.06.006

[53] Ng CG, Lai KT, Tan SB, Sulaiman AH, Zainal NZ. The effect of 5 minutes of mindful breathing to the perception of distress and physiological responses in palliative care cancer patients: A randomized controlled study. Journal of Palliative Medicine. 2016;**19**:917-924. DOI: 10.1089/jpm.2016.0046

[54] Thase ME, Simons AD, McGeary J, Cahalane JF, Hughes C, Harden T, et al. Relapse after cognitive behavior therapy of depression: Potential implications for longer courses of treatment. The American Journal of Psychiatry. 1992;**149**:1046-1052. DOI: 10.1176/ajp.149.8.1046

[55] Foa EB, Zoellner LA, Feeny NC, Hembree EA, Alvarez-Conrad J. Does imaginal exposure exacerbate PTSD symptoms? Journal of Consulting and Clinical Psychology. 2002;**70**:1022-1028

[56] Hembree EA, Foa EB, Dorfan NM, Street GP, Kowalski J, Tu X. Do patients drop out prematurely from exposure therapy for PTSD? Journal of

Traumatic Stress. 2003;**16**:555-562. DOI: 10.1023/B:JOTS.0000004078.93012.7d

[57] Speckens AE, Ehlers A, Hackmann A, Clark DM. Changes in intrusive memories associated with imaginal reliving in posttraumatic stress disorder. Journal of Anxiety Disorders. 2006;**20**:328-341. DOI: 10.1016/j.janxdis.2005.02.004

[58] Wells C, Kolt GS, Bialocerkowski A. Defining Pilates exercise: A systematic review. Complementary Therapies in Medicine. 2012;**20**:253-262. DOI: 10.1016/j.ctim.2012.02.005

[59] Anderson BD, Spector A. Introduction to Pilates-based rehabilitation. Orthopaedic Physical Therapy Clinics of North America. 2000;**9**:395-410

[60] Kloubec JA. Pilates for improvement of muscle endurance, flexibility, balance, and posture. The Journal of Strength & Conditioning Research. 2010;**24**:661-667. DOI: 10.1519/JSC.0b013e3181c277a6

[61] Sekendiz B, Altun Ö, Korkusuz F, Akın S. Effects of Pilates exercise on trunk strength, endurance and flexibility in sedentary adult females. Journal of Bodywork and Movement Therapies. 2007;**11**:318-326. DOI: 10.1016/j.jbmt.2006.12.002

[62] Cruz-Ferreira A, Fernandes J, Laranjo L, Bernardo LM, Silva A. A systematic review of the effects of Pilates method of exercise in healthy people. Archives of Physical Medicine and Rehabilitation. 2011;**92**:2071-2081. DOI: 10.1016/j.apmr.2011.06.018

[63] Barker AL, Bird ML, Talevski J. Effect of Pilates exercise for improving balance in older adults: A systematic review with meta-analysis. Archives of Physical Medicine and Rehabilitation. 2015;**96**:715-723. DOI: 10.1016/j.apmr.2014.11.021

[64] Lopes S, Correia C, Félix G, Lopes M, Cruz A, Ribeiro F. Immediate effects of Pilates based therapeutic exercise on postural control of young individuals with non-specific low back pain: A randomized controlled trial. Complementary Therapies in Medicine. 2017;**34**:104-110. DOI: 10.1016/j.ctim.2017.08.006

[65] Miyamoto GC, Costa LOP, Galvanin T, Cabral CMN. Efficacy of the addition of modified Pilates exercises to a minimal intervention in patients with chronic low back pain: A randomized controlled trial. Physical Therapy. 2013;**93**:310-320. DOI: 10.2522/ptj.20120190

[66] Kemp AH, Quintana DS, Gray MA, Felmingham KL, Brown K, Gatt JM. Impact of depression and antidepressant treatment on heart rate variability: A review and meta-analysis. Biological Psychiatry. 2010;**67**:1067-1074. DOI: 10.1016/j.biopsych.2009.12.012

[67] Chalmers JA, Quintana DS, Abbott MJ, Kemp AH. Anxiety disorders are associated with reduced heart rate variability: A meta-analysis. Frontiers in Psychiatry. 2014;**5**:1-11. DOI: 10.3389/fpsyt.2014.00080

[68] Lewinsohn PM, Sullivan JM, Grosscup SJ. Changing reinforcing events: An approach to the treatment of depression. Psychotherapy: Theory, Research & Practice. 1980;**17**:322-334. DOI: 10.1037/h0085929

[69] Jacobson NS, Dobson KS, Truax PA, Addis ME, Koerner K, Gollan JK, et al. A component analysis of cognitive-behavioral treatment for depression. Journal of Consulting and Clinical Psychology. 1996;**64**:295-304. DOI: 10.1037/0022-006X.64.2.295

[70] Cuijpers P, Straten AV, Warmerdam L. Behavioral activation treatments of depression: A meta-analysis. Clinical Psychology Review. 2007;**27**:318-326. DOI: 10.1016/j.cpr.2006.11.001

[71] Ekers D, Webster L, Straten AV, Cuijpers P, Richards D, Gilbody S. Behavioural activation for depression; an update of meta-analysis of effectiveness and sub group analysis. PLoS One. 2014;**9**:e100100. DOI: 10.1371/journal.pone.0100100

[72] Dimidjian S, Hollon SD, Dobson KS, Schmaling KB, Kohlenberg RJ, Addis ME, et al. Randomized trial of behavioral activation, cognitive therapy, and antidepressant medication in the acute treatment of adults with major depression. Journal of Consulting and Clinical Psychology. 2006;**74**:658-670. DOI: 10.1037/0022-006X.74.4.658

[73] Mori A, Okamoto Y, Okada G, Takagaki K, Jinnin R, Takamura M, et al. Behavioral activation can normalize neural hypoactivation in subthreshold depression during a monetary incentive delay task. Journal of Affective Disorders. 2016;**189**: 254-262. DOI: 10.1016/j.jad.2015.09.036

[74] Takagaki K, Okamoto Y, Jinnin R, Mori A, Nishiyama Y, Yamamura T, et al. Behavioral activation for late adolescents with subthreshold depression: A randomized controlled trial. European Child and Adolescent Psychiatry. 2016;**25**:1171-1182. DOI: 10.1007/s00787-016-0842-5

[75] Dichter GS, Felder JN, Smoski MJ. The effects of brief behavioral activation therapy for depression on cognitive control in affective contexts: An fMRI investigation. Journal of Affective Disorders. 2010;**126**:236-244. DOI: 10.1016/j.jad.2010.03.022

[76] Shiota S, Okamoto Y, Okada G, Takagaki K, Takamura M, Mori A, et al. Effects of behavioural activation on the neural basis of other perspective self-referential processing in subthreshold depression: A functional magnetic resonance imaging study. Psychological Medicine. 2017;**47**:877-888. DOI: 10.1017/S0033291716002956

[77] Shiota S, Okamoto Y, Okada G, Takagaki K, Takamura M, Mori A, et al. The neural correlates of the metacognitive function of other perspective: A multiple regression analysis study. Neuroreport. 2017;**28**:671-676. DOI: 10.1097/WNR.0000000000000818

[78] World Medical Association. World medical association declaration of Helsinki: Ethical principles for medical research involving human subjects. Journal of the Medical Association. 2013;**310**:2191-2194. DOI: 10.1001/jama.2013.281053

[79] Klatte R, Pabst S, Beelmann A, Rosendahl J. The efficacy of body-oriented yoga in mental disorders: A systematic review and meta-analysis. Deutsches Ärzteblatt International. 2016;**113**:195-202. DOI: 10.3238/arztebl.2016.0195

[80] Beauchemin J, Hutchins TL, Patterson F. Mindfulness meditation may lessen anxiety, promote social skills, and improve academic performance among adolescents with learning disabilities. Complementary Health Practice Review. 2008;**13**:34-45. DOI: 10.1177/1533210107311624

Advances in Decision Making

Edited by Fausto Pedro García Márquez

Published in London, United Kingdom

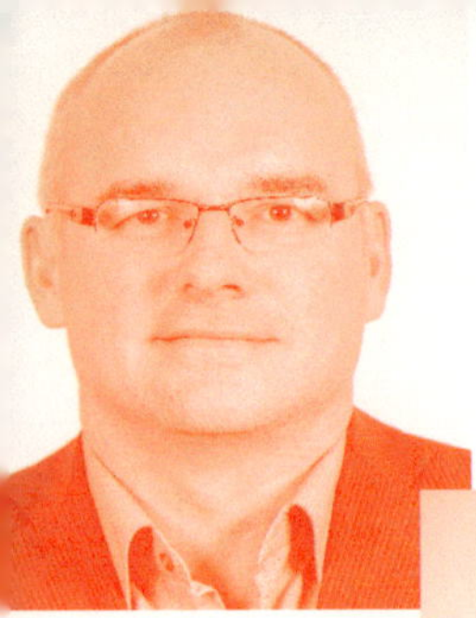
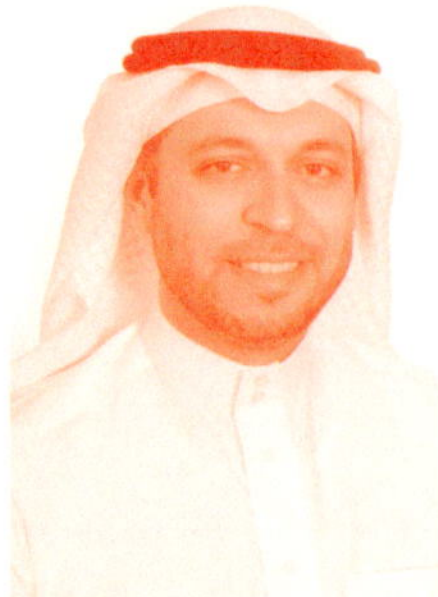
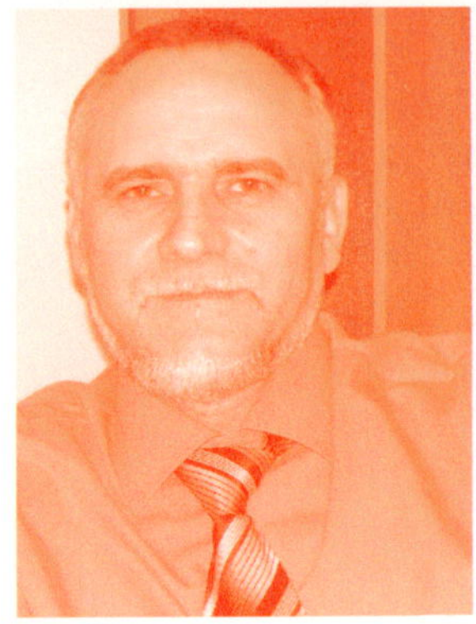
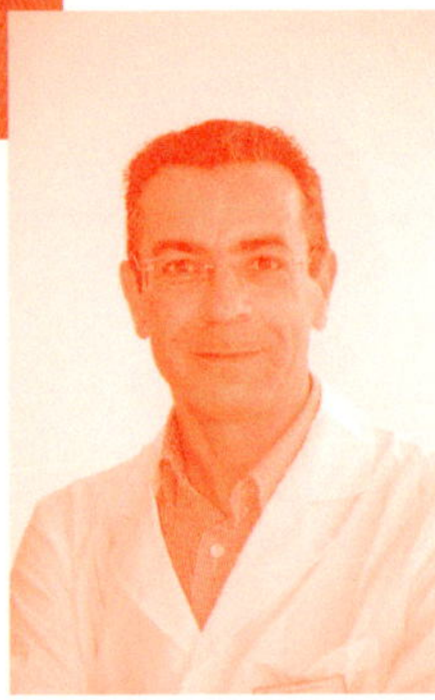
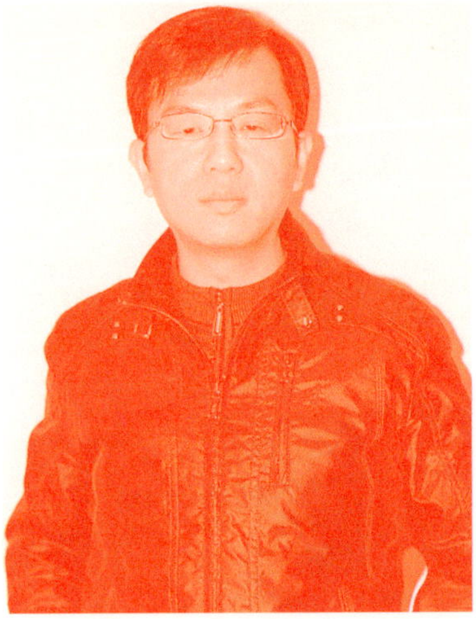
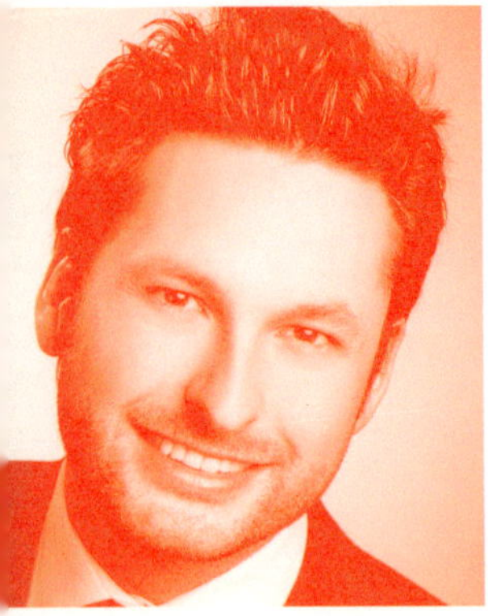
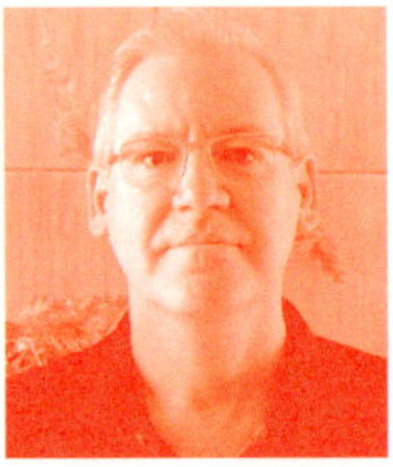

IntechOpen

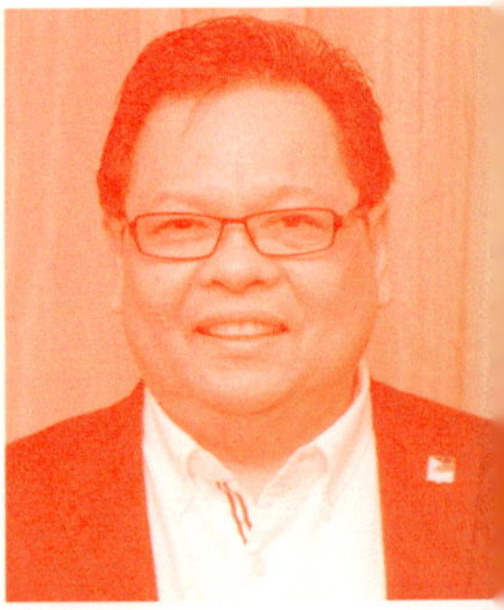
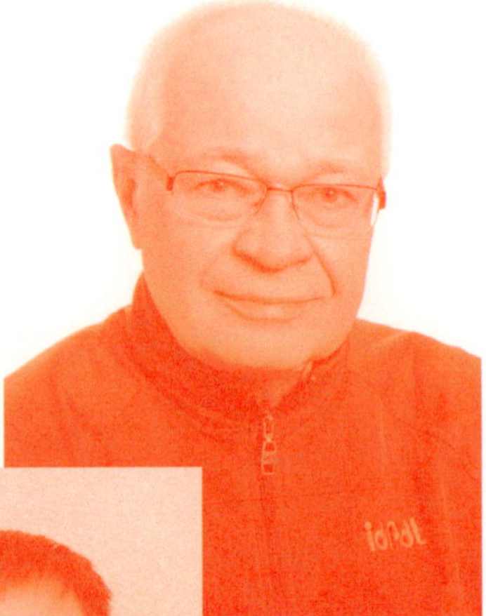
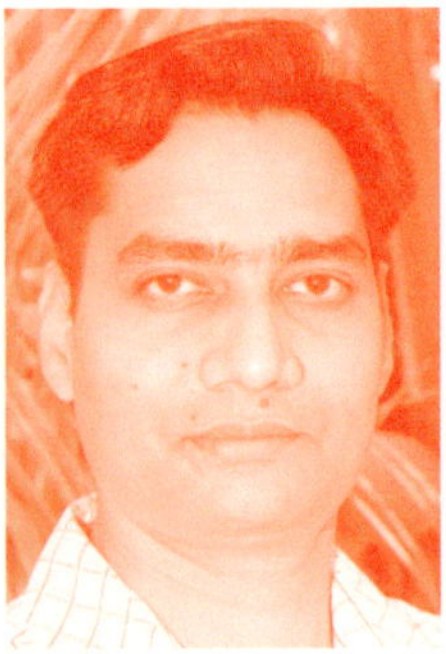
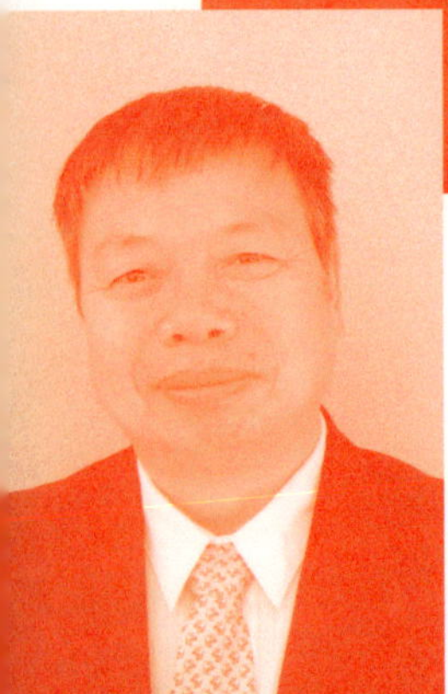
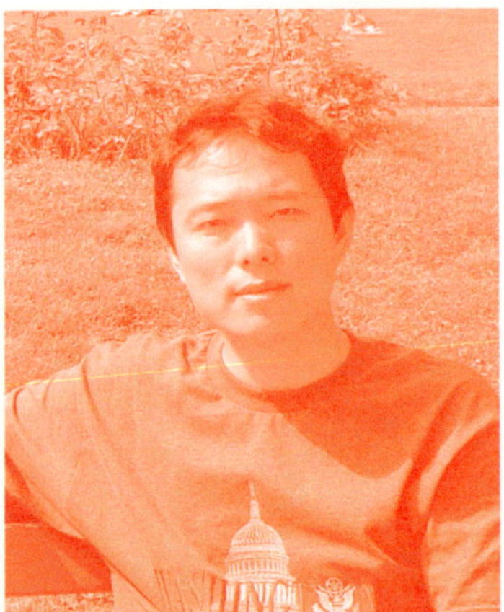
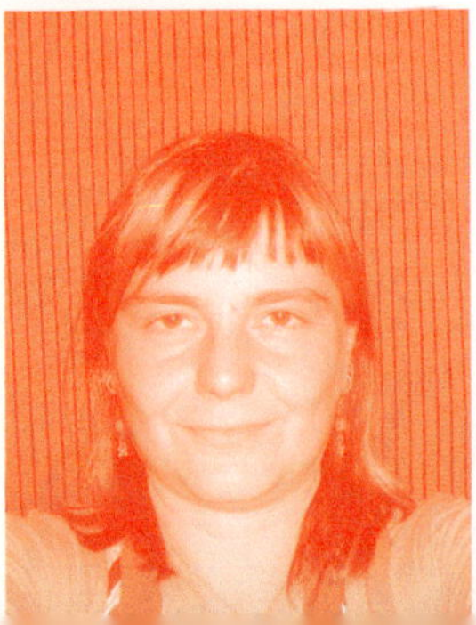

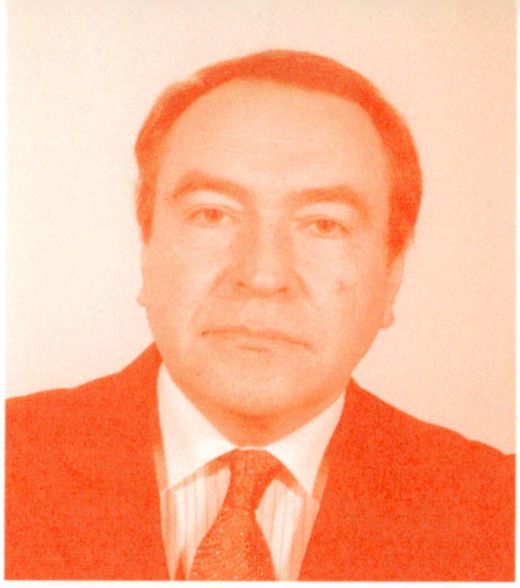
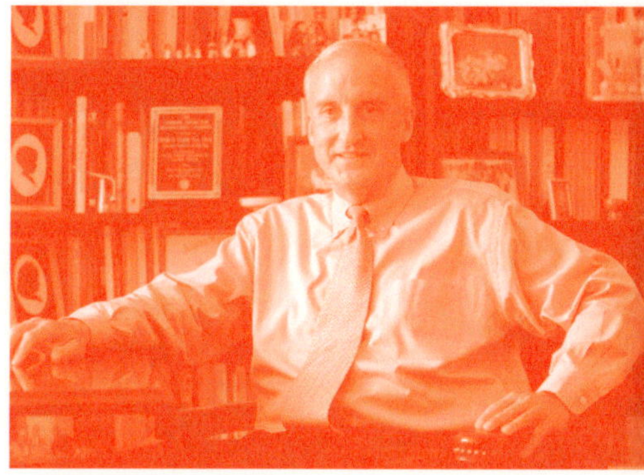
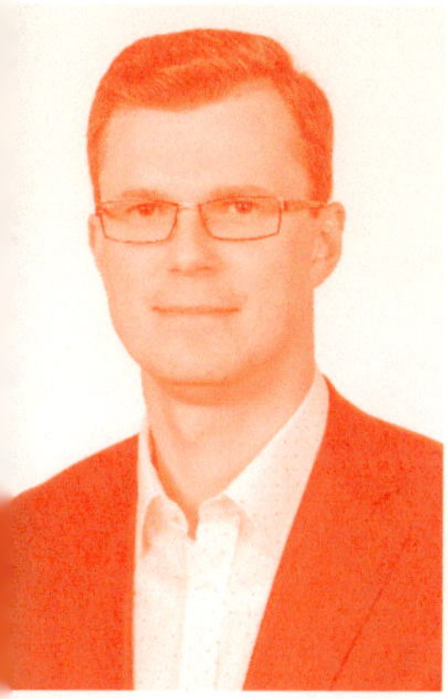
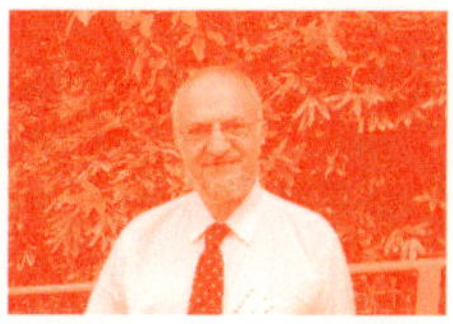
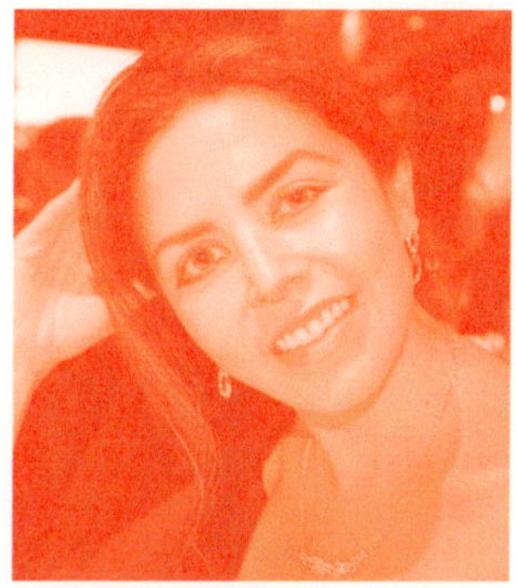

Supporting open minds since 2005

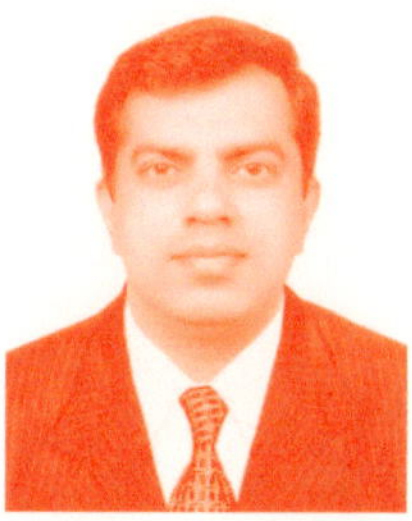
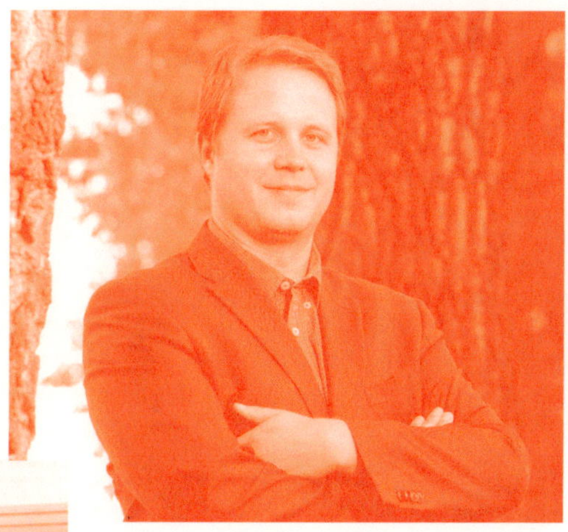
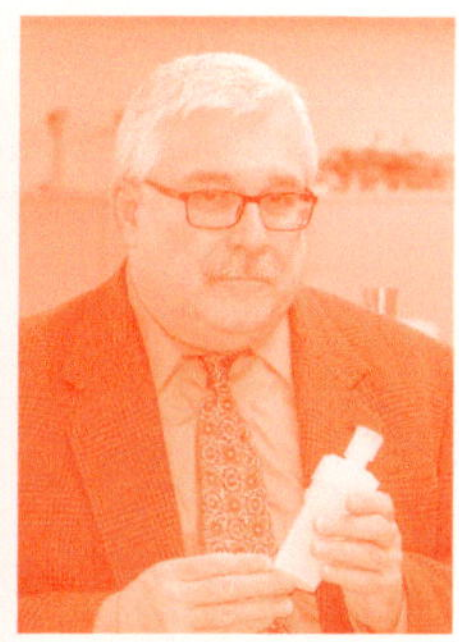
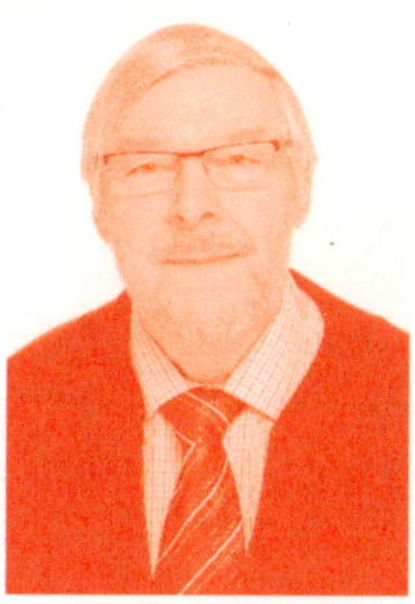
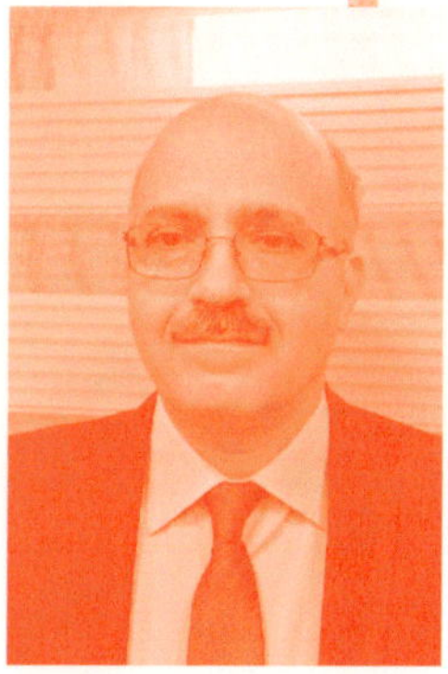
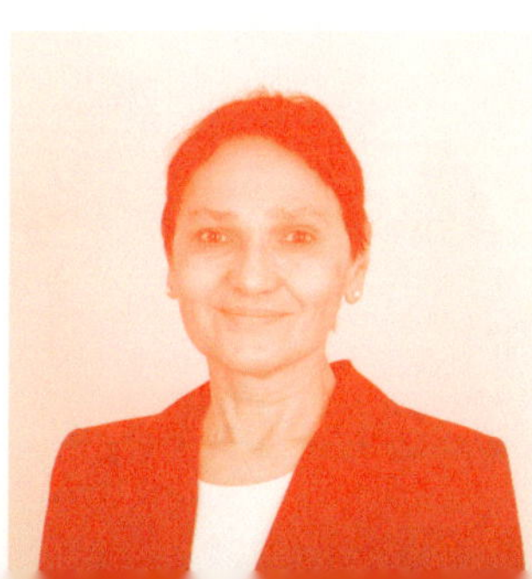
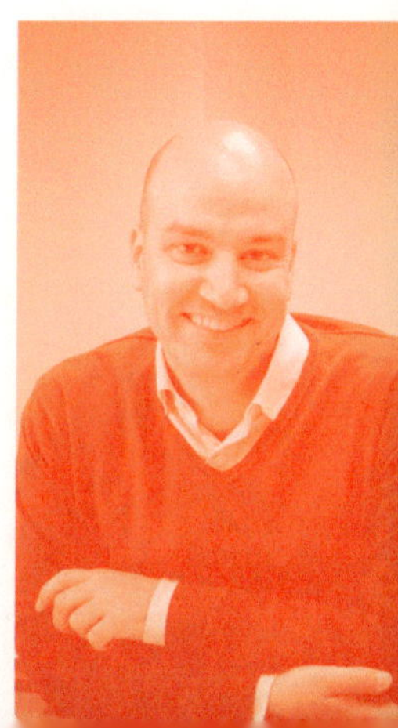

Advances in Decision Making
http://dx.doi.org/10.5772/intechopen.95217
Edited by Fausto Pedro García Márquez

Contributors
Daniels Aide Okun, Osama Ose Iyawe, Oluwatomi Adetunji, Xiaona Xia, Gérard de Boisboissel, Sangdo Choi, Aissa Bensattalah, Rachid Chalal, Tahar Hassaine Daouadji, Tayeb Bensattalah, Syed Abou Iltaf Hussain, Uttam Kumar Mandal, Himanshu Chandra, Bernard Cadet, Garazi Carranza Ruiz de Loizaga, Begoña Sanchez Gonzalez, Nivetha Martin, Fausto Pedro García Márquez

First published in London, United Kingdom, 2022 by IntechOpen
IntechOpen is the global imprint of INTECHOPEN LIMITED, registered in England and Wales, registration number: 11086078, 5 Princes Gate Court, London, SW7 2QJ, United Kingdom
Printed in Croatia

British Library Cataloguing-in-Publication Data
A catalogue record for this book is available from the British Library

Additional hard and PDF copies can be obtained from orders@intechopen.com

Advances in Decision Making
Edited by Fausto Pedro García Márquez
p. cm.
Print ISBN 978-1-83969-496-7
Online ISBN 978-1-83969-497-4
eBook (PDF) ISBN 978-1-83969-498-1

For EU product safety concerns:
IN TECH d.o.o., Prolaz Marije Krucifikse Kozulić 3, 51000 Rijeka, Croatia, info@intechopen.com or visit our website at intechopen.com.

Meet the editor

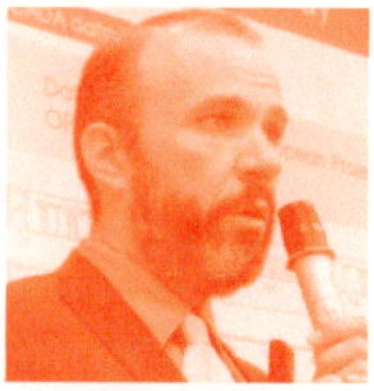

Fausto Pedro García Márquez is a full professor at the University of Castilla–La Mancha (UCLM), Spain. He is also an honorary senior research fellow at Birmingham University, United Kingdom, and a lecturer at the Postgraduate European Institute. During 2013–2014, he was a senior manager at Accenture. He obtained his European Ph.D. with a maximum distinction. He is the recipient of numerous awards, including prizes from the International Society of Management Science and Engineering Management (ICMSEM). He has published more than 170 papers in scientific journals and authored 40 books, 90 book chapters, and 6 patents. He is the editor of five international journals and a committee member for more than sixty conferences. He has been the Principal Investigator for more than 150 national and international projects. His main interests are artificial intelligence, maintenance, management, renewable energy, transport, advanced analytics, and data science.

Contents

Preface

Advances in Decision Making synthesizes the analytical principles with the business practice of decision making. Specifically, it provides an interface between the main disciplines of engineering/technology and the organizational, administrative, and planning abilities of decision-making. It is complementary to other sub-disciplines such as economics, finance, marketing, decision and risk analysis, and more. The chapters introduce and demonstrate decision-making theory using practical case studies. Discussions of the theory of decision-making are accompanied by relevant analysis techniques, progressing from simple theory to complex and dynamic decisions with multiple data points. Computational techniques, dynamic analysis, probabilistic methods, and mathematical optimization techniques are expertly blended to support the analysis of multi-criteria decision-making problems with defined constraints and requirements. The algorithms, approaches, and methods presented in each chapter can be applied to problems of all sizes. This book is useful for graduate students, researchers, professionals, engineers, and other interested readers.

Fausto Pedro García Márquez
Ingenium Research Group,
University of Castilla-La Mancha,
Ciudad Real, Spain

Chapter 1

Introductory Chapter: Introduction to Advances in Decision-Making

Fausto Pedro García Márquez

1. Introduction

The main principles of decision-making applied in business practice by advance analytics are summarized in this book [1]. The book is the compilation of chapters written by authors who are experts in the topic covered. Main disciplines, such as management, engineering/technology, economic, etc., are considered as interface with decision-making, being complementary to others, e.g., administrative, finance, risk analysis, marketing, etc.

Decision-making could be defined as the choosing process from several options. It can be done by simple or advanced analytics, by exact or not procedures, by the opinion of any, etc. [2]. The frequency at which the decision-making is done is also variable, from 1 to any. If the effect of decision is considered in a period, then decision-making is classified as operational (short period: daily, weekly, or monthly), strategic (long period: generally 1 year), and politic (very long period: usually more than 1 year).

Decision-making is gaining more importance because the new market scenario is being more competitive [3–6]. This leads the researchers to focus on this topic, together with new technologies and advanced analytics, generating new software and tools based on the Internet of Things [7, 8].

Triantaphyllou analyzed the best decision-making method according to the best decision-making method [9].

The measurement of the efficiency for decision-making units was done via linear and nonlinear programming methods [10]. The authors also took into account the economic and engineering relationship for decision-making.

Hwang and Masud [4] and White [11] showed a complete review of decision-making methods. New algorithms are appearing, for example, [12–14], where more robust and complex problems are being solved by employing artificial intelligence [15–17] and the most important ones are presented in this book.

The main theories are studied and presented in this book in different case studies. The main results are analyzed and discussed, suggesting new future works to continue working on that. Case studies are going from simple to complex cases, including big data, from static to dynamic problems, and also from offline to online cases, including the Internet of Things. Models, methods, and algorithms based on dynamic analysis, mathematical optimization, and computational techniques are designed and implemented to carry out the data analysis of decision-making, also considering the constraints.

IntechOpen

The book has been written to be used by students and professionals of multiple disciplines, e.g., industrial organization, applied microeconomics, business administration, among others, and, of course, decision science applied to simple problems to complex and large problems and for different case studies. The book is also written for academics and researchers on different disciplines.

Author details

Fausto Pedro García Márquez
Ingenium Research Group, University of Castilla-La Mancha, Spain

*Address all correspondence to: faustopedro.garcia@uclm.es

References

[1] Marugan AP, Marquez FPG. Decision-Making Management: A Tutorial and Applications. Cambridge, MA: Academic Press; 2017

[2] Marugán AP, Márquez FPG. Decision making approach for optimal business investments. In: Advanced Business Analytics. Berlin, Germany: Springer; 2015. pp. 1-20

[3] Pliego Marugán A, García Márquez FP, Lev B. Optimal decision-making via binary decision diagrams for investments under a risky environment. International Journal of Production Research. 2017;**55**:5271-5286

[4] Hwang C-L, Masud ASM. Multiple Objective Decision Making—Methods and Applications: A State-of-the-Art Survey. Vol. 164. Berlin, Germany: Springer Science & Business Media; 2012

[5] Pérez JMP, Asensio ES, Márquez FPG. Economic viability analytics for wind energy maintenance management. In: Advanced Business Analytics. Berlin, Germany: Springer; 2015. pp. 39-54

[6] Márquez FPG, Lev B. Advanced Business Analytics. Berlin, Germany: Springer; 2015

[7] Bose R. Advanced analytics: Opportunities and challenges. Industrial Management & Data Systems. 2009;**109**:155-172

[8] Barton D, Court D. Making advanced analytics work for you. Harvard Business Review. 2012;**90**:78-83

[9] Triantaphyllou E. Multi-criteria decision making methods. In: Multi-Criteria Decision Making Methods: A Comparative Study. Berlin, Germany: Springer; 2000. pp. 5-21

[10] Charnes A, Cooper WW, Rhodes E. Measuring the efficiency of decision making units. European Journal of Operational Research. 1978;**2**:429-444

[11] White D. Multiple attribute decision making—A state-of-the-art survey. Journal of the Operational Research Society. 1982;**33**:289-289

[12] Marugán AP, Márquez FPG. Improving the Efficiency on Decision Making Process via BDD. In: Proceedings of the Ninth International Conference on Management Science and Engineering Management. 2015. pp. 1395-1405

[13] Pliego Marugán A, García Márquez FP, Lorente J. Decision making process via binary decision diagram. International Journal of Management Science and Engineering Management. 2015;**10**:3-8

[14] Marugán AP, Márquez FPG, Lavirgen JL. Decision Making via Binary Decision Diagrams: A Real Case Study. In: Proceedings of the Eighth International Conference on Management Science and Engineering Management. Germany: Springer; 2014. pp. 215-222

[15] Chen S-J, Hwang C-L. Fuzzy multiple attribute decision making methods. In: Fuzzy Multiple Attribute Decision Making. Berlin, Germany: Springer; 1992. pp. 289-486

[16] Jiménez AA, Muñoz CQG, Marquez FPG, Zhang L. Artificial intelligence for concentrated solar plant maintenance management. In: Proceedings of the Tenth International Conference on Management Science and Engineering Management. Germany: Springer; 2017. pp. 125-134

[17] Marquez FPG, Pliego A, Lorente J, Trapero JR. A new ranking method

approach for decision making in maintenance management. In: Proceedings of the Seventh International Conference on Management Science and Engineering Management Lecture Notes in Electrical Engineering. Germany: Springer; 2013. pp. 27-38

Chapter 2

Cognitive Decision-Making in Dynamic Systems: When the Objectivity (of the Processing) Does Not Guarantee the Validity (of the Choice of Action)

Bernard Cadet

Abstract

Since around 1970, academic studies on decision-making have changed in nature. Whereas they used to be laboratory studies of selected situations giving rise to the expression of individual choices, nowadays studies focus on real situations. These situations are processed in their natural contexts at the time they occur. The decisions to be made concern generally social problems (for instance forest fires, maritime pollution or global warming). This mutation in the nature of situations studied requires a paradigm shift, which leads to elaborate decisions in complex, dynamic and evolving systems, even sometimes resilient to human actions implemented to control them. This chapter analyses, at individual and group level (crisis units), cognitive difficulties encountered by decision-makers in handling such situations. These situations consist in treating information by assigning them, from the outset, meanings (sometimes personal). This is done by looking for temporary interactions, while respecting the global nature of the situation, by focusing on knowing the properties of context as well as those of the temporal evolution of the system concerned. This chapter analyses a case study for which urgent and fundamental decisions could not be taken and proposes an interpretation in terms of paradigms. Previous studies noted that the decision in complex systems, could entail paradoxes. This study on the decision-making dynamic shows that seeking objectivity, as defined under its current intangible form, does not produce a significant increase in the validity of choices made.

Keywords: Decision-making, Complexity, Dynamism, Systems, Holism, Paradigm

1. Introduction

Since psychology has set as its main purpose the study of behaviour, decision-making behaviour represents a stimulating subject for studies and research. Not only are there numerous circumstances in which it proves necessary to make a choice, but they are also highly varied. This chapter analyses a quite specific category of decisions: those concerning the action choices in complex and dynamic systems. Highly different from other decisions studied in fixed environments, they lead us to explore the field of epistemology and cognitive psychology and offer the advantage of generating sensitive crossed interrogations in these two disciplines also required for the construction of knowledge.

This chapter will focus on one of these, in other words the relations between the choice of an objective epistemology and the absence, observed in the field, of relevant decisions. The argument has seven facets. The first describes the cognitive and epistemological specificities of decision-making in complex and dynamic systems. The second deals with the assignment of meaning to information, while the third describes a selection of real situations which led to decision-making difficulties. The fourth facet is dedicated to the examination of an investigation tool: the paradigm, and refers to a particular paradigm; the objective experimental paradigm (OEP) which underlies scientific progress in numerous disciplines. The fifth facet focuses on its transferability to decision-making in complex and dynamic systems and any resulting cognitive dilemmas. The sixth facet raises the question of the globality of the situations to be processed (rather than their breakdown into variables) by taking as guideline an attempt made to this effect in psychology. The seventh examines the epistemological position of the decision-makers faced with a paradox which seems to be related to valorisation at all costs of objectivation, at the expense of other characteristics of the decision.

2. Decision-making aimed at cognitive psychology

2.1 A decision-making proto-schema

The most concise characterisation of decision-making facing with uncertainty [1] consists in describing it as an approach prior to choosing one action [Ai] amongst a set of *n* actions [An] considered as being potentially relevant. In this characterisation, decision-making consists in generating what psychologists call a conduct (a behaviour in common language) in order to choose the action [Ai] amongst a set of **n** possible actions. This action is evaluated as being the most relevant to change an existing situation considered to be inappropriate or dangerous. For example: which action(s) should be chosen to stop the persistent financial losses of a company? However, the cognitive approach is not solely interested in the end result (the chosen action); it attempts to explain the characteristics which led to this conclusion. These characteristics must be found in the information present in the situation and with respect to the objective to be reached. The theoretical references used will therefore concern cognitive psychology, whose purpose is to study how to process the information which will lead to a judgement, then to a decision.

2.2 Decision-making as cognitive management of systems and networks

It can be observed that, in this conception, decision-making is not limited to initially selecting outcomes to create the set **n** and to making a limited number of binary comparisons. This type of limitation would exclude from the field of the decision any "surprise" which could arise from the reality of the situation processed. We will then observe that the informational characteristics of the environment and even more its ability to evolve, are largely or totally absent from this approach. While the condition that the set of **n** actions must be exhaustive is initially put forward, it is not always possible to meet this condition. All operational decision-makers are aware of the frequency of unexpected or unforeseen conditions in the initial plan [2]. Mental fixism, which consists in thinking that "everything is under control" and that everything has been planned, is often accepted too readily due to the sole fact that it confirms an earlier mental representation.

This type of difficulty is frequently encountered in situations where behavioural automation is important, for example when piloting an aircraft. While it undoubtedly reduces the mental effort, automation may nevertheless prove to be disconcerting faced with unplanned situations, especially if the level of concentration drops temporarily. Amongst the causes mentioned during "inappropriate decision-making", analysts estimate that "airline pilots do not receive sufficient training on manual piloting".

2.3 Epistemological characteristics of the chosen action

The chosen action [A1], also referred to as the dominant action, is that which, at the end of the decision-making process, is the one most likely to achieve the required effect. This first requirement applies to all decisions to define the objective to be reached but involves specificities in decisions qualified as complex. In such contexts, deciding is much more than choosing a subject or a procedure. Based on the dynamics of the systems concerned, we must consider that the decisions are taken to cause *state changes* in order to set up new operating balances in the systems: the health system, the economic system, the company, the emergency systems, etc.

Except in special cases, to obtain these state changes, the "decision" entity must itself be composite, i.e. must consist of a set of elementary actions (a1, a2, ... ak), where each individual action has an impact on the system and where the set of actions taken together forms a global action module. The decision as such is the equivalent of a vector.

Scientific knowledge requires that the epistemological characteristics of the chosen informations must be clearly defined. The most obvious are the validity (*v*), the generality (*g*) and the fidelity (*f*). The sequence of elementary actions must prove that it is composed in such a way that it can act on the system in the required direction (v), do so for all situations of the same type (g), with a stability of effect which is repeated over time (f). These qualities can be used to distinguish the daily information forming know-how from the scientific information which satisfied these requirements, substrate on which the theoretical systems are built.

3. Information, cognition, and assignment of meaning

3.1 Perception and interpretation

In the press and in the media, the discriminating power of the sensory functions is largely overestimated. Taking vision for example, the eye, compared with a camera, which would record events, is supposed to provide a faithful image of the external context sometimes called reality. However, the information that we will use to build an adapted our conduct is necessarily obtained by *interpretation*. It consists of dynamic entities to which meanings are assigned due to the mere fact they have transited via the neural networks of the brain. The retinal image therefore acquires, in the brain, a meaning related to the decision-maker's knowledge networks.

3.2 Two cognition modules (levels)

Decision-making thus appears as a mental task involving two different but complementary types of operation corresponding to two cognition levels, each one representing a homogeneous subset of operations and therefore deserving to be considered as a module.

3.2.1 The information sampling *process (module 1)*

The first cognitive operations consist in collecting information by performing a global inspection of the situation; the subsequent operations, carried out in successive steps, will then reduce the field explored.

All human-decision-makes absorb the situation to be processed using data supplied by their sensory functions. Two important points must nevertheless be specified. Firstly, the term "sensory functions" must be understood in a very broad sense not restricted to the well-known five senses but also including all the receptors involving movement, sensitivity and possibly intuition. The range of information available therefore extends far beyond the data processed in the specific areas traditionally mentioned. Secondly, we must stress, as said previously, that each sensory input is processed and *interpreted* by the brain. Apart from its physiological properties, we must therefore point out its main characteristic: being an element which brings meaning.

3.2.2 The information formatting *processes (module 2)*

The level-2 cognitive processes are referred to as executive functions. They differ from the previous functions by the fact that they regulate the scheduling (planning) of the behavioural construction sometimes as activation (useful information) and sometimes as inhibition (interfering information). The main functions concerned are attention, flexibility of thought, implementation of adaptive feedback loops, global reformulations, etc. They are involved in determining the behaviour at a global activation level. The most illustrative example is that of attention, which does not belong to any specific item of information but which can be applied to each one.

3.3 Complementarity

In line with the systemic outlooks, it is important to consider that these modules represent two entities which, far from being opposed, complement each other in numerous circumstances. It would be worthwhile considering them as inducing each other mutually. Module 1 samples information in situ whereas module 2 handles the formatting and organisation of the set so created. Module 2 is involved in the creation of the cognitive maps which will be described in greater detail in this document.

4. Epistemological characteristics of the situations studied

4.1 Structural data

To complete the data collection, it is necessary to mention a few real decision-making situations in complex systems which occurred since about 1960. The situations studied by the social sciences exhibit four properties:

- complex situations which include a large number of dimensions with non-linear relations, making it difficult to assess how the situations are going to evolve.

- systems organised in subsystems, not around variables. These subsystems represent activation "focal points" which create dynamisms.

- evolving entities which change state over time. Time must therefore be taken into consideration when determining the appropriate action.

- situations which often have a strong societal dimension. In numerous contexts, the action choices are designed to put an end to a damaging situation by controlling its effects and the situation itself (for example, controlling a technological accident such as the Chernobyl disaster). The decisions must be made rapidly, under the pressure of public opinion, in a context where stress is highly present.

4.2 Field data

In natural situations, this type of characterisation applies to events which appear to be quite different from the outside but which are relatively similar as regards their underlying architecture and organisation. The media report these events regularly when they have harmful effects.

The events most frequently encountered are:

- Forest fires, extremely difficult to control, whose recurrence and duration (sometimes lasting several months) are retrospective signs of decisions that are hard to take. Recently in California and Australia, despite major and appropriate firefighting measures, the fires lasted for several weeks, even several months, and caused serious human and material damage.

- Marine pollution due to oil spills from tankers. Coastal areas have been polluted by hydrocarbons from shipwrecks on numerous occasions. Those which received the most media attention, due to the scale of the damage caused, are remembered by the names of the oil tankers themselves. We may mention Amoco Cadiz (1978), Exxon Valdez (1989), Aegean Sea (1992), Erika (1999), Prestige (2002) and Hebei Spirit (2007).

- Global warming represents another complex and dynamic system for which decisions must be taken at large scale. Scientists quickly raised the alert on the need to "manage" the climate. The Swedish chemist Arrhenius (1859–1927) was the first to establish a link between energy production (coal at the time) and global warming. Over the next decades, however, there was such a gap between the perceived reality and the difficulties announced that these predictions were forgotten by the public opinion. More recently, a predominant political factor has been added to the initially scientific treatment given to this issue. Since 1995, the United Nations has organised in a different country every year a conference hosting some 185 nations. Known under the acronym COP (Conference of Parties), these meetings have already been held 25 times. COP 26 to be held in the United Kingdom in 2021 for about ten days has been postponed due to the Covid-19 pandemic but finally will take place, another example as disconcerting as the previous ones regarding the management of a complex system.

- The management of pandemics exhibits all the above-mentioned characteristics of a complex system. The objective to be reached is clearly determined and the means to change it from its current state to the final required state consist in setting up a decision-making sequence. This entity, which includes an evolving time dimension, comprises a series of successive decisions, each one being designed to make the system evolve in the required direction. The decision is built one step at a time, so as to preserve what has been achieved and validated and to duly validate the changes introduced. Examination of the strategies implemented in the countries of the European Community, federated around a common project, reveals, both in terms of time and structure, major differences in the way the situation is processed and the decisions made.

In all these categories (the types of situation which have just been mentioned), the decision-makers encounter major difficulties in managing the active systems not only individually but also as a committee: the collective intelligence so often proposed as the solution is temporarily inoperative. Some forest fires last for weeks, even months, damaged oil tankers continue to spill their cargoes for weeks and sometimes much longer, the issue of global warming proves difficult to manage, like the pandemic which, since the alert was raised in 2019, has not yet been controlled at the time this document was written.

In view of such obvious and recurrent difficulties, we must examine the methods and cognitive strategies involved in the decision-making process when faced with complex systems.

5. Decision-making in dynamic systems: the paradigm tool

5.1 Cognition and complex systems (reminder)

Historically, relations between cognition and complex systems have been difficult to manage. It was around the 1900s with the studies conducted by J.H. Poincaré (1854–1912) that the first evidence relating to a problem observed in astronomy was detected. It was only in the 1970s, however, probably out of despair, that the expression "chaos theory" was introduced. It was to experience a major impact in relation with the quasi-oxymoron characterising it. The project to theorise disorder is in fact the exact opposite of the deterministic conceptions on which scientific theories are built and based. In other words, chaos seemed to be a chance event.

When studying turbulences, Ruelle and Takens [3] indicate quite to the point that, beyond an apparent disorder, chaos is in fact "deterministic", but this observation introduces a new paradigm into the scientific research activity. Today the complexity of the situation and the dynamics that underlie it are no longer considered to be disruptive elements but as structuring characteristics of the situation and can be used to find the appropriate concrete action [4].

5.2 Roles and functions of the paradigm

Very broadly characterised, a paradigm, sometimes defined as a "school of thought" is the combination, within a given set, of theoretical and methodological notions with concrete cases which are compatible together so that there is no rupture in the approach to build a corpus of knowledge. For the last two centuries, the objectivity required to choose the relevant action has been related to the experimental method resulting in the construction of the objective experimental paradigm (OEP) which has witnessed major successes. OEP has led to the development of physical sciences, material sciences, life and health sciences. This paradigm underlies experimental medicine, as well as the progress made in the techniques which have accelerated its development.

5.3 Objective experimental paradigm and psychology

While the formalised sciences (virtually) never raise the question of which paradigm to use since the OEP is the obvious choice, in the human and social sciences, it must be chosen in a preliminary step. This is clearly the case of psychology where the OEP has been used for many years in laboratory studies (Wundt created the first experimental psychology laboratory at Leipzig in 1879. His initial training as a physiologist probably contributed to the transfer of skills and models to psychology). The central theme studied by this laboratory was in fact perception. More recently, from the 1960s, cognitive psychology has made extensive use of this OEP adding new technological tools in order to study the dynamics of the brain processes during information processing operations.

5.4 Characteristics and migrations of the PEO

The well-known OEP has become so dominant that it represents an idealised conception of research built around clearly defined options. The main ones, apart from the public nature of the investigation procedure, include the permanent concern for verification using a device conceived and/or built by the researcher. To meet these epistemological requirements, a workplace and clearly defined working conditions are necessary. The workplace is the laboratory, isolated from the influences of the outside world, to prevent unwanted influences - without really knowing what they are - from disturbing the network of relations between variables. The device used is a reconstruction simplified by means of the "scientific reductionism" of potential relations between certain (potentially causal) independent variables and (resulting) dependent variables. Validation tools, sometimes statistical, are used to check whether or not the links proposed are valid.

In view of the guarantees it offers regarding the objectivity of the conclusions and their applicability in real situations, the OEP has been adopted in numerous human and social science research studies [5], rarely in its canonical form and frequently in forms adapted to the situation being processed. The latter forms may be increasingly remote from the basic schema. From an epistemological point of view, it is interesting to consider these successive shifts. They highlight the existence of a compromise, in other words an attenuation of the generality and rigour of the method by considering the specific characteristics of each situation.

5.5 Epistemological functions of the paradigm

In addition to the intrinsic functions of the paradigm, those of information processing, Kuhn [6] adds a global, trans-situational function. This author points out that the results obtained during its applications to situations of different type but of similar architecture (organisation) are indicators of its validity (the generality requirement g is met). Due to scientific progress, all paradigms are superseded as soon as they are no longer able to provide answers to the questions raised. A new epistemological option and a new paradigm become necessary. Kuhn designated this moment of transition "a scientific revolution". The progress made in scientific knowledge is neither linear nor regular; it is built up discontinuously by a series of leaps separated by periods of stability, of irregular duration, but which shorten according to the degree of progress of science.

6. Cognitive dilemmas

6.1 Opposed characteristics

The most recent paradigmatic leap in the evolution of human sciences is that marking the transition from the objective experimental paradigm to the systemic paradigm. What are the consequences? The study of dynamic and complex situations using the OEP analysis grid is unable to determine the efficient decision which would bring the system to the required state (how to put out the forest fire, for example).

Due to the recurrence of difficulties and failures, a more in-depth epistemological analysis must be conducted. This could be explained, for example, by the fact that the characteristics of the complex and dynamic situation to be analysed (S) and those of the tool (paradigm O) used to do so, clearly appear to be contradictory in many respects. As regards the structuring units considered: dynamic subsystems (S) against variables (O); a problem *reconstructed* to be operationalised in a laboratory isolated from the outside world (O) faced with a *real* problem observed in natural environment (S); non-linear relations (S) translated by linear relations (O); dismissal of the temporal perspective (O) although the time of observation and evolution of the system is a determining factor for the decisional choice (S). This amounts to applying a tool built using properties which are rigorously opposed to the situations to which it is applied.

6.2 An epistemological choice and its consequences

Due to another source of malfunction, the scientific reductionism operation must be re-examined. In this case, the methodological reductionism will be considered differently from its ordinary meaning: we will consider it as a methodological approach aimed at condensing a real situation to reduce it to its most fundamental components. This type of operation, also used for a quite different purpose, has been called "eidetic reduction" by the phenomenologists, to shift, using their terminology, from the "existence" of things to their "essence".

Thus, a natural situation (i.e. outside the laboratory) is an instantiation surrounded by a "clutter" of temporal or circumstantial particularisms, which prove secondary for those wanting to isolate *general* information to be used for theorising and modelling. Moreover, this reduction also takes a material form when it allows researchers to build the device mentioned above in order to select from the flow the information which must be kept and then test the information which seems important, in particular that used to satisfy the objectivity.

6.3 Cognitive map / heuristic map

The cognitive map, sometimes also referred to as the heuristic map, is a mental model or representation that a human individual makes of the arrangement of steps, methods or conditions which he/she considers necessary to decide what to do. In other words, it is an organised representation of knowledge. It indicates the time required to identify a task (about one minute), in forms that are sometimes rather basic, it transmits, when necessary, the information to the long-term memory which stores it for future reuse.

Like numerous cognitive productions, this map is subject to the heuristic approaches identified by Kahneman, Slovic and Tversky [7]. While numerous occurrences exist, they all have the same objective: introduce simplicity into a situation which, due to its complexity, appears to be disconcerting. We may mention again the initial lack of understanding conveyed by the term "chaos theory", direct reflection of a cognitive failure. As confirmed subsequently by the research studies in cognitive psychology on judgement, as part of the basic need of every human being to understand the present world, individuals will perform heuristic reductions of this complexity which will then be used to produce simplified cognitive maps. However, although the mental representation is simplified, the reality of the situation nevertheless remains complex. Applying the simplified mental models to the reality of the situation fosters errors of judgement and therefore inappropriate decisions. (A very similar approach in the field of perception underlies the development of conspiracy "theories".)

7. Management of globality: counterproductive simplifications

7.1 An essential requirement

In the decision-making concerning the complex situations mentioned in 2.2, the decision is more complex than choosing a single action directly. The term "decision-making" means determining a *sequence of actions* meeting the characteristics stated at the start of this study. Each situation chosen must be considered as a reactive systemic globality. Trying to isolate the elements, separate them from the set means simultaneously altering the system and fragmenting the relations between elements. Unlike the device built in the laboratory whose architecture is intangible and where only the intensities vary, the complex system is an evolving and reacting entity: a forest fire does not have the same characteristics when it has just broken out as when it has lasted for several days. The temporal dynamic aspect becomes preponderant.. Assessing the potential of a complex system implies being able to quantify a global index that expresses its evolutionary power. Entropy represents a reference often used although in different forms: quantified when the data allow it [8], cognitive in other cases [9].

7.2 Consider the globality: the example of gestalt psychology

How to conceive the processing of globality? A first option mainly consists in not breaking it down according to the Cartesian and Newtonian analysis methods, which are highly attractive since they have demonstrated their usefulness for the construction of numerous highly attractive disciplinary corpuses. The recommended strategy in this case is not to discard them but to examine, when analysis tools are concerned, the conditions and benefits of preserving the globality.

The Gestalt Psychology initiated by German researchers working in the United States, and pioneered by Lewin (1890–1947), attempted to do so. The Gestalt movement does not refer to the laboratory and adopts the principle based on the analysis of global entities. These terms designate the situation as such (often referred to as the figure) and the informational field in which it is immersed (often referred to as the ground). According to this epistemological movement, trying to distinguish between the elements is pointless since "the whole is more than the sum of its parts". The whole has its own characteristics (we might be tempted to say its own "personality") which is more than the sum of the elements taken individually.

7.3 Dynamisms

Another extremely important property of the Gestalts is their dynamism. This can be easily observed by examining the reversible figures widely published in magazines, designed in such a way that the figure and the ground can be interchanged. It takes a few moments to observe the dynamism of the phenomenon which globally and suddenly modifies the nature of what is perceived.

When attempting to sketch out an epistemology of globality, Lewin, who developed the concept of group techniques, strived to study each situation, each type of behaviour, inserted in its natural context. One well-known example is that of purchasing behaviour. So no isolation and no more or less successful reconstruction. In his book entitled "Principles of Topological Psychology", Lewin [10] studies social behaviour and is the first one to analyse psychological behaviour. His project consists in modelling the analysis approaches used in psychology on those of mathematics but mainly of the physics of his time, in other words in terms of forces and force resultants. Lewin also introduces the concept of psychological life space including space, time and forces as dynamic elements; entities which prepare the way for the distribution of dynamic complex systems in human sciences.

8. Structural differences between the object and the tool

8.1 The decision-maker's locus of control in situation

Psychologists use the term "locus of control" to designate: "*the degree to which people believe that they, as opposed to external forces (beyond their influence), have control over the outcome of events in their lives*."[1] In this case, the control concerns the choice of the action which would bring the system to the required objective.

8.2 Means underlying the locus of control

What means are available to decision-makers to consider that they can control the development of the situation? In actual fact, these decision-makers implicitly or clearly perceive that their resources are limited. They are not in a position to use a previous professional experience or an apprenticeship since, in most cases, the situations to be processed are both complex and infrequent; in human sciences, they have in fact given rise to very few conceptualised approaches. In terms of decision-making, the only "scientific" data regarding the action choices are determined based on case studies and generally to analyse errors or malfunctions. In such a context, few cognitive resources are assigned to the locus of control, based at best on "degrees of belief", i.e. at best on subjective probabilities. The resulting uncertainty experienced has a negative effect on the action choices, especially if the stakes are high.

8.3 A transition

To reduce this uncertainty in order to choose the best actions, the decision-makers will opt for a strategy different from that of collecting ever more information. Although the PEO guarantees objectivity, this is at the cost of reducing the field of study. In addition, being a typical laboratory paradigm, it does not apply to the situations we have qualified as natural. Being unable to determine the action required with a sufficient guarantee of validity, the decision-makers will switch to type 2 information. They will build their decision using the properties of type 2 information, in other words giving priority to structuring a set rather than accumulating information (type 1). This emphasis placed on the tool before processing the informational context reminds us of the "toolbox" of Gigerenzer's concepts ("The mind as an adaptive toolbox") [11].

[1] Wikipedia

8.4 Existence and consequences of a paradox

Not all the difficulties have been resolved, however. In view of the difficulties arising in the field situations, the verdict of reality suggests the potential existence of future obstacles. We will make the assumption, currently only supported by observations, that application of this toolbox depends on a cognitive map and that the map is a simplified representation of the reality of field data, which remain complex.

It is therefore not unreasonable to mention the underlying existence of a paradox for the decision-makers. Since [12] they are all scientists, engineers and high-level technicians experienced in traditional scientific procedures, they will seek to be objective in the decisional choices by applying, naturally one might say, the PEO via the cognitive map to data which are above all complex and dynamic. This paradigmatic tool, imported from the experimental paradigm, too fixist and too simplified and which, finally, provides quality (objectivity) but which in these situations considerably limits the validity. The PEO proves to be poorly adapted to the characteristics of complex systems.

9. Conclusion

What can be concluded from the decisional inabilities identified in this document? We observe firstly the importance of the internal consistency of the paradigm, in particular that required between the characteristics of the information and the tools used to process it. We then note that all subjective references involving the personal knowledge and experience of the decision-makers have been carefully avoided. The Italian statistician de Finetti (1906–1985) proposes abandoning the objective definition of probability without this affecting the quality of the judgements. The method used is that of the odds applied to bets on racecourses. This type of quantification known as "subjective probability" is considered as expressing the "degrees of belief" which are clearly cognitive.

List of acronyms

DMCS	Decision making in complex systems
OEP	Objective experimental paradigm
COP	Conference of parties

Author details

Bernard Cadet[1,2]

1 Cognitive Psychology, University of Normandy Caen, France

2 GRIE, University of Estremadura, Badajoz, Spain

*Address all correspondence to: bernard.cadet50@gmail.com

References

[1] Khosravi, F., Jha-Takur, U. (2019). Managing uncertainties through scenario analysis in strategic environnemental assessment. Journal of Environnemental Planning and Management, 62, 6, 979-1000.

[2] Harrison, J.R., March, J.G. (1984). Decision making and postdecision surprises. Science Quarterly, 29, 1, 26-42.

[3] Ruelle, D., Takens, F. (1971). Sur la nature de la turbulence. Mathematical Physics 20 3, 167- 192.

[4] Fernandez Campos, P., Trucco, P., Huaccho Huatuco L. (2019). Managing structural and dynamic complexity in supply chains. Insights from four cases studies. Production, Planning and Control, 30, 8, 611-623.

[5] Byrne, D.; Callaghan, G. (2013). Complexity Theory and Social Sciences. The State of the Art. London: Routledge.

[6] Kühn, T.S. (1970). The structure of scientific revolutions. In: International Encyclopedia of Unified Science. Chicago; Chicago University Press. 2nd edition.

[7] Kahneman, D.; Slovic, P.; Tversky, A. (Eds). (1982). Judgment under Uncertainty: Heuristics and Biases. Cambridge: Cambridge University Press.

[8] Fuyuan, X., Xiao-Guang Y. (2021). Complex entropy and its application in decisión making for medical diagnosis. Journal of Healthcare Engineering, 21, 1-10.

[9] Williams, N. (2011). The Concept of Psychological Entropy. The Negative Psychologist. Internet. Retrieved on May 27, 2021.

[10] Lewin, K. (1936). Principles of Topological Psychology. New York: Mc Graw Hill.

[11] Gigenrenzer, G., Silben, R. (2001). Bounded Rationality. The Adaptative Toolbox. Cambridge: MIT Press.

[12] Ferdman, B.M. (2017). Paradoxes of inclusion. Understanding and managing the tensions of diversity and multiculturalism. Journal of Applied Behavioral Science, 53,2, 235-263.

Chapter 3

Single-Period Capacity and Demand Allocation Decision Making under Uncertainty

Sangdo Choi

Abstract

The newsvendor model deals with a single-period capacity allocation problem under uncertainty. The real world examples include perishable products (e.g., fish, vegetable), holiday-related products (e.g., Easter, Christmas, Halloween), seasonal products (e.g., fashion), and promotional products. This section addresses three newsvendor models: traditional newsvendor, inverse newsvendor, and sequential newsvendor models. The main decision under the traditional newsvendor setting is capacity allocation (i.e., how much to order), whereas the main decision under the inverse newsvendor setting is demand allocation (i.e., how many customers to be served) under the fixed capacity. This section demonstrates how to compare profit maximization approach to customer-oriented approach under the traditional newsvendor. The inverse newsvendor applies to revenue management for the hospitality industry. The sequential newsvendor model determines the optimal sequence when the number of customers to be served (determined by the inverse newsvendor model) is given. Normal distribution is considered for analytical solution and numerical studies. In addition, a discrete distribution is considered for numerical studies.

Keywords: Capacity Allocation, Demand Allocation, Newsvendor, Inverse Newsvendor, Sequential Newsvendor

1. Introduction

How can an operations manager make a one-time decision that covers a fixed future period if the manager cannot adjust the decision afterwards? A typical approach to this question is the single-period newsvendor model [1–4]. Suppose the operations manager herein is a newsvendor who would like to maximize profit or to satisfy a probability of not running out of newspaper. The newsvendor must place and receive an order before the start of each day to put on the newspaper stand. All left-over newspapers will be salvaged through paper-collection companies after the day, because nobody is interested in out-dated newspapers. The newsvendor is supposed to know all demand history and is able to forecast demand distribution properly, but not exact demand quantity on certain date. The newsvendor will not be able to match supply with demand exactly, unless the newsvendor is lucky [1], because only one demand scenario is realized during the selling period, i.e., $P(\textit{demand quantity} = \textit{order quantity}) = 0$ for a continuous demand distribution. Similar examples include grocery products (e.g., fish, vegetable), holiday-related products (e.g., Christmas, Easter, Halloween), seasonal products (e.g., fashion), and promotional products (e.g., T-shirts for a championship basketball or football game) [3]. These products also have a single selling period and will be deeply discounted after the selling season. If the newsvendor orders too much, left-over (overage) inventory is salvaged or steeply discounted. Otherwise, the newsvendor will forgo net profit because of lack of inventory (underage). Erlebacher et al. [5, 6] address the multi-item newsvendor model for inventory optimization problem with a capacity constraint. The newsvendor would like to keep balance between overage and underage, depending on the importance of two opposing directions.

The main decision variable for the traditional newsvendor is how many orders to be placed, which is a capacity allocation problem. Inversely, the newsvendor can also make decision on demand size to take full advantage of capacity [7–11]. If the newsvendor allocates too many demand, the resource is over-utilized (overusage). Otherwise, the resource is under-utilized (underusage). The inverse newsvendor would like to keep balance between overusage and underusage. A sequential newsvendor can make sequencing decision, when the demand size is determined by the inverse newsvendor [12]. Each customer is assigned to a slot in a sequence and the expected service start time should be scheduled. The sequential newsvendor would like to keep balance between earliness and lateness.

This chapter is organized as follows. Section 2 explains the traditional newsvendor model. Section 3 addresses the inverse newsvendor model. Section 4 addresses the sequential newsvendor model. Section 5 concludes this chapter.

2. The traditional newsvendor model

The traditional newsvendor is supposed to deal with inventory control. The newsvendor has to decide the order quantity to maximize the expected profit. If the newsvendor orders one less than the desired quantity, the newsvendor will forgo unit net profit owing to the lost sales. If the newsvendor order one more than the desired quantity, the newsvendor will loose unit net loss owing to the left-over inventory. Through the marginal analysis, the critical fractile determines the desired (or optimal) quantity and is regarded as the customer service level (CSL) [1–4].

On the contrary, the newsvendor may be interested in improving CSL than maximizing internal profit. For example, the newsvendor might want to make 90 percent sure of not running out of inventory, even though the critical fractile to maximize the expected profit is 0.7. The newsvendor would expand the market size in the long run while sacrificing the short-term maximum profit.

2.1 Mathematical model and solution approach

Let p be price; c order cost; s salvage, respectively. Demand D has mean of μ and standard deviation σ. Our decision variable is order quantity, q. The objective function is to maximize the expected profit. The profit function $\pi(q)$ is defined as follows:

$$\max_{q} \pi(q) = pE[\min(q, D)] - cq + sE\left[(D-q)^{+}\right], \tag{1}$$

where $\min(q, D)$ is the realized sales out of demand and $(D-q)^{+}$ is left-over inventory, respectively. The profit maximization problem $\pi(q)$ reduces to the equivalent problem $\tilde{\pi}(q)$ to minimize the expected sum of underage and overage as follows:

$$\min_{q} \tilde{\pi}(q) = c^o E\left[(q - D)^+\right] + c^u E\left[(D - q)^+\right], \tag{2}$$

where $c^u = p - c$, net profit and $c^o = c - s$, net loss, respectively. The optimal solution to either $\pi(q)$ or $\tilde{\pi}(q), q^*$ can be obtained by first and second necessary conditions or through marginal analysis as follows [1, 2, 4]:

$$F(q^*) = \frac{c^u}{c^u + c^o}, \tag{3}$$

where $F(\cdot)$ is the cumulative distribution function of demand D. In addition, $F(q^*)$ is the probability that you are able to cover all demand up to q^*, CSL for order quantity, q^*.

2.2 Numerical example of discrete demand

The newsvendor is supposed to sell Christmas trees between Halloween and Christmas Eve, this year. Suppose that the newsvendor has such a long sales history to build a reasonable demand forecast. **Table 1** shows the demand forecast based upon the historical data.

The newsvendor has to place and receive an order before Halloween, which is supposed to be the first day of selling season. The newsvendor sets the selling price to $25 per unit and promises to pay $10 per unit to a farmer. A local mulch firm will collect left-over trees for $3 per unit to cut them into small pieces for mulch after Christmas. Note that the underage penalty $c^u = 25 - 10 = 15$ per unit and the overage penalty $c^o = 10 - 3 = 7$ per unit. The newsvendor tends to order more than the average 260, which is close to median, because $c^u > c^o$, i.e., the newsvendor wants to avoid underage rather than overage. The critical fractile is $\frac{15}{15+7} = 0.68$. The optimal order quantity should be 300 because of $F(250) < 0.68 < F(300)$. However, if the newsvendor sets CSL to 90 percent, the order quantity should be 350 because of $F(350) > 0.9$, of which profit is lower than the profit of the optimal order quantity 300.

Table 2 provides the expected profit of three order quantities: 250, 300, and 350. Order quantity of 300 is (at least) a local optimum. Note that the profit function $\pi(q)$ is convex function, i.e., increasing-then-deceasing [1, 2, 4]. If the newsvendor would compute the expected profit for all other order quantities, the newsvendor can recognize that order quantity of 300 is global optimal. If the newsvendor orders too much (e.g., 350), salvages are larger than the optimal

Demand quantity	Probability	Cumulative probability
100	0.03	0.03
150	0.07	0.10
200	0.10	0.20
250	0.25	0.45
300	0.30	0.75
350	0.20	0.95
400	0.05	1.00

Table 1.
Demand forecast with probability and cumulative probability for Christmas tree.

Demand	Probability	Revenue	Cost	Salvage	Profit
Order = 250					Exp. Profit = 3,387
100	0.10	100 × 25	250 × 10	150 × 3	450
150	0.10	150 × 25	250 × 10	100 × 3	1,550
200	0.15	200 × 25	250 × 10	50 × 3	2,650
250	0.15	250 × 25	250 × 10	0 × 3	3,750
300	0.25	250 × 25	250 × 10	0 × 3	3,750
350	0.15	250 × 25	250 × 10	0 × 3	3,750
400	0.10	250 × 25	250 × 10	0 × 3	3,750
Order = 300					Exp. Profit = 3,642
100	0.10	100 × 25	300 × 10	200 × 3	100
150	0.10	150 × 25	300 × 10	150 × 3	1,200
200	0.15	200 × 25	300 × 10	100 × 3	2,300
250	0.15	250 × 25	300 × 10	50 × 3	3,400
300	0.25	300 × 25	300 × 10	0 × 3	4,500
350	0.15	300 × 25	300 × 10	0 × 3	4,500
400	0.10	300 × 25	300 × 10	0 × 3	4,500
Order = 350					Exp. Profit = 3,567
100	0.10	100 × 25	350 × 10	250 × 3	−250
150	0.10	150 × 25	350 × 10	200 × 3	850
200	0.15	200 × 25	350 × 10	150 × 3	1,950
250	0.15	250 × 25	350 × 10	100 × 3	3,050
300	0.25	300 × 25	350 × 10	50 × 3	4,150
350	0.15	350 × 25	350 × 10	0 × 3	5,250
400	0.10	350 × 25	350 × 10	0 × 3	5,250

Table 2.
Expected profit for three order quantities: 250, 300, and 350.

quantity and revenues are also larger than the optimal quantity. However, larger ordering cost affects more on the expected profit. The expected profit of 350 is lower than the maximum. If the newsvendor orders too little (e.g., 250), the newsvendor can save salvages compared to the optimal quantity and revenue is not large.

2.3 Numerical example of normally distributed demand

Now take into account a continuous demand distribution. Suppose that the demand distribution is normally distributed with mean of 275 and standard deviation of 50. It is hard to compute the revenue and salvage for each order, because there are infinite scenarios of order quantity. The newsvendor can compute the expected profit, starting from the expected lost sales, which is expressed as follows:

$$E\left[(D-q)^{+}\right] = \sigma L(z), \tag{4}$$

Step	Item	Profit-based	CSL-oriented
1	Critical Fractile (or CSL)	0.68	0.9
2	Order Quantity	298.6	339.1
3	Expected Lost Sales	7.4	5.0
4	Expected Sales	267.6	270.0
5	Expected Left-over	31.0	69.1
6	Expected Profit	3,797.5	3,566.0

Table 3.
Expected profit for two approaches: Profit maximization vs. CSL-oriented.

where $L(z) = \phi(z) - z(1 - \Phi(z))$ [2]. Note that $\phi(z)$ is normal probability distribution and $\Phi(z)$ is cumulative distribution, respectively.

1. Compute the critical fractile, or CSL.
2. Compute the associated quantity with CSL, $norm.inv(CSL, \mu, \sigma)$.
3. Compute the expected lost sales, $\sigma L(z)$.
4. Compute the expected sales: = expected demand - expected lost sales.
5. Compute the expected left-over: = order quantity - expected sales.
6. Compute the expected profit: = $c^u \times$ expected sales - $c^o \times$ expected left-over.

The newsvendor can take two perspectives: internal profit maximization vs. higher CSL. **Table 3** shows computational steps to get the expected profits of both profit-based and CSL-oriented approaches, respectively. For profit-based approach, the critical fractile is computed and its associated order quantity is determined accordingly. The expected profit is $3,797.5. For CSL-oriented approach, the newsvendor is supposed to determine the desired CSL first. Suppose that the newsvendor would like to guarantee 90% probability of not running out, i.e., 90% of demand will be covered by the order quantity. Because of higher CSL, the order quantity is far larger than the optimal order quantity; lower expected lost sales; larger left-over. Henceforth, the expected profit is lower. The newsvendor can choose either order quantity based on your strategic direction.

3. The inverse newsvendor model

The inverse newsvendor model applies to revenue management, which deals with fixed capacity and has to determine demand allocation [7, 8, 10, 11]. Airline industry uses quantity (i.e., number of seats) for capacity, whereas hospital may use time unit for capacity. Time-based inverse newsvendor model can be addressed for time-sensitive service industries such as hospital and law-firm.

The inverse newsvendor can take into account both identical and non-identical service durations. When the inverse newsvendor takes into account all identical service durations, the decision reduces to the number of allocation, i.e., how many customers will be assigned. When the inverse newsvendor takes into account heterogeneous service durations, the decision reduces to setting priority problem. Who should be allocated first and who can be next on? [9].

3.1 Mathematical model for identical service durations

Let h be the given and fixed capacity in hour. Each customer requires service duration, T which follows normal distribution with mean of μ and standard deviation σ. Assume that all customers are homogeneous, i.e., they have the same mean and standard deviation. The inverse newsvendor has to decide the number of customers to be served, x to minimize the sum of expected overusage and underusage. Consider the unit overusage penalty, c^g and unit underusage penalty, c^ℓ. The objective function $\rho(x)$ is defined as follows:

$$\min_x \rho(x) = c^g E\left[\left(\sum_{k=1}^{x} T_k - h\right)^+\right] + c^\ell E\left[\left(h - \sum_{k=1}^{x} T_k\right)^+\right]. \tag{5}$$

$\sum_{k=1}^{x} T_k$ also follows normal distribution with mean of $x\mu$ and variance of $x\sigma^2$. Let $z = \frac{h - x\mu}{\sqrt{x}\sigma}$. Overusage $E\left[\left(\sum_{k=1}^{x} T_k - h\right)^+\right]$ and underusage $E\left[\left(h - \sum_{k=1}^{x} T_k\right)^+\right]$ are defined as follows [12]:

$$E\left[\left(\sum_{k=1}^{x} T_k - h\right)^+\right] = (\phi(z) - z(1 - \Phi(z)))\,\sigma, \tag{6}$$

$$E\left[\left(h - \sum_{k=1}^{x} T_k\right)^+\right] = (\phi(z) + z\Phi(z))\,\sigma. \tag{7}$$

Figure 1 depicts a graphical representation of an inverse newsvendor problem with $\mu = 2, \sigma = 0.8$, and $h = 9$. The optimal solution to (5), x^* is defined as follows [9]:

$$x^* = \lfloor \hat{x} \rfloor \text{ or } \lceil \hat{x} \rceil, \tag{8}$$

$$\text{where } \hat{x} = \left(\frac{-z\sigma + \sqrt{z^2\sigma^2 + 4\mu h}}{2\mu}\right)^2. \tag{9}$$

$$F_N\left(h; x^*, x^{*2}\right) = \frac{c^g}{c^\ell + c^g} = \Phi(z), \tag{10}$$

For the case of **Figure 1**, the optimal allocation can be either 4 or 5 by visualization and analytical solution, (8) and (9).

3.2 Numerical example for identical service durations

Consider an operating room (OR) with 8 or 9 hour capacity. When each patient requires 2 hour service durations on average, how many patients would be assigned in the OR daily? Overusage penalties would cover overtime pay to the attending surgeon(s), nurses, anesthesiologist, and other staff. Underusage penalties would cover opportunity cost when the OR is under-utilized, but be hard to measure. The inverse newsvendor can determine the optimal demand size if the newsvendor knows parameters of service duration and two penalties. Numerical studies show

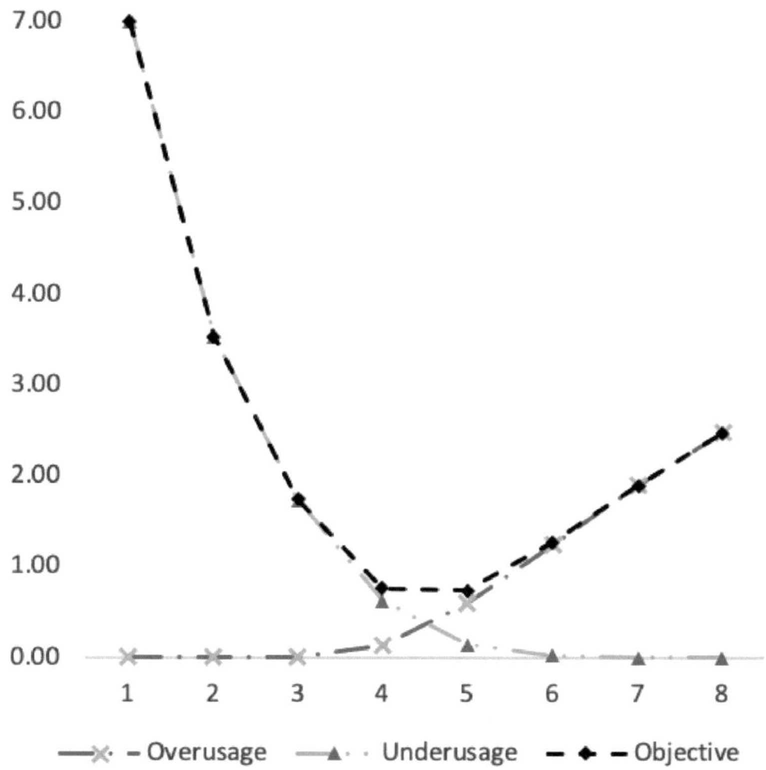

Figure 1.
Graphical representation of an inverse newsvendor model. The objective function for the case of $\mu = 2, \sigma = 0.8$, and $h = 9$. The overusage is an ever-increasing function of x, whereas the underusage is an ever-decreasing function of x. Hence, the objective function is a decrease-then-increase function.

Scenario	1	2	3	4	5	6	7	8
μ	2	2	2	2	3	3	3	3
σ	0.2	0.2	0.8	0.8	0.3	0.3	1.2	1.2
h	8	8	8	8	9	9	9	9
$c^g : c^\ell$	0.1:0.9	0.9:0.1	0.1:0.9	0.9:0.1	0.1:0.9	0.9:0.1	0.1:0.9	0.9:0.1
x	4.26	3.75	5.17	3.10	3.23	2.79	4.03	2.23
$\rho(\lfloor x \rfloor)$	0.16	0.20	0.32	0.25	0.21	0.30	0.42	0.33
$\rho(\lceil x \rceil)$	0.20	0.16	0.41	0.64	0.30	0.21	0.61	0.83
x^*	4	4	5	3	3	3	4	2

Table 4.
Patient allocation under different cost ratios, service durations and capacity.

impact of cost ratio and parameters on patient allocation. Consider the following data set in **Table 4**.

Table 4 summarizes numerical studies with varying mean, standard deviation, cost ratios, and capacity values. The inverse newsvendor can take into account two capacity levels: 8 or 9. Hospital may operate 8 hours each day or 9 hours if the inverse newsvendor expects high possibility of overtime. Each surgery duration requires 2 or 3 hours. Take into account two levels of standard deviation for each service duration. Two extremely different cost ratios are considered.

The ratio of capacity to the mean service duration, $\frac{h}{\mu}$ can be a base scenario. Actual allocation can be the base scenario, one more allocation, or one less allocation from the base scenario. For example, scenarios 1–4 have the ratio of 4 and scenarios 5–8 have the ratio of 3. When the inverse newsvendor has a non-integer value of ratio, the newsvendor can use either floor or ceiling value of the ratio. Actual allocations are 3, 4, or 5 for scenarios 1–4; 2, 3, or 4 for scenarios 5–8, respectively.

When $c^g > c^l$ (i.e., overusage is more penalized than underusage), the inverse newsvendor tends to allocate less patients (than the base) to avoid overusage penalty. On the contrary, when $c^l > c^g$ (i.e., underusage is more penalized than overusage), the inverse newsvendor tends to allocate more patients (than the base) to avoid underusage penalty. Allocating one more patient or one less patient would affect a lot on the objective function. As a matter of fact, allocating more (less) patients means ONE more (less) patient than the base scenario.

Variance may amplify impact of cost-ratio, which means there must exist interactive effect between variance and cost-ratio. When $c^g < c^l$ (e.g., scenarios 1, 3, 5 and 7), the larger variance, the more allocated patients. When $c^g > c^l$ (e.g., scenarios 2, 4, 6, and 8), the larger variance, the less allocated patients. For lower variance examples (scenarios 1, 2, 5, and 6), cost-ratio would not affect on allocation much.

3.3 Mathematical model for non-identical service durations

Suppose that there are N customers, of which index is $i = 1, 2, \cdots, N \in \mathcal{I}$, respectively and that individual service time T_i of customer i has mean of μ_i and standard deviation σ_i. New decision variable x_i is a binary variable, 1 if customer i is served, 0 otherwise. The number of customers to be served is $\sum_i x_i$. The total service time is defined as $\sum_i x_i T_i$. The inverse newsvendor problem with non-identical service durations can be represented as follows:

$$\min_{x_i, i \in \mathcal{I}} c^g E\left[\left(\sum_{i=1}^{N} x_i T_i - h\right)^+\right] + c^\ell E\left[\left(h - \sum_{i=1}^{N} x_i T_i\right)^+\right]. \tag{11}$$

The inverse newsvendor should evaluate $2^N - 1$ possible combinations to find the optimal number of customers to be served. To find the optimal solution based on numerical evaluation of (11), the inverse newsvendor can reformulate it using Stochastic Programming with discrete scenarios $\omega \in \Omega$. The inverse newsvendor can adopt the sample average approximation (SAA) approach to get a close approximation [13]. Let T_i^ω be the service time for customer i under scenario ω; u^ω underusage under scenario ω; o^ω overusage under scenario ω; p^ω probability of scenario ω, respectively. SAA formulation is given as follows:

$$\min \quad c^l u^\omega p^\omega + c^g o^\omega p^\omega \tag{12}$$

$$s.t. \sum_{i=1}^{N} x_i T_i^\omega + u^\omega \geq h, \omega \in \Omega \tag{13}$$

$$\sum_{i=1}^{N} \mathrm{x}_i T_i^\omega - o^\omega \leq h, \omega \in \Omega \tag{14}$$

The inverse newsvendor can get the optimal solution of the SAA approach [9]. However, it is hard to derive a certain (intuitive) rule for the optimal allocation of customers. A heuristic to get a near-optimal solution in a reasonable time limit is prescribed: smallest-variance (SV) first, which is close to the optimal solution [9]. The heuristic is based on the discussion that partial expected values are associated with variability rather than central location measure such as mean or median.

Take advantage of the results from the case of identical service durations from Subsection 3.1. Suppose that n customers are about to be served. Let $\overline{\mu}$ be the sample average service time for n customers; $\overline{\sigma}$ the standard deviation of the sample average service times for n customers, respectively. If n is equal to the solution of (8) and (9) with $\overline{\mu}$ and $\overline{\sigma}$, the inverse newsvendor can stop adding customers to be served. The detail procedure of the heuristic with the SV selection rule is described as follows [9]:

- **Initialization.** Let $\mathcal{A} = \mathcal{A}^* = \{\}, \mathcal{N} = \{1, 2, \cdots, N\}$, and $Z_{opt} = \infty$.
- **Step 1.** Select i with the smallest variance. Remove i from $\mathcal{N}$ and add i to $\mathcal{A}$.
- **Step 2.** Compute the sample mean $\overline{\mu}$ and sample standard deviation $\overline{\sigma}$ of the set $\mathcal{A}$.
- **Step 3.** Plug $\overline{\mu}$ and $\overline{\sigma}$ into (8) and (9) to compute the optimal number of customers to be served, say x^*.
- **Step 4.** Compute the objective function value, say Z_{curr}. If $Z_{curr} < Z_{opt}$, let $\mathcal{A}^* \leftarrow \mathcal{A}$ and $Z_{opt} \leftarrow Z_{curr}$.
- **Step 5.** If $x^* \leq |\mathcal{A}^*|$ and $\mathcal{N} \neq \{\}$, go to Step 1. Otherwise, go to Step 6.
- **Step 6.** Let $\mathcal{A}^*$ be the set of optimally assigned customers and Z_{opt} be the heuristic results.

The inverse newsvendor can show how the SV heuristic works with the following example. The inverse newsvendor can use cost ratio of 0.5:0.5; 120 min blocks without loss of generality. **Table 5** shows all parameter values of ten customers: μ and σ. The SV heuristic will select customers as the following order: $10 \rightarrow 7 \rightarrow 9 \rightarrow 6 \rightarrow 8 \rightarrow \cdots \rightarrow 2$.

The followings are detail steps resulted from the SV selection rule.

- Initial Step. $\mathcal{A} = \mathcal{A}^* = \{\}; \mathcal{N} = \{1, 2, 3, \cdots, 10\}; Z_{opt} = \infty$
- Iteration 1. $\mathcal{A} = \{10\}; \overline{\mu} = 10.3; \overline{\sigma} = 1.80; x^* = 12 > |\mathcal{A}^*| = 1; Z_{curr} = 54.87; Z_{opt} = 54.87; \mathcal{A}^* = \{10\}$
- Iteration 2. $\mathcal{A} = \{10, 7\}; \overline{\mu} = 18.79; \overline{\sigma} = 3.07; x^* = 6 > |\mathcal{A}^*| = 2; Z_{curr} = 41.21; Z_{opt} = 41.21; \mathcal{A}^* = \{10, 7\}$
- Iteration 3. $\mathcal{A} = \{10, 7, 9\}; \overline{\mu} = 16.38; \overline{\sigma} = 4.09; x^* = 7 > |\mathcal{A}^*| = 3; Z_{curr} = 35.43; Z_{opt} = 35.53; \mathcal{A}^* = \{10, 7, 9\}$

Customer	1	2	3	4	5	6	7	8	9	10
μ_i	18.5	27.9	24.9	28.5	26.8	27.5	27.3	19.8	11.6	10.3
σ_i	6.5	21.7	17.3	7.5	18.8	5.7	3.9	6.4	5.6	1.8

Table 5.
Customer service duration information.

- Iteration 4. $\mathcal{A} = \{10, 7, 9, 6\}; \overline{\mu} = 19.16; \overline{\sigma} = 4.55; x^* = 6 > |\mathcal{A}^*| = 4; Z_{curr} = 21.67; Z_{opt} = 21.67; \mathcal{A}^* = \{10, 7, 9, 6\}$

- Iteration 5. $\mathcal{A} = \{10, 7, 9, 6, 8\}; \overline{\mu} = 19.3; \overline{\sigma} = 4.97; x^* = 6 > |\mathcal{A}^*| = 5; Z_{curr} = 11.82; Z_{opt} = 11.82; \mathcal{A}^* = \{10, 7, 9, 6, 8\}$

- Iteration 6. $\mathcal{A} = \{10, 7, 9, 6, 8, 1\}; \overline{\mu} = 19.16; \overline{\sigma} = 5.27; x^* = 6 = |\mathcal{A}^*|; Z_{curr} = 5.53; Z_{opt} = 5.53; \mathcal{A}^* = \{10, 7, 9, 6, 8, 1\}$

- Iteration 7. $\mathcal{A} = \{10, 7, 9, 6, 8, 1, 4\}; \overline{\mu} = 20.51; \overline{\sigma} = 5.64; x^* = 6 < |\mathcal{A}^*| = 7; Z_{curr} = 12.15; Z_{opt} = 5.53; \mathcal{A}^* = \{10, 7, 9, 6, 8, 1\}$. Stop.

4. The sequential newsvendor model

A sequential newsvendor has to determine the sequence of assigned customers and their arrival times, when the newsvendor already knows the total number of customers to be served in a fixed duration [12]. Once the sequential newsvendor determines the sequence, the arrival time of each customer can be the cumulative expected service time of all prior customers without loss of generality. Basically, this is a block scheduling problem that determines the starting times of blocks.

The sequential newsvendor model applies to time-sensitive service industries as the inverse newsvendor. The inverse newsvendor may decide the strategic level decision, whereas the sequential newsvendor decides the tactical level decision and relies on the inverse newsvendor decision. The newsvendor may use identical service durations for the strategic decision (e.g., capacity size, demand size) and non-identical durations for the tactical decision (e.g., setting priority).

4.1 Mathematical model and solution approach

Suppose that the sequential newsvendor has to serve $|I|$ customers (or customer groups) and that each customer $i \in I$ requires different service duration T_i, of which mean is μ_i and its standard deviation is σ_i. The sequential newsvendor has to determine its sequence and starting time of each patient i.

Use map $\Delta : I \to K$ to represent a set of sequences (or permutations), each of which $\delta \in \Delta$ assigns each customer to one and only one sequence position, hence $|K| = |I|$. Use subscripts $[k]$ for k^{th} block sequence position and i for customer to avoid potential confusion.

Decision variables must prescribe planned block durations and block sequence, δ. The sequential newsvendor determines the planned end time of block in the kth position, given a sequence δ, prescribed by $y^{\delta}_{[k]}$. The planned end time of the block corresponds to the end of service durations and is important in deciding the number of hours that the server will be required to work. Define $B^{\delta}_{[k]} := T^{\delta}_{[1]} + \cdots + T^{\delta}_{[k]}$ as the random end time to complete all services assigned to blocks [1] through $[k]$ and compare it with the decision variable $y^{\delta}_{[k]}$.

Assume that one service begins as soon as the previous one ends [14–16]. This assumption appears to be reasonable because each customer can be prepared well in advance of his/her scheduled start time and successive services within each block is likely to be performed by the same server so that s/he would be available as well. However, expediting efforts is required if a planned service ends earlier than the planned end time. The sequential newsvendor can penalize the earliness.

The objective function penalizes the expected earliness $E\left[\left(y_{[k]}^{\delta}-T_{[k]}^{\delta}\right)^{+}\right]$ and expected lateness $E\left[\left(T_{[k]}^{\delta}-y_{[k]}^{\delta}\right)^{+}\right]$ of each block $k\in K$. The sequential newsvendor imposes earliness penalty c^{e} and lateness penalty c^{l}, respectively. The former represents the cost of expediting the start time of the next surgery; and the letter, the cost of delaying the start time of the next surgery. The sequential newsvendor can build a schedule that balances the expected costs of earliness and lateness associated with each block, defining objective function $f_{[k]}\left(y_{[k]}^{\delta}\right), k\in K, \delta\in\Delta$

$$f_{[k]}\left(y_{[k]}^{\delta}\right)=c^{e}E\left[\left(y_{[k]}^{\delta}-T_{[k]}^{\delta}\right)^{+}\right]+c^{l}E\left[\left(T_{[k]}^{\delta}-y_{[k]}^{\delta}\right)^{+}\right]. \tag{15}$$

The sequential newsvendor has to determine the optimal planned end time $\hat{y}_{[k]}^{\delta}$ of the kth block, $k\in K$ and the optimal block sequence $\hat{\delta}$. **Figure 2** depicts a graphical representation of the sequential newsvendor model. For each sequence $\delta\in\Delta$, the objective function $\sum_{k\in K}f_{[k]}\left(y_{[k]}^{\delta}\right)$ should be minimized. The sequential newsvendor has to find the best solution out of all minimized solutions. The sequential newsvendor problem can be defined as follows:

$$\min_{\delta\in\Delta}\ \min_{y_{[k]}^{\delta}:k\in K}\sum_{k\in K}f_{[k]}\left(y_{[k]}^{\delta}\right) \tag{16}$$

$$s.t.\quad y_{[k-1]}^{\delta}\le y_{[k]}^{\delta}\ k=2,\cdots,|K|,\delta\in\Delta \tag{17}$$

$$y_{[k]}\ \ge 0\qquad k\in K,\delta\in\Delta \tag{18}$$

Fix a sequence δ to find the optimal planned end time. Suppress this superscript for the sake of simplicity. (16) is separable with respect to $y_{[k]}$ [12]:

$$\min\left\{f_{[1]}\left(y_{[1]}\right)+f_{[2]}\left(y_{[2]}\right)+\cdots+f_{[|K|]}\left(y_{[|K|]}\right)\right\} \tag{19}$$

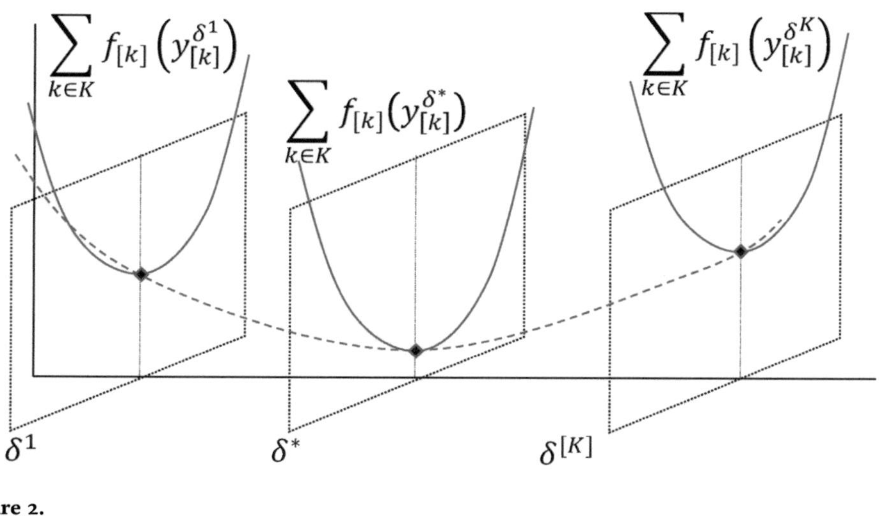

Figure 2.
Graphical representation of a sequential newsvendor model. For each sequence $\delta\in\Delta$, the objective function should be minimized.

$$\equiv \min f_{[1]}\left(y_{[1]}\right) + \min f_{[2]}\left(y_{[2]}\right) + \cdots + \min f_{[|K|]}\left(y_{[|K|]}\right). \tag{20}$$

Let $\overline{\mu}_{[k]} = \mu_{[1]} + \mu_{[2]} + \cdots + \mu_{[k]}$ be the mean of the random end time $B_{[k]}$ and $\overline{\sigma}_{[k]} = \sqrt{\sigma_{[1]}^2 + \sigma_{[2]}^2 + \cdots + \sigma_{[k]}^2}$ be the standard deviation of $B_{[k]}$, respectively. Random end time $B_{[k]}, k \in K$ is also normally distributed as follows:

$$B_{[k]} = T_{[1]} + T_{[2]} + \cdots + T_{[k]} \sim N\left(\overline{\mu}_{[k]}, \overline{\sigma}_{[k]}^2\right) \tag{21}$$

Henceforth, the optimal planned end time $\hat{y}_{[k]}$ of kth block can be obtained as follows [17]:

$$\hat{y}_{[k]} = \overline{\mu}_{[k]} + z\overline{\sigma}_{[k]} \tag{22}$$

$$\Phi(z) = \frac{c^l}{c^e + c^l}. \tag{23}$$

The optimal objective function value for k^{th} block is given as follows [12]:

$$f_{[k]}\left(\hat{y}_{[k]}\right) = \left(c^e + c^l\right)\frac{\overline{\sigma}_{[k]}}{\sqrt{2\pi}}e^{-z^2}. \tag{24}$$

(24) is an increasing function of $\overline{\sigma}_{[k]}$. Hence, smallest-variance first rule is the optimal sequencing rule.

5. Conclusions

Three newsvendor models are addressed to match supply with demand, or vice versa. The traditional newsvendor model can answer how much to order, given that the newsvendor knows demand distribution. The inverse newsvendor model applies to the strategic level decision, e.g., how many customers should be allocated in a fixed capacity. Time-based newsvendor model has been used for service-oriented settings (e.g., operating rooms, law firm). The sequential newsvendor model determines the sequence of the assigned customers by the strategic inverse newsvendor model, and prescribes the corresponding expected arrival times of the customers. The optimal sequence should be a variability-based rule, because the objective function elements involve partial expected values: overage vs. underage, overusage vs. underusage, or earliness vs. lateness. The smallest-variance-first assignment rule is optimal to minimize the expected earliness and lateness when the newsvendor takes into account normally distributed service durations.

All newsvendor models keep balance between surplus (i.e., supply > demand) and deficit (supply < demand), accepting the fact that the newsvendor cannot match supply with demand all the time. Supply chain professionals may face with either case of surplus or deficit, not matched. When a product is highly profitable (or net profit is greater than net loss), the newsvendor tends to order more than the average to avoid the lost sales in the long run. On the contrary, when net loss is greater than net profit, the newsvendor tends to order less than the average in the long run. However, if the newsvendor is myopic, the newsvendor tends to order average demand without respect to cost structure or demand shape, so-called pull-to-center [18]. To avoid pull-to-center bias, supply chain professionals must understand how to get optimal decision considering cost structure and demand parameters for long-term perspective.

Abbreviations

CSL	Customer Service Level
OR	Operating Room
SAA	Sample Average Approximation
SV	Smallest Variance

Author details

Sangdo Choi
Bloomsburg University of Pennsylvania, Bloomsburg, PA, USA

*Address all correspondence to: sangdo.choi@snu.ac.kr

References

[1] Cachon GP, Terwiesch C (2004) *Matching supply with demand: An introduction to operations management* (New York: McGraw-Hill Custom Publishing).

[2] Chopra S, Meindl P (2014) *Supply Chain Management, Strategy, Planning, and Operation* (New York: Pearson).

[3] Jacobs FR, Chase RB (2014) *Operations and Supply Chain Management* (New York: McGraw-Hill Irwin).

[4] Silver EA, Peterson R (1985) *Decision Systems for Inventory Management and Production Planning* (New York: John Wiley & Sons).

[5] Erlebacher SJ (2000) Optimal and heuristic solutions for the multi-item newsvendor problem with a single capacity constraint. Production and Operations Management 9:303 – 318.

[6] Punia S, Singh SP, Madaan JK (2020) From predictive to prescriptive analytics: A data-driven multi-item newsvendor model. *Decision Support Systems* 136:113340.

[7] Bakal IS, Geunes J, Romeijn EE (2008) Market selection decisions for inventory models with price-sensitive demand. *Journal of Global Optimization* 41:633 – 657.

[8] Carr S, Lovejoy W (2000) The inverse newsvendor problem: Choosing an optimal demand portfolio for capacitated resources. *Management Science* 46:912–927.

[9] Choi S, Ketzenberg M (2018) An inverse newsvendor model to set the optimal number of customers in a capacitated environment. *International Journal of Production Economics* 1:1–12.

[10] Merzifonluoglu Y, Geunes J, Romejin H (2012) The static stochastic knapsack problem with normally distributed item sizes. *Mathematical Programming* 134:459 – 489.

[11] Taaffe K, Geunes J, Romeijn HE (2008) Target market selection and marketing effort under uncertainty: The selective newsvendor. *European Journal of Operational Research* 189:987 – 1003.

[12] Choi S, Wilhelm WE (2014) An approach to optimize master surgical block schedules. *European Journal of Operational Research* 235:138–148.

[13] Birge JR, Louveaux F (1997) Introduction to Stochastic Programming. Springer, New York

[14] Blake J, Donald J (2002) Mount sinai hospital uses integer programming to allocate operating room time. Interface 32:63 – 73.

[15] Denton BT, Miller AJ, Balasubramanian HJ, Huschka TR (2010) Optimal allocation of surgery blocks to operating rooms under uncertainty. Operations Research 58:1 – 15.

[16] Fei H, Chu C, Meskens N (2009) Solving a tactical operating room planning problem by a column-generation-based heuristic procedure with four criteria. Annals of Operations Research 166:91 – 108.

[17] Porteus E (2002) Foundations of Stochastic Inventory Theory. Stanford University Press, Stanford

[18] Schweitzer M, Cachon G (2000) Decision bias in the newsvendor problem with a known demand distribution: Experimental evidence. *Management Science* 46:404–420.

Chapter 4

Decision Making in the Context of Natural Disasters Based on a Geographic Information System and the Internet of Things (IoT)

Aissa Bensattalah, Rachid Chalal,
Tahar Hassaine Daouadji and Tayeb Bensattalah

Abstract

Decisions within the company, managers in countries or regions are made by one or more groups of decision-makers. The management of natural disasters involves several specialized decision-makers (experts, firefighters, police officers, drivers,). The aim of the chapter is to improve decision making in the context of natural disasters situation. Zero risk in the world does not exist due to natural phenomena that occur randomly and appear suddenly. It is essential to manage the risks in the situation of natural disasters and also to confront the influence of natural disasters on the phenomenon of Soil-Structure Interaction. For this, this chapter presents a conceptual architecture of a knowledge base to manage the risks of natural disasters remotely by a Geographic Information system (GIS) and embedded systems. This architecture is based on the integration of data via different sources of information (GIS, satellites, electronic sensors and comments from experts). To properly manage this information, this chapter uses the ontology of Soil-Structure Interaction With Agents External (OSSIWAE) in the context of the Internet of Things (IoT). A case study is conducted on a prototype of a model for building a structure three-story for testing the usability of the proposed architecture.

Keywords: Risks of natural disasters, Soil-Structure Interaction; Geographic Information system, Ontologies, Internet of Things (IoT)

1. Introduction

Natural disasters (Flood, Storm, Earthquake, Extreme temperature, Landslide, wind...) are phenomena that occur every time and humans must find appropriate solutions to minimize the damage. With the increase in the use of embedded system and the web technologies in all fields. These technologies have enabled us to help find solutions that were not possible previously or it is difficult to access a certain types of disasters by decision makers. The aim of the chapter is to improve decision making in the context of natural disasters. Zero risk in the world does not exist due to natural phenomena that occur randomly and appear suddenly. It is essential to manage the risks of natural disasters and to inform the people concerned, the leaders, the citizens, firefighters, police officers, drivers... etc. However, the phenomenon of Soil-Structure Interaction poses real and important problems for the design of new structures that resist to natural disasters because of the heterogeneous mechanical behavior of the soil, which changes through the influence of external agents such as: temperature, water, rain snow (freeze–thaw phenomenon) earthquake (dynamic effect). For this purpose, this chapter presents a conceptual architecture of a knowledge base to manage the risks of natural disasters. The architecture of the system is based on the use of ontology, a Geographic Information system (GIS), a sensors electronic system and the documents of experts in the context of Internet of Things (IoT) in order to build a knowledge base on the influence of external agents on the phenomenon of Soil-Structure Interaction. In this chapter an ontology of Soil-Structure Interaction With Agents External (OSSIWAE) was proposed to capitalize the information on agents external in a real time in order to fully understand, analyze and estimate this phenomenon. The proposed ontology was validated by experts in civil engineering, who helped us to build this ontology. In order to validate the proposed architecture, a web application is developed that supports this architecture. The rest of this chapter is organized as follows. First the related works on the Geographic Information System and the ontologies for the management of natural disasters are detailed in Section 2. In Section 3, the ontology for representing the phenomenon of Soil-Structure Interaction with the connection of natural disasters (OSSIWAE) is presented. In Section 4, the architecture of a knowledge base of natural disasters is presented. Finally, the chapter ends with the implementation of a web platform applied on the prototype of a model for building a structure three-story in the context of Internet of Things (IoT) for testing the usability of the proposed architecture.

2. Related work

This section describes the proposed related work that used the Geographic Information System and the ontologies for the management of natural disasters.

2.1 Geographic information system for the management of natural disasters

[1, 2] Geographic Information Science is developed to manage and analyze spatial data, which is based on geomatics technologies, Geographic Information Science as a technology/system allows the storage of spatial information in the relational database. According to [3] Geographic information system (GIS) has emerged as a dominant tool for accumulating, analyzing and displaying spatial data and using this data for decision making in several areas. In addition to [3] Geographic Information System (GIS) is one the technologies that evolves to allow people to solve many geographic problem quickly, effectively and easily with the abilities to make analysis, especially location analysis in combination with traditional database systems.

There are several computer systems that manipulate geographic databases such as ArcGis, QGIS, MapInfo, SuperGis, Surfer...etc. and at the same time there are GIS web applications to make GIS accessible through web technologies.

Several works have shown the interest of GIS for the study of floods and risks. In [4], authors proposed a methodology by using the SAR data along with GIS for flood water mapping, monitoring and analyzing the propagation of flood water in a flood prone area. In [5], authors proposed an approach based on GIS for flood management strategy in a river basin; this approach consists of two main interlinked components the first is a proper flood management strategy, and the second is the determination of the flood-hazard areas. This work [6] demonstrated the importance of the use of earth observation (EO) products and geographic information systems (GIS) in disaster-risk management. [7] used the data collection methods and GIS applications to develop a detailed mapping of the main natural and human factors responsible for the flooding phenomenon. [8] used remote sensing and GIS to reduce flood damage in the study area by improving flood forecasting and flood defense. In [9], authors developed a flood sensitivity spatial decision support system (SDSS) that integrates the spatial analytical strengths of a GIS platform with the structured analytical hierarchy process (AHP).

This section demonstrates the importance of using a GIS for flood risk management, however, but few works that integrate embedded sensors and the semantic web with a GIS to effectively manage natural disasters.

2.2 The ontologies for the management of natural disasters

An ontology can be defined as an explicit specification of a conceptualization [10]. In recent years ontologies have been used in various fields of application to create knowledge bases (search engines, e-commerce, electronic library, etc.). Applications not only need to exchange data and information with each other but also need to agree on the semantics of that data and information. Knowledge can describe and explain its meaning using the following elements (class, instance, attribute, relation, etc.). The organization of these elements of description of knowledge can be done in the form of ontology. So an ontology is the set of individual instances of classes, specifying the specific values of the attributes as well as the restrictions on the attributes to constitute a knowledge base. According to Noy [11] there is not just one correct way to model a knowledge domain there are always varying alternatives, the best solution generally depends on the application carried out and the anticipated developments. In the context of the creation of ontologies in the field of soil science, in the field of structure and the field of disaster risk management, we mention: In [12], authors proposed an Ontology-Based Knowledge Network of soil/water physicochemical & biological properties (soil/water concepts) for the semantic representation of infiltration/percolation process of contamination water through soil structure and porous media. According to [13] Pile foundation is a basic form that can adapt to complex geological conditions and is widely used in high-rise buildings, bridges, ports, and other important structures, this work proposed an integrated evaluation system that can make reasonable evaluations of pile integrity where specific measured reflective wave curves. The evaluation system based on the ontology of pile integrity evaluation (OntoPIE), this ontology used for quantitative identification of pile defects and qualitative evaluation of pile integrity. THE OntoPIE represent the essential terms of the pile integrity evaluation system which includes the degree, length, depth, and integrity category of the pile defects. In [14], authors proposed an ontology of soil properties and processes for representing soil properties, processing and their interaction in order to make integrated decisions, and to combine the knowledge and expertise in multiple areas, such as roads, soil, buried assets, sensing, etc. [15, 16] proposed an ontology-based simulation environment in agriculture and natural resources for constructing models and representing equations and symbols in a formal ontology language, the utility of the approach by building moderately complex models of soil–water and nutrient management. This approach has the advantage of making models more explicit and better defining the meaning of symbols used in a model. [17] Proposed ontology of the flood domain and describes how they can be benefited to access, analyze, and visualize flood-related data with natural language queries. Flood ontology developed under three major ontological branches (i.e. Natural Hazard, Instrument, and Environmental Phenomena) Geological Hazards (e.g. earthquake), Meteorological Hazards (e.g. tornado), Diseases, Wildfires, and Floods. Flood ontology utilized in cyberinfrastructure systems for natural hazard preparedness, monitoring, response, and recovery. And to allow visual, intuitive, and collaborative development for domain experts who may have a limited technical background [18]. Aims to use the data from different sources to reason on them. Data comes from water sensors, satellite images, field studies, hydrological models, GIS, etc. to model risk management for flash floods. [19] proposed integrated watershed flood risk assessment ontology based on different perceptual models of watershed flood risk. This ontology represents the complex process involving physical systems and organizational systems in flood risk assessment [20]. Proposed the ontology named FloodOntology for floods forecasting based on continuous measurements of water parameters gathered in the watersheds and in the sewers and simulation models. FloodOntology is used for obtaining a structured and unified knowledge-base on the flooding risk forecasting. Three main domains are used hydrological, hydraulic and sensor networks. In [21], the authors identify the core literature available on flood ontologies and present a review on these ontologies from various perspectives [22]. Proposed the Ontology for River Flow and Flood Mitigation (ORFFM) for semantic knowledge formalization with semantic understandability of irrigation, disaster management, related administrative and agricultural domain concepts. This ontology allows the effective coordination, collaborative response activities leads to reduce the impact of a disaster and improve information representation among stakeholders.

The phenomenon of Soil-Structure Interaction poses real and important problems for the design of structures in order to resist to the natural disasters due to heterogeneous mechanical behavior of soil which changes through the influence of external agents such as: temperature, water, rain snow (freeze–thaw phenomenon) earthquake (dynamic effect). However the cited works are not considered this knowledge in ontology. For this purpose, we based on the existing ontologies and the Soil-Structure Interaction model proposed in literature in order to propose a new ontology to represent the phenomenon of Soil-Structure Interaction with the connection of external agents named OSSIWAE.

3. Ontology of soil-structure interaction with external agents proposed

In this chapter, the Protégé tool 5.2 is used to realize the ontology of OSSIWAE. There are several methods for developing ontology. To design this ontology, the iterative method for the development of the ontology, proposed by [11] is followed.

The development of the ontology is started by defining its domain and scope by answering the following questions:

What is the field that ontology will cover? The domain of the ontology is the concepts used in the domain of Soil-Structure Interaction and natural disasters, this ontology conceptualizes the concepts in different domain Soil, Natural Disasters, Structures and the relations between them. The relations which represent the interactions between Soil, natural disasters and structures are taken into consideration with sensors. The ontology therefore includes all the concepts of the external agents which influence on the structures such as the temperature, water, rain snow (phenomenon of freeze–thaw) the earthquake (the dynamic effect) ... etc. And describe the concepts which link heterogeneous soil and structure information.

What are the development goals of ontology? The ontology is designed with the aim of formalizing and clarifying the semantics of the collection of information by electronic sensors. This formalization allows us to implement the semantics of information in Web tool dedicated to the actors involved in the decision process. And also to ensure the sematic integration of data via different sources of information (GIS, satellites, electronic sensors and comments of experts).

Reuse of existing ontologies:

The objective of this step is to reuse existing ontologies even if they have a different objective from ours. We can reuse all or part of these ontologies after having adapted them to our needs. Some concepts proposed by [12–14, 17] are reused.

Identification and structuring of ontology concepts:

To identify the main concepts of ontology, the concepts proposed by [12–14, 17] are extracted and enriched them with the concepts analyzed in the Soil-Structure Interaction model proposed in literature and the concepts proposed by civil engineering experts. These concepts are organized and structured in an ontology called "OSSIWAE". Finally, the Protégé editor is used to define this ontology (**Figure 1**).

This ontology has been validated by experts in civil engineering who have helped us to build and enrich the concepts of ontology.

We explain below some of the concepts identified in this ontology.

The top-level classes of the OSSIWAE ontology are Soil, natural disasters, structures (superstructure and infrastructure) and we have hierarchized each class with its subclass.

The class Soil its subclass are physical characteristics, mechanical characteristics and chemical characteristics. For example the class of physical characteristics its subclass are sand, silt and clay.

The class structures its subclass are superstructure and infrastructure, the class superstructure its subclass are column, beam, slab and wall, the infrastructure is foundation.

The class natural disasters its subclass are temperature, Humidity, Rain, water, Wind, snow, freeze–thaw (freeze–thaw phenomenon) earthquake (dynamic effect), volcano. And each class has the values for example the concept of Humidity (has value), Temperature (has value), Wind (has frequency and has direction).

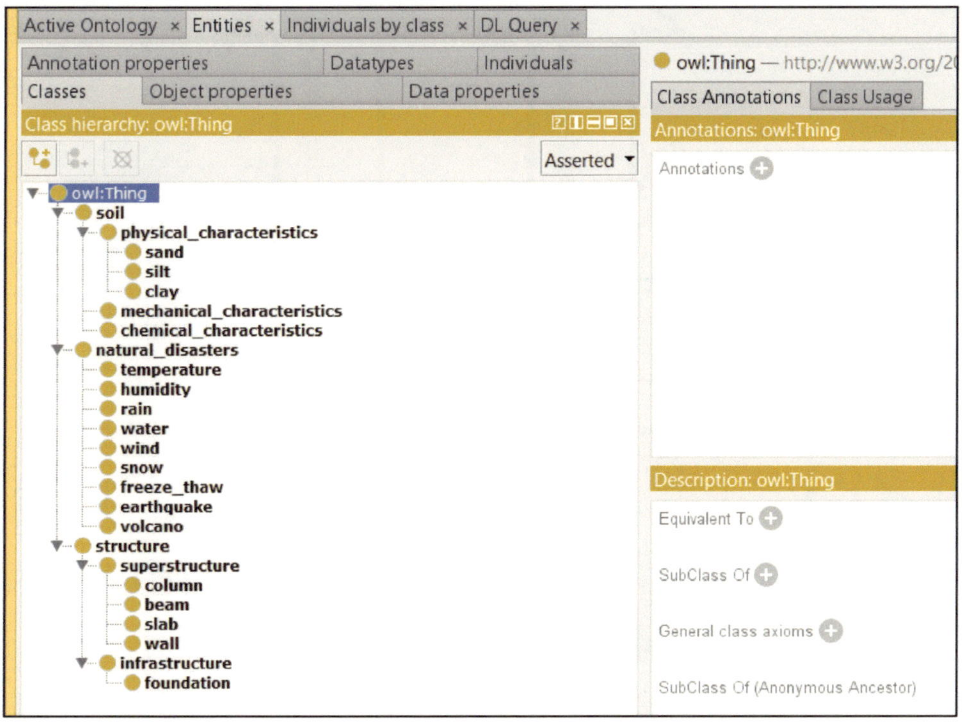

Figure 1.
The OSSIWAE ontology.

The impedance in Soil-Structure Interaction is the most important parameter, which represents the interaction between the structure and the soil, for this, this parameter is represented by relations in order to clarify the knowledge in ontology. Then these relationships used to capture useful information by sensors installed in different places in the soil and the structure. We have used the following four relationships for linking between the classes of ontology: soil liquefaction, Structural vibration, soil compaction and Structure dilatation.

4. Proposed architecture of a knowledge base of natural disasters

The proposed architecture is illustrated in **Figure 2**. The conceptual architecture is made up of four parts:

The first part is the Information gathering; this part uses GIS to map areas and so uses electronic sensors to collect information. It uses a set of sensors installed in

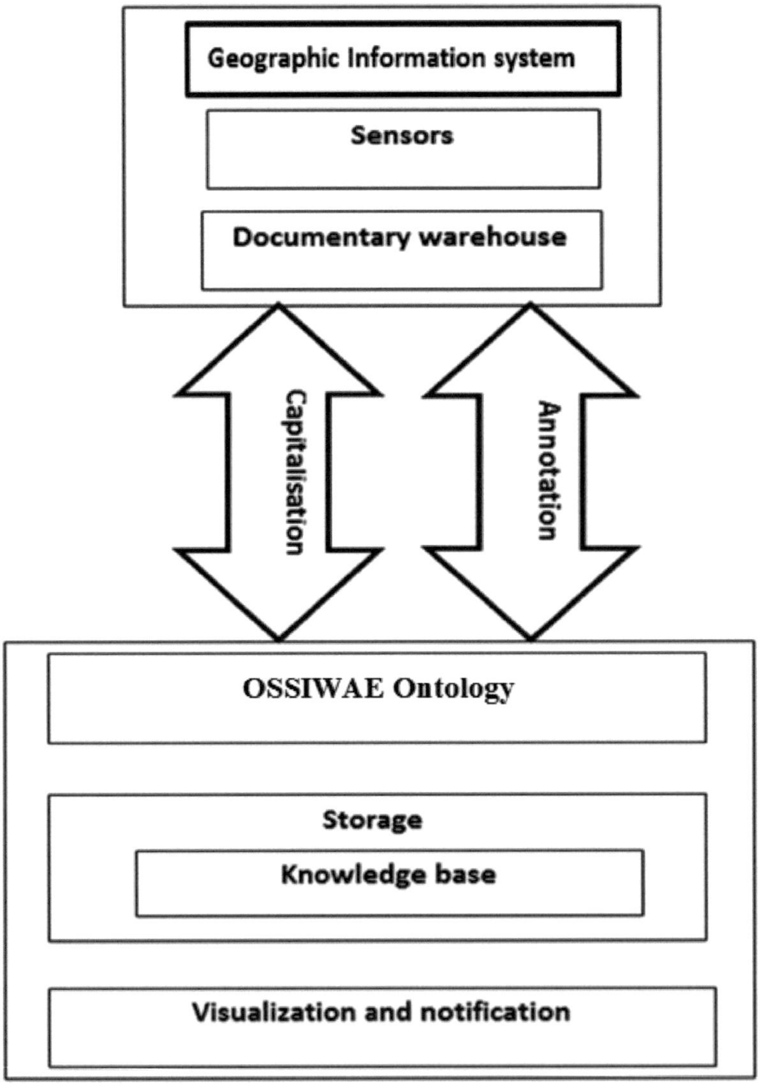

Figure 2.
Architecture of a knowledge base of natural disasters.

well-defined places in the structure and in the Soil. These sensors can communicate with each other. The collection of information also uses a documentary warehouse for the collection of documents (expert report, opinions, etc.). These documents are annotated by the ontology in order to extract additional information. Documentary warehouse allows experts to record the events produced in order to make the right decisions. In the previous work [23, 24] we have demonstrated the importance of annotating documents handled during the process of decision making.

The second part is the knowledge base, it is used to store the information sent automatically by the electronic sensors (high water level, vibration, temperature, humidity, rotation, acceleration, inclination, force, etc.) and linked this information to graphical information mapped by GIS and information annotated by experts. **Figure 3** gives the class diagram of the knowledge base. The validation phase for the classification of knowledge according to the criteria of value and veracity of knowledge for the group is important. According to [25] there are three categories of knowledge among the knowledge to be certified (validated, not validated and rejected), we used these three categories as annotative acts between the actors of the group to certify and validate their knowledge and the data collected. In this function the following annotative acts are used: a validated annotation, a rejected annotation and an invalidated annotation.

The third part is the OSSIWAE ontology. The ontology used to conceptualize the interaction between structure and soil. The ontology is used to semantically capture the information sent by the sensors and also to annotate the documents stored in the document repository. The OSSIWAE ontology described in Section 3.1.

The fourth part is the user interface, which allows users to view the evolution in real time of the graphs for each mapped area and send them the Short Message (SMS) of notifications to mobile phones for decision makers to inform themselves

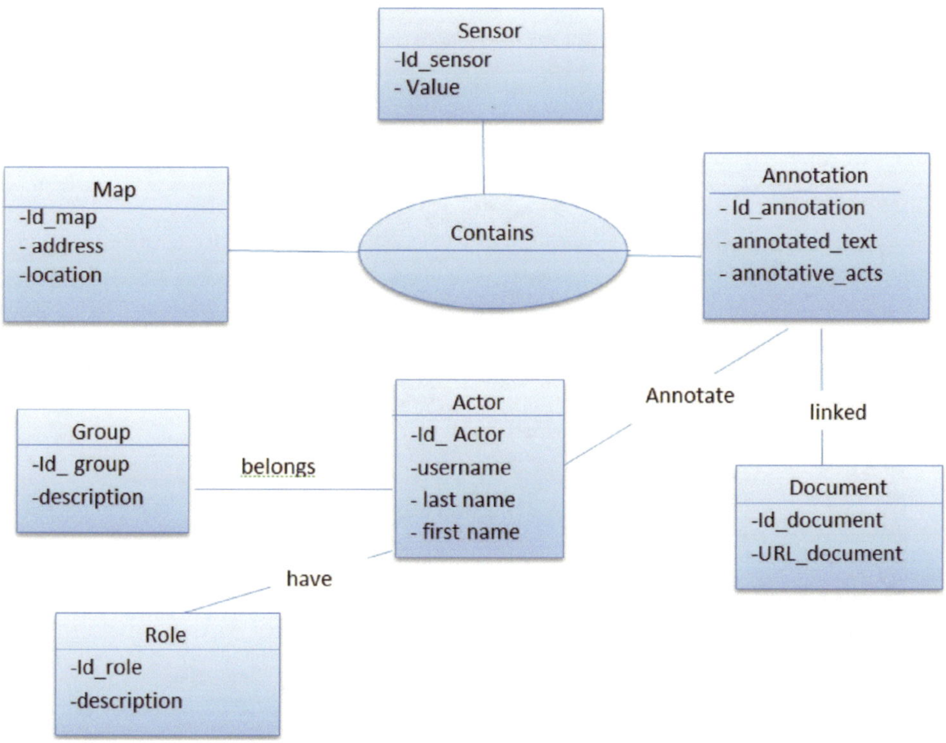

Figure 3.
The class diagram of the knowledge base.

and take the necessary measures. And also allows fully understanding, analyzing and estimating this phenomenon by experts.

5. Implementation

The main technologies used to develop this application are: jQuery it is a JavaScript library is used to facilitate the development of user interface. PHP language it is used for manipulation of data in the data base. Asynchronous JavaScript and XML (AJAX) is used to send data to server. MySQL server it is used for the creation of the database to store the information.

For the Geographic Information system (GIS) a web cartographic server was developed which allows for managing maps and data. This server makes it possible to share data and to link with the data via sensors and annotations. The HTML canvas element it is used to draw graphics, with using the JavaScript to add annotation, draw a line, draw a circle, draw a Text... on cards.

For the electronics system, the Arduino nano and uno with the different sensors used to capture the data in real time. The programming software of the Arduino board is used, which serves as a code editor in a language close to C to program this part.

For document annotation, an annotator was developed to annotate word and excel documents via ontology. These annotations are linked with the areas mapped by the GIS and the information collected by the sensors.

A model for building a structure three-story was prepared and then put on the soil. Vibrations are applied to simulate data collection via sensors (**Figure 4**) then these data are processed and display it in a web page to link with the relevant geographic map.

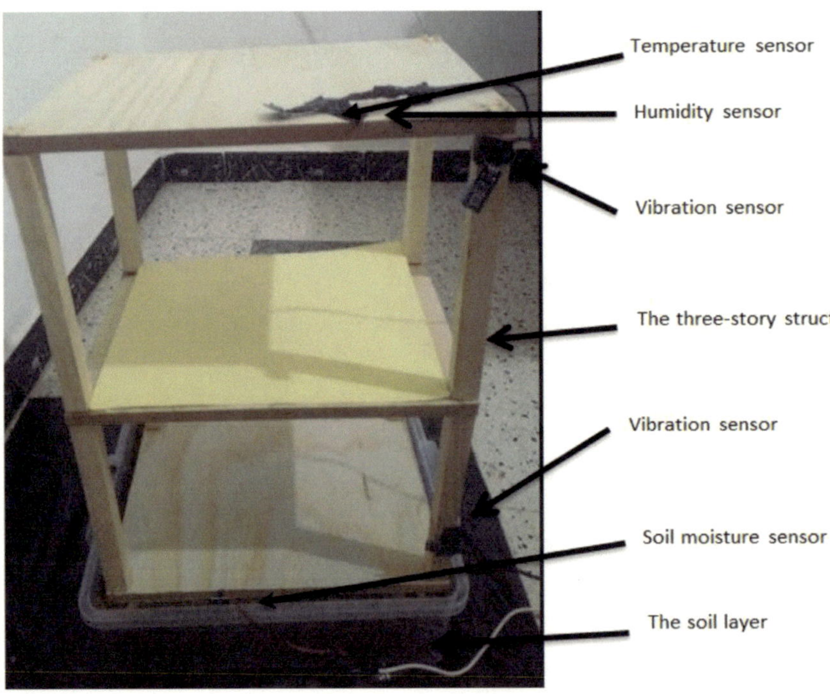

Figure 4.
Model of soil-structures interaction with sensors.

6. Conclusion

The risk management of natural disasters becomes a necessity to take the necessary measures at the right time and in the right place and for the construction of new structures weak and resistant to natural disasters. This chapter presents a conceptual architecture based on ontology, embedded systems and Geographic Information system for the creation of a knowledge base on the phenomenon of soil-structures interaction with the connections of external agents in real time in order to fully understand, analyze and estimate this phenomenon by experts. Considering that the ontologies play a critical role to solve the problem of the heterogeneity of external and multi-source information. An Ontology of Soil-Structure Interaction With Agents External (OSSIWAE) was proposed for managing and integrating the data coming from different sources of information (GIS, satellites, electronic sensors and comments from experts). To validate this architecture, a web platform was developed in the context of Internet of Things (IoT), which supports the different technologies used. Then, a case study is conducted on a prototype of a model for building a structure three-story to simulate data collection. Given the large number of mapping areas, in this chapter some sensors are installed. As a perspective we want to increase the number of sensors to capture other parameters.

List of acronyms and abbreviations

IoT	Internet of Things
GIS	Geographic Information system
OSSIWAE	Ontology of Soil-Structure Interaction With Agents External
SAR	Synthetic Aperture Radar
EO	Earth Observation
SDSS	Spatial Decision Support System
AHP	Analytical Hierarchy Process
ORFFM	Ontology for River Flow and Flood Mitigation
AJAX	Asynchronous JavaScript and XML
HTML	HyperText Markup Language
SMS	Short Message Service

Author details

Aissa Bensattalah[1,2*], Rachid Chalal[2,3], Tahar Hassaine Daouadji[1,4] and Tayeb Bensattalah[1,4]

1 Faculty of Applied Sciences, University of Tiaret, Algeria

2 Laboratoire des Méthodes de Conception des Systèmes (LMCS), Algiers, Algeria

3 Ecole Nationale Supérieure d'Informatique (E.S.I), Algiers, Algeria

4 Laboratory of Geomatics and Sustainable Development, University of Tiaret, Algeria

*Address all correspondence to: a_bensattalah@esi.dz

References

[1] Liu, X.; Wang, X.Y.; Wright, G.; Cheng, J.C.P.; Li, X.; Liu, R. A State-of-the-Art Review on the Integration of Building Information Modeling (BIM) and Geographic Information System (GIS). ISPRS Int. J. Geo-Inf. 2017, 6, 53. [CrossRef].

[2] Adimalla N, Taloor AK. Hydrogeochemical investigation of groundwater quality in the hard rock terrain of South India using Geographic Information System (GIS) and groundwater quality index (GWQI) techniques. Groundwater for Sustainable Development. 2020; (10),100288.

[3] Okan ERAY. Application of geographic information system (GIS) in education. Journal of Technical Science and Technologies. 2012; p. 53-58

[4] Rahman MR, Thakur PK. Detecting, mapping and analysing of flood water propagation using synthetic aperture radar (SAR) satellite data and GIS: A case study from the Kendrapara District of Orissa State of India. The Egyptian Journal of Remote Sensing and Space Science. 2018; 21, p.S37-S41.

[5] Kourgialas NN, Karatzas GP. Flood management and a GIS modelling method to assess flood-hazard areas—a case study. Hydrological Sciences Journal. 2011; 56(2), 212-225.

[6] Van Westen CJ. Remote sensing and GIS for natural hazards assessment and disaster risk management. Treatise on geomorphology. 2013; (3), 259-298.

[7] Zogning MMO, Tsalefac M, Ursu A, Lațu C. Contribution of geographic information systems for the mapping of flooding factors in Yaoundé: The case study of Mfoundi upstream watershed. Present Environment and Sustainable Development. 2016; (1), 217-234.

[8] Stancalie G. Contribution of satellite remotely sensed data to flood risk mapping. In: Geophysical Research Abstracts. 2005; (7), 315.

[9] Balogun AL. Developing a flood susceptibility model for real estate site optimization and planning using Spatial Decision Support System (SDSS). In: The 12th GIS Symposium in Saudi Arabia. 2018.

[10] Gruber TR. A translation approach to portable ontologies. Knowledge Acquisition. 1993; 5 (2), 199-220.

[11] Noy NF, McGuinness DL. Ontology Development 101: A Guide to Creating Your First Ontology. Knowledge Systems Laboratory. Technical Report, Stanford University. 2001.

[12] Giakoumatos SDV, Gkionakis AKT. Development of an Ontology-Based Knowledge Network by Interconnecting Soil/Water Concepts/Properties, Derived from Standards Methods and Published Scientific References Outlining Infiltration/Percolation Process of Contaminated Water. Journal of Geoscience and Environment Protection. 2021; 9(1), 25-52.

[13] Meng K, Cui C, Li H. An Ontology Framework for Pile Integrity Evaluation Based on Analytical Methodology. IEEE Access. 2020, (8), 72158-72168.

[14] Du H, Dimitrova V, Magee D, Stirling R, Curioni G, Reeves H, Clarke B, Cohn A. An ontology of soil properties and processes. In International Semantic Web Conference, Springer, Cham. 2016; p. 30-37.

[15] Beck H. Evolution of database designs for knowledge management in agriculture and natural resources. Journal of Information Technology in Agriculture. 2008;3 (1), 23.

[16] Beck H, Morgan K, Jung Y, Grunwald S, Kwon HY, Wu J. Ontology-based simulation in agricultural systems modeling. Agricultural Systems. 2010; 103(7), 463-477.

[17] Sermet Y, Demir I. Towards an information centric flood ontology for information management and communication. Earth Science Informatics. 2019; 12(4), 541-551.

[18] Stolf P, Pierson JM, Sayah A, Da Costa G, Renaud-Goud P. e-Flooding: Crisis Management Through Two Temporal Loops. In: Proceedings of the 52nd Hawaii International Conference on System Sciences. 2019.

[19] Yi S, Xiao Y .The development of integrated watershed flood risk assessment ontology. In : the 23rd International Conference on Geoinformatics. IEEE, 2015; p. 1-6.

[20] Agresta A, Fattoruso G, Pollino M, Pasanisi F, Tebano C, De Vito S, Di Francia G. An Ontology Framework for Flooding Forecasting. In : International Conference on Computational Science and Its Applications. Springer, Cham. 2014; p. 417-428.

[21] Sinha P K, Dutta B. A systematic analysis of flood ontologies: A parametric approach. Knowledge Organization. 2020; 47(2), 138-159.

[22] Mughal MH, Shaikh ZA, Wagan AI, Khand ZH, Hassan S. ORFFM: An Ontology-Based Semantic Model of River Flow and Flood Mitigation. IEEE Access. (9), 2021; 44003-44031.

[23] Bensattalah A, Nader F, Chalal R. Collective memory based on semantic annotation among economic intelligence actors. International Journal of Collaborative Intelligence. 2014; 1(1), p. 18-32.

[24] Bensattalah A, Azouaou F, Nader F, Chalal R. EI-Annotate: An adaptive collective memory based on annotation ontology and context for decision making in economic intelligence. International Journal of Business Information Systems. 2018; 29(2), 207-232.

[25] Chalal R . An approach for the cooperative capitalization of knowledge on product risks in the initial phase of an industrial project. [thesis]. The National Higher School of Computer Science (ESI, Ex-INI), Alger. Algeria; 2007.

Chapter 5

Comparison of Cross-Entropy Based MCDM Approach for Selection of Material in Sugar Industry

Syed Abou Iltaf Hussain, Himanshu Chandra and Uttam Kumar Mandal

Abstract

One of the major problems faced in engineering is the selection of the material which is most suitable for the product. Material selection from a large number with diverse mechanical, physical and chemical properties and choosing the best material which is the most satisfying for making the job is a very complex process. Material selection is important as it determines durability, reliability and cost of the product. Selection of suitable material which gives maximum performance with minimum cost is often observed to be a multi-criterion decision-making (MCDM) problem with different objectives. This chapter presents an integrated approach to select the suitable material to be used as base of induction cookware which can give maximum performance with minimum cost. In the integrated approach the weights of the criteria are computed using the cross-entropy method and ranking of the alternatives is done using the different MCDM methods. The methods are further illustrated with an example and the result obtained from different cross-entropy MCDM methods are compared for finding the most suitable method for serving the purpose.

Keywords: Cross Entropy method, Different MCDM methods, Comparison, Spearman's Rank correlation coefficient, Coefficient of Determination

1. Introduction

In this present techno-economic scenario material selection poses one of the major challenges in industries. Selection of the improper material adversely affects the reputation of an organization and also reduces the profitability. Selection of the proper material is a step in the process of product design where it aims in increasing the performance with minimum cost. Material selection is also important from the perspective of sustainability of industries [1, 2].

In the recent years, traditional materials were replaced by more advance materials due to their mechanical and chemical properties. The materials were used for manufacturing from complex geometry to long lasting products. With the large number of readily available materials the process of material selection is done with the help of multi-criteria decision-making (MCDM) process.

Moreover, MCDM is the study concerned with optimal decision making and the modelling of deterministic systems. Its focus in the interdisciplinary field of application, clutching a wide range of quantitative techniques. Whereas, Industrial Engineering is about the enhancement, refinement, and installation of integrated systems of personnel, material, and equipment. Industrial engineering is also about processing of the information. MCDM integrated industrial engineering provide a rational approach to engineering and managerial problem solving through deliberate application of scientific methods. In the MCDM model, the set of available materials are called alternatives among which the best material is selected on the basis of the certain properties called criteria.

In practical scenario MCDM addresses the performance of different alternatives on the basis of information and resource limitations of a company or industry or organization, working towards the establishing of beneficial policies. The function of the decision maker is to guide the engineers, managers and administration by processing the information available in the industries.

1.1 Entropy based Multi-Criteria Decision Making (MCDM)

In today's hi-tech engineering world, MCDM have evolved as one of the most important tools of decision making in a complex situation. MCDM also help in taking decisions in a situation where there is little or no chance of any altercation. In the present socio-economic world where a decision of selecting the best is effected by a large number of criteria, MCDM plays a very important role in such aspects. Decision making is done based on various criteria which might be important equally or not. From the last statement it can be said that every criterion are weighted which help the decision maker in taking the decision. One of the major problems faced in MCDM problem is the assigning of weights to the criterion. Some of the different techniques of assigning weights to the criteria are 5Ws and H method, fuzzy method, cross-entropy method etc. Cook [3] and Vesna Čančer [4] used 5Ws and H technique; Kumar and Gag , Amiri *et al.*, Kemal Vatansever and Yiğit Kazançoğlu , Keshavarz Ghorabaee *et al.*, used fuzzy for determining the weights of different criteria. ZOU Zhi-hong *et al.* [5], Wei Liu and Jin Cui [6], Chia-Chang Hung and Liang-Hsuan Chen [7], Farhad Hosseinzadeh Lotfi and Reza Fallahnejad [8], Yuguo Qi *et al.* [9], Peiyue *et al.* [10], Kshitij Dashore *et al.* [11], Deepa Joshi and Sanjay Kumar [12], Anhai Li *et al.* [13], Harish Garg *et al.* [14], Zhang-peng Tian *et al.* [15], Elham Ebrahimi *et al.* [16], Harish Garg [17], Javier Martínez-Gómez *et al.* [18] used cross-entropy method for determining the weightage of the criteria for solving MCDM problem.

1.2 Application of MCDM in material selection

With increasing choice of materials and large number of manufacturing process available to the designers, the selection of an optimal material have become more complex and more challenging than before [19]. In order to address the issue of material selection researchers like Ashby proposed MCDM as one of the best tools. Ashby *et al.* [20] have identified three material selection strategies which are (a) free searching based on quantitative analysis, (b) checklist/questionnaire based on expertise capture, and (c) inductive reasoning and analog procedure. A large number of literature exist for selecting the suitable material for a product. Based on the Ashby work a lot of researches is carried out in this respect. Out of which some are reviewed. Milani *et al.* [21] studied the ways in which different criteria transformation techniques effects the result in TOPSIS method for selecting gear material. In the year 2006, R.V. Rao and J.P. Davim [22] developed a combined AHP-TOPSIS model for selecting material to be used in non-heat-treatable cover material. Shanian A and Savadogo O. [23, 24], successfully applied TOPSIS in selecting material for a particular product design with maximum performance and minimum cost. Again in the same year Shanian A and Savadogo O. implemented the ELECTRE-I method for selecting material to be used in Bipolar Plates for Polymer Electrolyte Fuel Cells Applications. In this chapter, ELECTRE-I gave the same result with or without negative criterion. In 2008, Sharif Ullah and Harib [25] proposed an intelligent method for selecting material where informations regarding the design configurations, working conditions and design-relevant information were not known. According to Karande and Chakraborty [26], material selection is also an important factor for a product to strive in the competition in market because improper material selection may result in failure to fulfil customer and manufacturer requirements. In 2013a, 2013b, Shankar Chakraborty and Prasenjit Chatterjee [27, 28], observed that in case of material selection the ranking performance of VIKOR is far better than the TOPSIS and PROMETHEE methods. In the chapter the authors also concluded that the best and the worst is solely dependent on the weights of the criteria. They further added that time for selecting the most suited material could be reduced by identifying the criterion with maximum weight. In their second chapter COPRAS and ARAS methods were termed as the most appropriate method for gear material selection as the result obtained from both the method are quite similar and also both the techniques are fool proof techniques.

1.3 Motivation

Decision making theory plays a vital role where decisions have to be taken in cases the performance parameter differs from each other by a very small margin. There are different decision making methods which takes in account different mathematical concepts such as the best alternative is one which in a best way can compromise the conflicting scenario (VIKOR), the alternative which is farthest from the non-benefit criteria is the best alternative (MOORA), the alternative having the highest relative weightage for the benefit criteria is the best alternative (COPRAS) and so on. Hence when a decision is taken with different MCDM methods, the result may differ for each method. Alternative which is best by one method may not be the best by some other method. In problems like material selection each wrong decision is associated with some penalty. For such cases the weights of the criteria are so calculated that it reduces the penalty for not choosing the actual best alternative instead of choosing the predicted best alternative. Moreover, selecting materials in sugar industry is well known MCDM problem. But, the literatures fail to answer which method to apply for material selection and the risk involved for choosing a method. The literatures also do not explain the accuracy degree to which two or more selection methods would agree to the same decision. The main aim of this chapter is find a material suitable for manufacturing equipment in the sugar industry by different MCDM methods and also to find the degree to which all the methods would agree to the decision.

1.4 Novelties

Lot of researchers have worked in the field of MCDM and developed novel approaches for precisely selecting alternatives. Some of the novelties developed in this chapter are as follows:

1. Application of CE integrated MCDM approaches are used for selecting material in sugar industry.

2. Comparison between the results obtained from CE based MCDM techniques.

3. Based on the comparison a predictive model is developed that can forecast the result by different CE integrated MCDM approaches.

1.5 Structure of the chapter

The chapter is organized into 7 sections. The first section is introduction which describes the importance of the material selection and the comprehensive literature related to the topic. Section 2 describes the preliminary concept of the methodologies used for the study. Section 3 summarises the steps of the MCDM methods and section 4 describes the case study that is considered for the present study. Section 5 is the comparative study of the result obtained from various MCDM methods. Section 6 discusses the summary of the findings and section 7 concludes the chapter.

2. Preliminaries

2.1 Multi-criteria decision making (MCDM)

Definitions 1: Decision can be defined as the rationale conclusions after evaluating the circumstances.

Definition 2: In perspective of cognitive science, selection of a particular action or a certain belief that is a subset of the alternatives is knows as Decision Making.

The process of selection of an action that belong to the subset of the alternatives is done by considering all criteria's which can either alter the judgement of same or dissimilar extent is called as Multi-Criteria Decision Making. In MCDM technique, the existing possibilities are the subset of alternatives or else, these are the choices out of which the finest possibility is to be selected by analysing various factors which could influence the outcome. All the alternatives are ranked in ascending order beginning from the finest to the worst and on the basis of factors which can influence the conclusions, these factors are known as criteria. Criteria can be defined as the factors which have direct influence on decision. In MCDM technique, there are number of criteria and which each of them effects the judgement and conclusion either to the similar or dissimilar extent.

2.2 Steps involved in decision making

2.2.1 GOFER method for taking decision

During 1980s, psychologist Leon Munn and some of his colleagues developed a technique called GOFER specifically for decision making [29]. The acronym for GOFER stands for a 5 decision making steps.

G: Goal - Selection of material
O: Options - Set of readily available materials
F: Facts - Performance with respect to the criteria
E: Effect - How the material selection are effected?
R: Review - Reviewing distinct facts and data associated to the options.

2.2.2 DECIDE method for taking decision

In the year 2008, another decision making technique was developed by Kristina Guo known as DECIDE [30]. This method consist of six parts namely:

D: Define the problem i.e. selection of material.

E: All the criteria and factors are established on basis of which the decision is made i.e. enlisting the criteria.

C: Enlisting the various available materials.

I: Discard the materials having high cost to benefit ratio.

D: A plan is developed for selecting the finest alternative.

E: Select the best material.

2.2.3 Working principle

All MCDM methods share some similar working principles upto certain extent, which are as follows:

1. Selection of Criteria:
    - All noted criteria must be in correlation to the alternatives.
    - The criteria are to be well-prepared along with the decision.
    - The criteria must have some relevance either equally or alike.
    - The criteria must not be dependent on each other in any sort of way.
2. Selection of Alternatives:
    - The alternatives which have been selected must be real in nature.
    - The alternatives which have been selected must be available.
3. Selection of method to provide weightage to the criteria:
    - Outranking Method – An outranking relation is to be built using a series of pairwise assessments of the alternatives.
    - Compensatory Method – Here, strengths and capabilities are embraced over the weakness.

2.2.4 Flowchart for decision making

See **Figure 1**.

2.3 Cross entropy (CE) method

In problems related to MCDM technique, the hardest job is to accurately assign weights to the various criteria with respect the ranked alternatives. Therefore, Cross Entropy Methods is often used to assign weights to the criteria. The cross entropy methods is nothing else but a generic form of a well-known Monte Carlo simulation that is used in complex estimation and optimization problems for error minimization. Y. R. Rubinstien was the first to suggest this approach in 1999 by extending his previous work done in 1997.

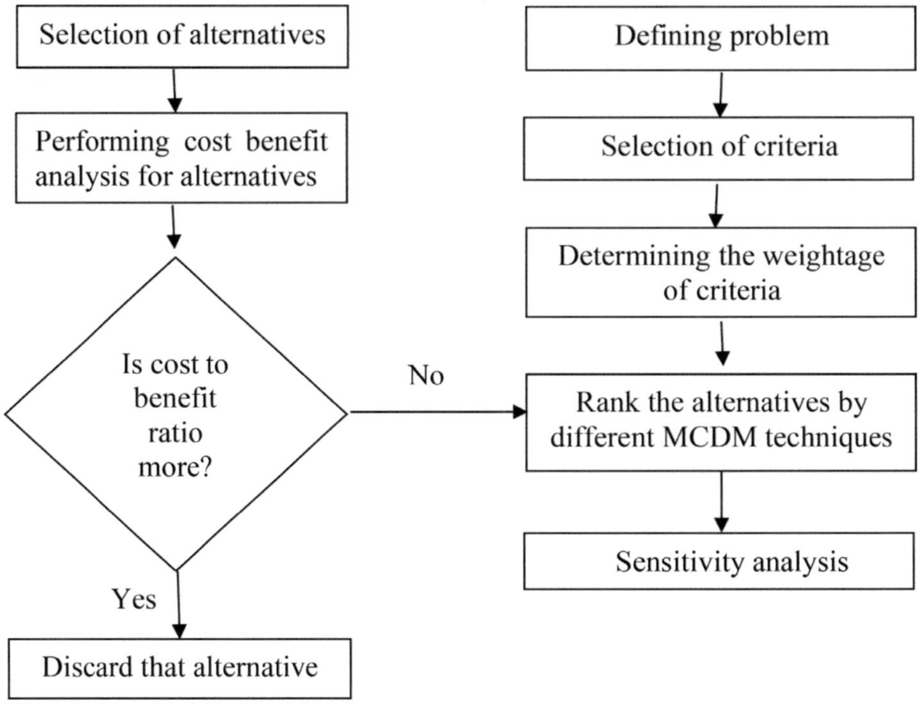

Figure 1.
Flowchart for decision making.

2.3.1 Algorithms for cross entropy method

Step 1: Feature weight β_{ij} is calculated for i^{th} alternative and j^{th} criterion as

$$\beta_{ij} = \frac{a_{ij}}{\sum_{i=1}^{m} a_{ij}^2}, (1 \leq \mathrm{i} \leq \mathrm{m}, 1 \leq \mathrm{j} \leq \mathrm{n})$$

Step 2: The output entropy ε_j of the jth factor

$$\varepsilon_j = -\kappa \sum_{i=1}^{m} \left(\beta_{ij} ln \beta_{ij}\right), (1 \leq \mathrm{j} \leq \mathrm{n})$$

$$\kappa = \frac{1}{\ln m}$$

Step 3: Calculation of variation coefficient of jth factor ξ_j

$$\xi_j = \left|1 - \varepsilon_j\right|$$

Step 4: Calculation of weight of the entropy w_j

$$w_j = \frac{\xi_j}{\sum_{j=1}^{n} \xi_j}$$

2.4 Application of CE based MCDM techniques in engineering problem

Cross Entropy is an important method for determining the weights of the criteria. The penalty for selecting a non-best alternative over the best is less when criteria are weighted using the Cross Entropy method. In the year 1997, Y. R. Rubinstein first developed an adaptive variance minimization algorithm for estimating probabilities of rare events for stochastic networks which was later in the year 1999 was modified for solving combinatorial optimization problems. Then later the Cross Entropy method was used along with the MCDM problems for minimizing the penalty for not choosing the best alternative.

A lot of researches have been conducted where Cross Entropy method is used along with the MCDM method for decision making. Some of the literatures are reviewed and presented. In the year 2006, ZOU Zhi-hong *et al.* [5] applied CE method to determine the weightage of different criteria for evaluating water quality in a fuzzy environment. Wei Liu and Jin Cui [6], applied CE method along with MCDM model for evaluation of sustainable development of China's sport. Farhad Hosseinzadeh Lotfi and Reza Fallahnejad [8], proposed a method where entropy method can be used for for weighting different criteria of non-deterministic data such as interval valued data. Chia-Chang Hung and Liang-Hsuan Chen [7] developed a fuzzy TOPSIS decision model where weights of the criteria are calculated with the entropy method and the alternative are represented by intuitionistic fuzzy sets. In the year 2010, Yuguo Qi *et al.* [9] proposed a model where evaluation of power network structure is done by entropy based MCDM method under fuzzy environment. This method is a combination of both subjectivity and objectivity, and provides good platform for quantitative as well as qualitative analysis. Kshitij Dashore *et al.* [11] compared the results obtained from different MCDM techniques where the weights of the criteria are evaluated using CE method. The authors concluded that the same best alternative is obtained from TOPSIS, SAW and WPM methods.

2.5 Recent work of CE based MCDM

Some of the recent CE based MCDM works that have been reviewed are also presented in this chapter. In the year 2015, Anhai Li *et al.* [13] in their chapter applied entropy based MCDM methodsfor optimal selection of cutting tool material. Harish Garg *et al.* proposed a CE based Multi-Attribute Group Decision Making (MAGDM). The model thus proposed gives a useful way for dealing fuzzy MAGDM within attribute weights efficiently and effectively. Zheng-peng Tian *et al.* [15], developed a CE based decision making model to deal with interval valued neutrosophic sets. In the year 2016, Elham Ebrahimi *et al.* [16] compared the result obtained from fuzzy COPRAS and CE-COPRAS to evaluate the customer-company relationship. Javier Martínez-Gómez *et al.* [18] developed a MCDM model which includes compromised weighting method composes of Analytical Hierachy Process and Entropy method. The authors successfully applied CE- based MCDM method for material selection.

3. Different CE-MCDM techniques

From a set of alternatives, best quantitative solution is evaluated using ranking solution and is provided by MCDM process. In this research work, cross entropy method is applied due to the reason that is highly reliable for measuring information and deliver good accuracy while evaluating the weights of the feature attribute. MCDM problem can thus be expressed as a matrix:

$$M = \begin{array}{c} \\ A_1 \\ A_2 \\ A_3 \\ \vdots \\ A_m \end{array} \begin{array}{c} \begin{array}{ccccc} C_1 & C_2 & C_3 & & C_n \end{array} \\ \begin{bmatrix} a_{11} & a_{12} & a_{13} & \cdots & a_{1n} \\ a_{21} & a_{22} & a_{23} & \cdots & a_{2n} \\ a_{31} & a_{32} & a_{33} & \cdots & a_{3n} \\ \vdots & \vdots & \vdots & \ddots & \vdots \\ a_{m1} & a_{m2} & a_{m3} & \cdots & a_{mn} \end{bmatrix} \end{array}$$

$$W = \begin{bmatrix} w_1 & w_2 & w_3 & \cdots & w_n \end{bmatrix}$$

Here, A_1, A_2, A_3 ... ... A_m are the alternatives which are available and supposed to be ranked by decision maker C_1, C_2, C_3 ... ... C_n are the criteria which will govern ranking of the alternatives. a_{ij} shows the performance of alternative A_i on the basis of C_j and w_j is the weight of the criterion.

3.1 The complex proportional assessment (COPRAS) method

In 1994, Zavadskas and Kaklauskas presented the COPRAS method which is a reference ranking method for ranking different alternatives [28]. Alternative's performance is primarily considered in COPRAS method with respect to various criteria. Therefore, the method aims to select the finest decision considering the ideal-best as well as the ideal-worst solutions. Steps used to rank those alternatives by using COPRAS method are as follows:

Step 1: Calculation of normalized decision matrix (n_{ij}):

$$n_{ij} = \frac{a_{ij}}{\sum_{i=1}^{m} a_{ij}}$$

Step 2: Calculation of weighted normalize decision matrix (W_{ij}):

$$W_{ij} = n_{ij} * w_j$$

Where w_j is the weightage of criterion C_j.

Step 3: Calculation of S^+ and S^-:

S^+ and S^- are the summation of weighted normalized value that are evaluated for benefit criteria as well as non-benefit criteria.

$$S_i^+ = \sum_{j=1}^{n} W_{ij}.(\mathrm{i} = 1, 2, 3 \ldots \mathrm{m})$$

Where W_{ij} is the weighted normalize elements for all the benefit criteria

$$S_i^- = \sum_{j=1}^{n} W_{ij}.(\mathrm{i} = 1, 2, 3 \ldots \mathrm{m})$$

Where W_{ij} is the weighted normalize elements for all the non-benefit criteria

Step 4: Evaluating relative weightage of each alternative Q_i:

$$Q_i = S_i^+ + \frac{\sum_{i=1}^{m} S_i^-}{S_i^- \quad \sum_{i=1}^{m} \frac{1}{S_i^-}}$$

Step 5: Determining the priority order (Pr_i):

$$Pr_i = \frac{Q_i}{max \quad Q_i}$$

Maximum value of Pr_i is given maximum priority and ranked 1, second largest value of Pr_i is given second priority and ranked 2 and so on.

3.2 The MOORA method

MOORA (Multi Objective Optimization on the Basis of Ratio Analysis) was developed by Brauers in 2004 for solving different complex and conflicting decision matrix. Performance measures of alternatives with respect to different criteria are represented by the decision matrix of MOORA. Steps governing the ranking of different alternatives by MOORA methods are:

Step1: Calculation of normalized decision matrix (n_{ij}):

$$n_{ij} = \frac{a_{ij}}{\sqrt{\sum_{i=1}^{m} a_{ij}^2}}$$

Step 2: Calculation of weighted normalize decision matrix (W_{ij}):

$$W_{ij} = w_j \times n_{ij}$$

Step 3: Evaluating of Priorities (Q_i):

$$Q_i = \sum_{j=1}^{n} W_{ij}$$

Priorities is the difference between the sum of benefit criteria and non-benefit criteria.

Step 4: Ranking of alternatives:

Maximum value of the variable Q_i is provided the maximum priority and ranked 1, second largest of Q_i is provided the second priority and ranked 2 and so on.

3.3 The VIKOR method

VIKOR method, developed for evaluating decision making problems with conflicting as well as non-commensurable criteria by Serafim Opricovic. This method assumes accepts compromise with conflicting resolution. VIKOR methods ranks various alternatives and evaluates the solution called as compromise which is the closest value to the ideal.

Step 1: Calculation of f_j^* *and* $f_j^\wedge$

$$f_j^* = Min(a_{ij}), (\ j = 1, 2, 3, \ldots n)$$

$$f_j^{\Lambda} = Max(a_{ij}), (j = 1, 2, 3, \ldots n)$$

Where a_{ij} stands for elements of decision matrix

Step 2: Calculation of relative matrix (R_{ij})

$$R_{ij} = \frac{f_j^{*} - a_{ij}}{f_j^{*} - f_j^{\Lambda}}$$

Step 3: Calculation of weighted normalized decision matrix (W_{ij})

$$W_{ij} = R_{ij} \times w_j$$

Step 4: Calculation of γ_j by the concept of Manhattan distance.

$$\gamma_j = \sum_{j=1}^{n} W_{ij}, (i = 1, 2, 3, \ldots m)$$

Step 5 : Calculation of δ_j by the concept of Chebyshev distance.

$$\delta_j = Max(W_{ij}), (i = 1, 2, 3 \ldots m)$$

Step 6: Calculation of priority values ρ_j.

$$\rho_j = \frac{V(\gamma_j - \gamma^{*})}{(\gamma^{\Lambda} - \gamma^{*})} + (1 - V)\frac{(\delta_j - \delta_j^{*})}{(\delta_j^{\Lambda} - \delta_j^{*})}$$

Where, $\gamma^{*} = min(\gamma_j)$

$\gamma^{\Lambda} = max(\gamma_j)$

$\delta_j^{*} = \min(\delta_j)$

$\delta_j^{\Lambda} = \max(\delta_j)$

$V = \frac{n+1}{2n}$, n is the no. of criterion

Step 7: Ranking of various possible alternatives

According to values of ρ_j, the alternative values are ranked from ascending order. Here, the smallest is the best alternative and the largest is considered as the worst alternatives.

3.4 The TOPSIS method

Technique for Order Preference by Similarity to Ideal Solution (TOPSIS) was developed in 1981 by Hwang and Yoon. The primary objective of TOPSIS was to determine the finest alternatives by minimizing the positive-ideal solution's distance and maximizing the negative-ideal solution's distance [31]. All the various alternative solutions shall be ranked on the basis of their closeness to ideal solution i.e., the closest alternative to the ideal is considered as the best solution whereas, the least close alternative to the ideal is considered as the worst solution. Steps governing the ranking of the alternatives by TOPSIS method are:

Step 1: Calculation of normalized decision matrix (n_{ij})

$$n_{ij} = \frac{a_{ij}}{\sqrt{\sum_{i=1}^{m} a_{ij}^2}}$$

Step 2: Calculation of weighted normalize decision matrix (W_{ij})

$$W_{ij} = w_j \times n_{ij}$$

Where w_j is the weight of the criterion C^j .

Step 3: Calculation of Positive Ideal Solution (P_{is}) and Negative Ideal Solution (N_{is})

$$P_{is} = \begin{cases} Max(W_{ij}), (j = 1, 2, 3, \dots .n) \, for \; benefit \; criteria \\ Min(W_{ij}), (j = 1, 2, 3, \dots .n) \, for \; non - benefit \; criteria \end{cases}$$

$$N_{is} = \begin{cases} Max(W_{ij}), (j = 1, 2, 3, \dots .n) \, for \; non - benefit \; criteria \\ Min(W_{ij}), (j = 1, 2, 3, \dots .n) \, for \; benefit \; criteria \end{cases}$$

Step 4: Calculation of separation measures (S_m^+) for P_{is} and (S_m^-) for N_{is}

$$S_m^+ = \sqrt{\sum_{j=1}^{n} (W_{ij} - P_{is})^2}, (1 \le i \le m, 1 \le j \le n)$$

$$S_m^- = \sqrt{\sum_{j=1}^{n} (W_{ij} - N_{is})^2}, (1 \le i \le m, 1 \le j \le n)$$

Separation measures are measured using Euclidean distance method.

Step 5: Calculation of relative closeness to the ideal solution (RC_{is})

$$RC_{is} = \frac{S_m^-}{S_m^+ + S_m^-}$$

Step 6: Arrangment of the RC_{is} values in descending order and ranking from the largest value to the smallest value.

3.5 The modified TOPSIS method

The Modified TOPSIS method is a revised version of the TOPSIS model. In the Modified TOPSIS model the Pis and Nis do not depends on the weighted decision matrix. Steps for ranking alternatives by Modified TOPSIS method is as follows:

Step 1: Calculation of normalized decision matrix (n_{ij})

$$n_{ij} = \frac{a_{ij}}{\sqrt{\sum_{i=1}^{m} a_{ij}^2}}$$

Where a_{ij} is the performance of value of alternative A_i on the basis of criterion C_j.

Step 2: Calculation of Positive Ideal Solution (P_{is}) and Negative Ideal Solution (N_{is})

$$P_{is} = \begin{cases} Max(n_{ij}), (j = 1, 2, 3, \dots .n) \, for \; benefit \; criteria \\ Min(n_{ij}), (j = 1, 2, 3, \dots .n) \, for \; non - benefit \; criteria \end{cases}$$

$$N_{is} = \begin{cases} Max(n_{ij}), (j = 1, 2, 3, \dots .n) \, for \; non - benefit \; criteria \\ Min(n_{ij}), (j = 1, 2, 3, \dots .n) \, for \; benefit \; criteria \end{cases}$$

Step 3: Calculation of separation measures $\left(S_m^+\right)$ for P_{is} and $\left(S_m^-\right)$ for N_{is}

$$S_m^+ = \sqrt{\sum\nolimits_{j=1}^{n} w_j \left(n_{ij} - P_{is}\right)^2}, (1 \le i \le m)$$

$$S_m^- = \sqrt{\sum\nolimits_{j=1}^{n} w_j \left(n_{ij} - N_{is}\right)^2}, (1 \le i \le m)$$

Separation measures are measured using Euclidean distance method.
Step 4: Calculation of relative closeness to the ideal solution (RC_{is})

$$RC_{is} = \frac{S_m^-}{S_m^+ + S_m^-}$$

Step 5: Arrangment of the RC_{is} values in descending order and ranking from the largest value to the smallest value.

4. Application

4.1 Material selection in sugar industry

A few researchers and product designer have studied the failure rate in the sugar industrial equipment. From their study they have found that in India, the failure due to corrosion of the equipments' cost a sum of about US$250 million [32]. A comparison of better corrosion resistance material was done in [33]. [34] has suggested the use anti-corrosive medium such as sulphanilamide, sulphapyridine and sulphathiazole for better performance. The corrosion effect of the sugar-cane juice on the carbon steel roll was studied in [35] along with the effect of austenitic stainless steel on the welded carbon steel roll. In [36], the authors studied the characteristics and corrosion behaviour of high Chromium White Iron. [37] studied the abrasion corrosion test for Iron-Chromium-Carbon shielded metal arc wielding for its used in the sugar industry whereas [38] studied the wear mechanism ploughed by silica in sugar cane roller shell.

4.2 The problem

The problem that mostly faced by the designers is to choose the suitable material for manufacturing equipment in the sugar industry. The different materials and the selection criteria are taken from [39] which are given in the form of **Table 1**.
The different criteria used for selecting the alternatives are as follows:

1. Yield strength (C^1): Yield strength is the most important criteria for material selection. It is a positive criterion. Yield strength does not allow the equipment to deform plastically.

2. Ultimate tensile strength (C^2): It is a measure of material's toughness. It is a positive criterion.

3. % of Elongation (C^3): It is the measure to withstand the operating load. It is a positive criterion.

Alternatives	Criteria	
J4 (A^1)	Yield strength (C^1)	Ultimate tensile strength (C^2)
JSLAUS (A^2)	Percentage of elongation (C^3)	Hardness (C^4)
204Cu (A^3)	Cost (C^5)	Corrosion resistance (C^6)
409M (A^4)	Wear resistance (C^7)	
304 (A^5)		

Table 1.
List of alternatives and the selection criteria.

4. Hardness (C^4): It is the measure to resist plastic deformation due to the applied force. It is a positive criterion.

5. Cost (C^5): It is the monetary value for purchase of the material. More the cost of material, lesser the chance to buy the material. Hence, it is a negative criterion.

6. Corrosion resistance (C^6): It is the measure of the material ability to reduce the binding energy in metals. It is a positive criterion.

7. Wear resistance (C^7): It is the measure of the material ability to resist the wearing. It is a positive criterion

The value of the properties is listed in **Table 2** and it acts as the decision matrix for selection of materials.

4.3 Weighting of criteria

Criteria are weighted by Cross Entropy method (**Table 3**).

4.4 Ranking by COPRAS method

According to COPRAS method alternative 4 i.e. 409M carbon alloy is the best alternative for manufacturing of equipment in sugar industry (**Table 4**).

Alternatives	Criteria						
	C^1	C^2	C^3	C^4	C^5	C^6	C^7
A^1	382	728	48	98	112	0.16	2.75
A^2	420	790	58	97	210	0.31	2.63
A^3	415	795	55	96	120	0.05	2.50
A^4	270	455	32	78	184	0.40	4.00
A^5	256	610	60	86	89	0.01	2.59

Table 2.
Decision matrix.

Criteria	C^1	C^2	C^3	C^4	C^5	C^6	C^7
Weight	0.09872	0.09669	0.09926	0.08166	0.1261	0.4034	0.09418

Table 3.
Table of weights of the criteria.

Material	S_i^+	S_i^-	Q_i	Pr_i	Rank
A^1	0.16619	0.0197534	0.19027	70.72	3
A^2	0.23815	0.0370377	0.25098	93.28	2
A^3	0.12303	0.0211644	0.14549	54.08	4
A^4	0.25441	0.0324521	0.26906	100.00	1
A^5	0.09213	0.0156969	0.12242	45.50	5

Table 4.
Table for ranking of alternatives by COPRAS method.

4.5 Ranking by MOORA method

According to the MOORA method alternative 4 i.e. 409M carbon alloy is the best alternative for manufacturing of equipment in sugar industry (**Table 5**).

4.6 Ranking by VIKOR method

According to the VIKOR method alternative 5 i.e. 304 carbon alloy is the best alternative for manufacturing of equipment in sugar industry (**Table 6**).

4.7 Ranking by TOPSIS method

According to TOPSIS method alternative 4 i.e. 409M carbon alloy is the best alternative for manufacturing of equipment in sugar industry (**Table 7**).

Material	Q_i	Pr_i	Rank
A^1	0.292	70.94	3
A^2	0.384	93.25	2
A^3	0.216	52.41	4
A^4	0.412	100.00	1
A^5	0.167	40.65	5

Table 5.
Table for ranking of alternatives by MOORA method.

Material	γ_j	δ_j	ρ_j	Rank
A^1	0.487	0.155	0.360	3
A^2	0.808	0.310	0.870	5
A^3	0.421	0.097	0.218	2
A^4	0.605	0.403	0.815	4
A^5	0.182	0.099	0.004	1

Table 6.
Table for ranking of alternatives by VIKOR method.

Material	S_m^+	S_m^-	RC_{is}	Rank
A^1	0.183	0.123	0.401	3
A^2	0.084	0.230	0.732	2
A^3	0.266	0.058	0.179	4
A^4	0.052	0.296	0.850	1
A^5	0.297	0.052	0.150	5

Table 7.
Table for ranking of alternatives by TOPSIS method.

Material	S_m^+	S_m^-	RC_{is}	Rank
A^1	0.183	0.123	0.599	3
A^2	0.084	0.230	0.268	2
A^3	0.266	0.058	0.821	4
A^4	0.052	0.296	0.150	1
A^5	0.297	0.052	0.850	5

Table 8.
Table for ranking of alternatives by modified TOPSIS method.

4.8 Ranking by modified TOPSIS method

According to Modified TOPSIS method alternative 4 i.e. 409M carbon alloy is the best alternative for manufacturing of equipment in sugar industry (**Table 8**).

5. Comparative analysis

The 5 different MCDM techniques are compared using the Spearman's rank correlation coefficient (r_s).

5.1 Comparison by r_s

Spearman's rank correlation coefficient (r_s) is the method of comparing the ranks of alternatives obtained from different test. Using r_s, the similarity between two sets of rankings can be measured. The value of r_s usually lies between -1 and 1, where the value of 1 denotes a perfect match between two rank orderings. **Table 10** shows the Spearman's rank correlation coefficient values when the rankings of the material alternatives as obtained employing all the considered MCDM methods are compared between themselves and also with respect to the rank ordering.

From the table it is observed that the value of r_s varies from -0.9 to 1.0. The value of $r_{s\ for}$ a MCDM method when compared with itself is always 1. Hence from the **Table 10** we can conclude the rank obtained from different MCDM models may or may not be in agreement with each other.

5.2 Comparison by R^2

R^2 is a statistic that will give some information about the goodness of fit of a model. In regression analysis, the coefficient of determination is a statistical measure of how well the regression line approximates the real data points. R^2 lies in between 0 to 1. If the value R^2 is 1 then it interprets that the predicted value is exactly equal to the actual value. When the result obtained from different MCDM methods are compared with each other the value of R^2 is shown in **Table 11**.

When the results obtained from different MCDM techniques are compared using regression analysis the maximum value of R^2 obtained is 1 among different combinations of COPRAS, MOORA, TOPSIS and Modified TOPSIS and the least value is 0.81 between VIKOR and COPRAS, MOORA and Modified TOPSIS. From the **Table 11** it can be concluded that there is some penalty for choosing a wrong MCDM method for ranking of alternatives. **Figures 2–11** are the comparative figure of different MCDM techniques.

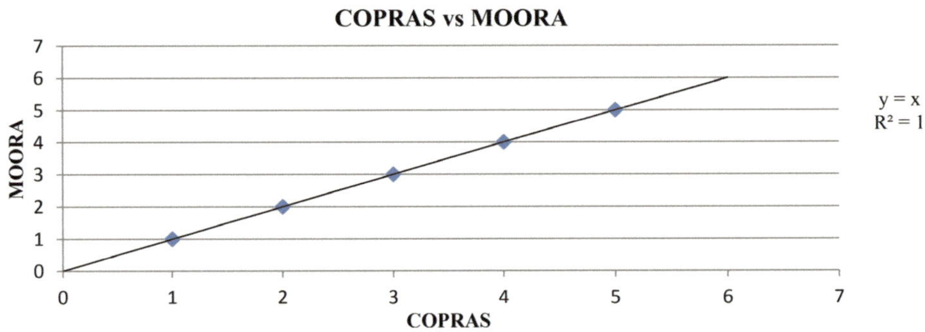

Figure 2.
Comparison of result obtained from COPRAS and MOORA.

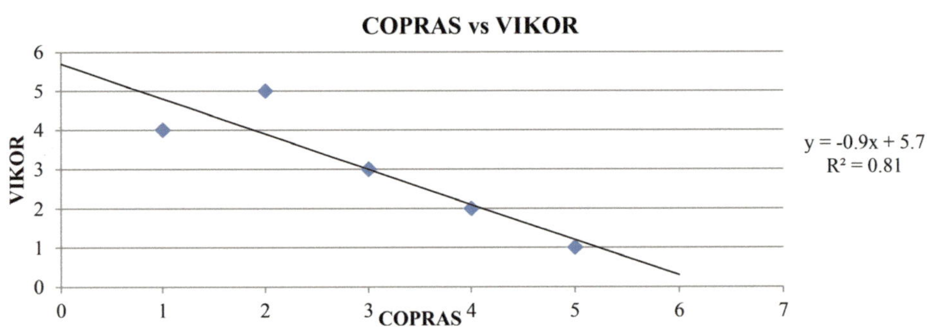

Figure 3.
Comparison of result obtained from COPRAS and VIKOR.

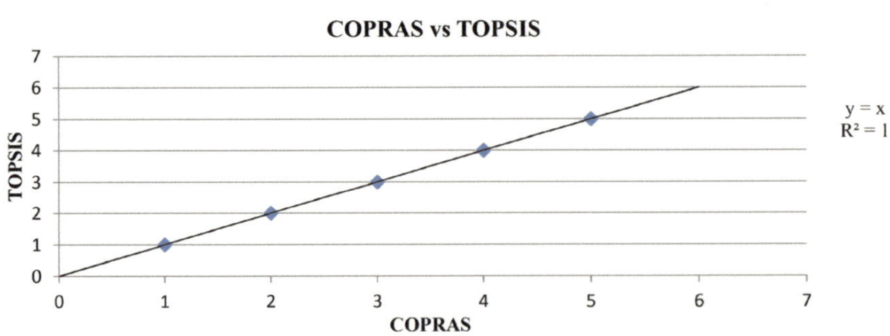

Figure 4.
Comparison of result obtained from COPRAS and TOPSIS.

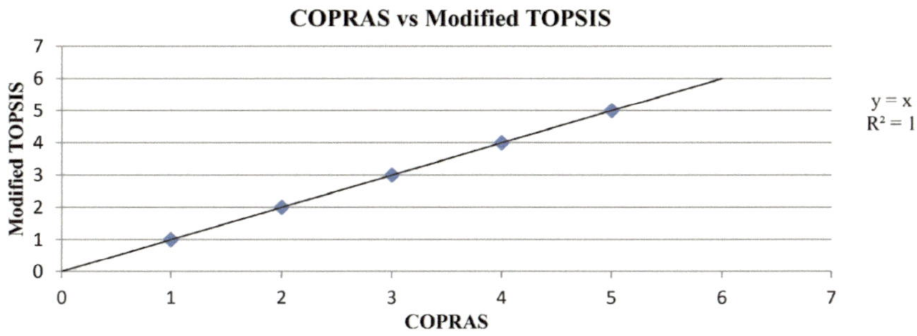

Figure 5.
Comparison of result obtained from COPRAS and modified TOPSIS.

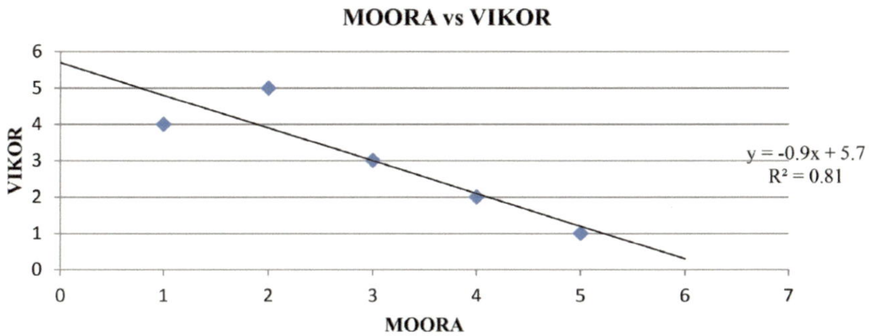

Figure 6.
Comparison of result obtained from MOORA and VIKOR.

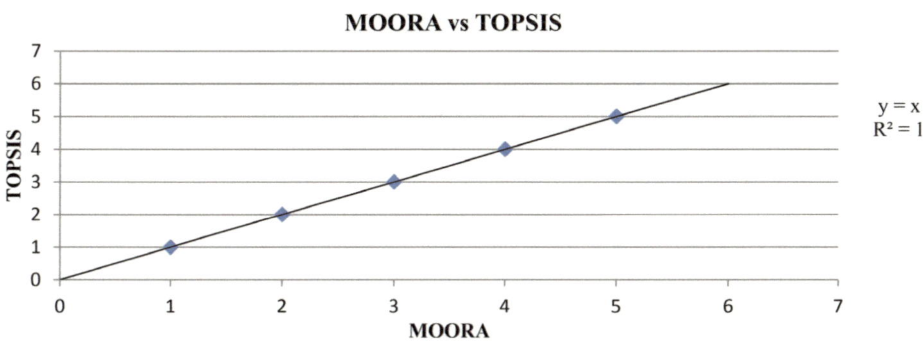

Figure 7.
Comparison of result obtained from MOORA and TOPSIS.

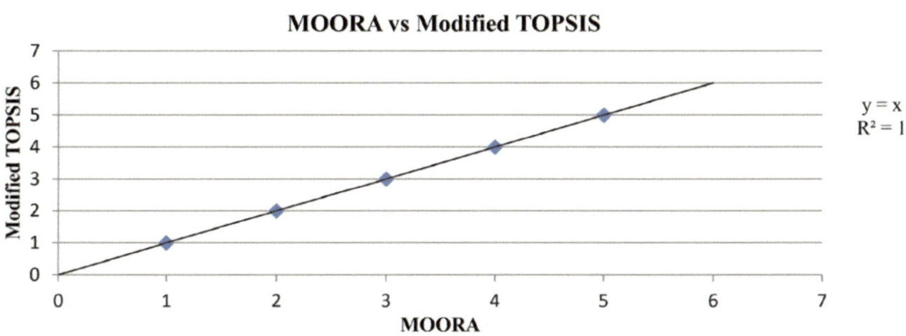

Figure 8.
Comparison of result obtained from MOORA and modified TOPSIS.

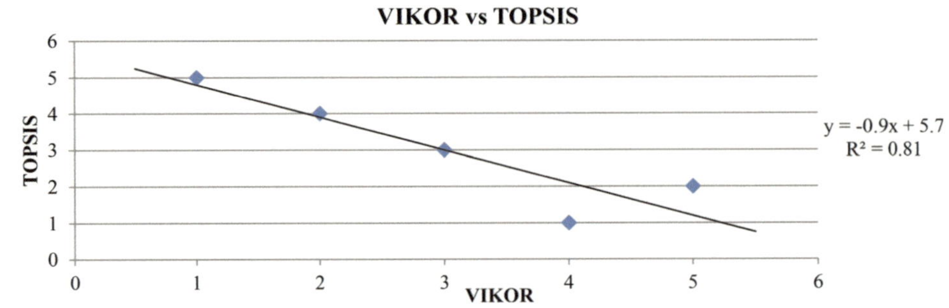

Figure 9.
Comparison of result obtained from VIKOR and TOPSIS.

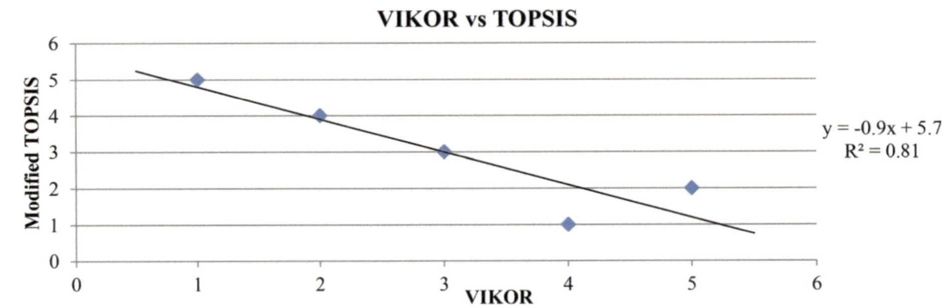

Figure 10.
Comparison of result obtained from VIKOR and modified TOPSIS.

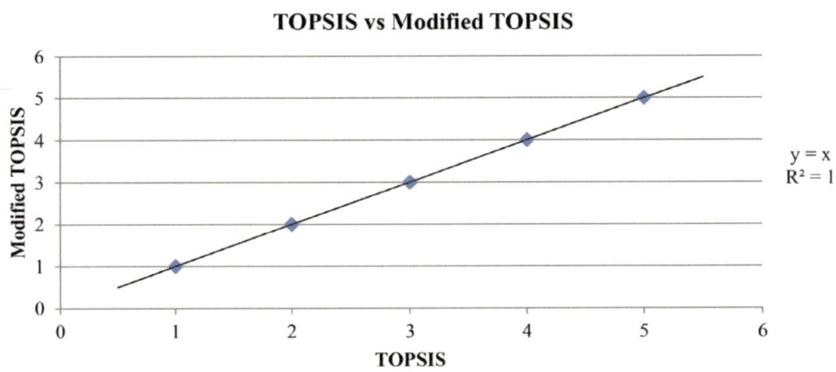

Figure 11.
Comparison of result obtained from TOPSIS and modified TOPSIS.

6. Discussion

As the weights of criteria is the most important parameter for the decision maker to choose the best alternative from a bunch of alternatives. So, in order to compute the best alternative, different integrated cross entropy based MCDM are implemented. The result obtained from different MCDM techniques is then compared with the existing result [39]. The result thus obtained from VIKOR method matches with the existing literature whereas the result obtained from other methods fail to match. From the **Table 9** and **Figure 12**, it was observed that the 4 out of the 5 Multi-Criteria Decision Making methods except VIKOR gives exactly the same result. Hence, it is validated and it can be conclude that 80% of the time alternative 4 is the best alternative for the given problem. But, result obtained from VIKOR

Material	COPRAS	MOORA	VIKOR	TOPSIS	Modified TOPSIS
A^1	3	3	3	3	3
A^2	2	2	5	2	2
A^3	4	4	2	4	4
A^4	1	1	4	1	1
A^5	5	5	1	5	5

Table 9.
Ranking of alternatives by different MCDM methods.

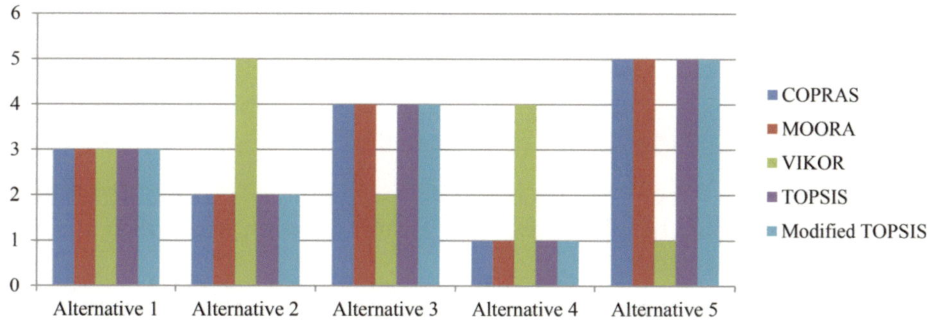

Figure 12.
Ranking by different MCDM methods.

	COPRAS	MOORA	VIKOR	TOPSIS	Modified TOPSIS
COPRAS	1	1	-0.9	1	1
MOORA		1	-0.9	1	1
VIKOR			1	-0.9	-0.9
TOPSIS				1	1
Modified TOPSIS					1

Table 10.
Spearman's rank correlation coefficient.

matches with the [39]. Therefore, a need of comparative analysis arose. The different cross entropy based MCDM methods are compared using Spearman's Rank Correlation Coefficient. From the comparative analysis, the value of r_s is tabulated in the **Table 10**. The regression coefficient value R^2 is tabulated in **Table 11**. From both the table it was found that the result obtained from the VIKOR method strongly disagrees with the result that obtained from the COPRAS, MOORA, TOPSIS and modified TOPSIS. Whereas the result obtained from COPRAS, MOORA, TOPSIS and modified TOPSIS are a perfect match. The reason behind this is that ranking of alternatives totally based on the values of the criteria of the alternatives. If the values of the criteria are changed then there is huge probability of the change in rank of the alternatives.

6.1 Benefits of the present study in industrial information

Benefits of implementing the present study in the industry

	COPRAS	MOORA	VIKOR	TOPSIS	Modified TOPSIS
COPRAS	1	1	0.81	1	1
MOORA		1	0.81	1	1
VIKOR			1	0.81	0.81
TOPSIS				1	1
Modified TOPSIS					1

Table 11.
Table of value of R^2.

- Decisions regarding operational research could be made with confidence.
- The present study can provide opportunities for improvement.
- Archive critical historical data for analysis and reference
- When everyone has unfettered access to the exact and precise predictive model then decision could be taken easily and in short duration which shall act in the favour of the industry.

7. Conclusion

In the present study, an approach to select the best material from a bunch of materials under different criteria is implemented. Although many researches have been conducted in this field, yet no literature exist which can pin point the method to be used for a certain problem. In the present study with the aim of choosing the best alternative, the criteria are weighted using the cross entropy method. Based on their weights the alternatives are ranked and it was observed that the ranking of alternatives is the same for 4 methods out of the 5. From the present study it can be concluded that the alternative 4 i.e 409M carbon alloy is the best alternative.

Acknowledgements

The authors like to extend their heartiest gratitude to the reviewers for their valuable advises and would also like to thank Production Engineering Department of N.I.T Agartala for helping in all possible ways to carry out the work.

List of abbreviations

MCDM	Multi-criteria decision-making
MAGDM	Multi-Attribute Group Decision Making
AHP	Analytical hierarchy process
CE	Cross entropy
COPRAS	Complex Proportional Assessment
MOORA	Multi Objective Optimization on the Basis of Ratio Analysis
VIKOR	VlseKriterijumska Optimizacija I Kompromisno Resenje
TOPSIS	Technique for Order Preference by Similarity to Ideal Solution

Author details

Syed Abou Iltaf Hussain*, Himanshu Chandra and Uttam Kumar Mandal
Production Engineering Department, National Institute of Technology, Agartala, India

*Address all correspondence to: syedaboui8@gmail.com

References

[1] Shanian, A., Savadogo O., 2006. "TOPSIS multiple-criteria decision support analysis for material selection of metallic bipolar plates for polymer electrolyte fuel cell", Journal of Power Sources 159, 1095-1104.

[2] Karande P., Chakraborty S., 2012. "Application of multi-optimization on the basis of ratio analysis (MOORA) method for material selection", Materials and Design 37, 317-324.

[3] Cook, P. (1998). Best Practice Creativity, Aldershot, Gower Publishing Limited.

[4] Čančer, V. (2012). "*Criteria weighting by using the 5Ws & H technique*", Business Systems Research, Vol. 3, No. 2, pp. 41-48.

[5] ZOU Zhi-hong, YUN Yi, SUN Jing-nan (2006). "*Entropy method for determination of weight of evaluating in fuzzy synthetic evaluation for water quality assessment indicators*", Journal of Environmental Science, Vol 18, No. 5, pp. 1020-1023

[6] Wei Liu , Jin Cui (2008). "*Entropy Coefficient Method to Evaluate the Level of Sustainable Development of China's Sports*", International Journal of Sports Science and Engineering Vol. 02 (2008) No. 02, pp. 72-78

[7] Chia-Chang Hung and Liang-Hsuan Chen (2009), "*A Fuzzy TOPSIS Decision Making Model with Entropy Weight under Intuitionistic Fuzzy Environment*", Proceedings of the International MultiConference of Engineers and Computer Scientists, 2009, Vol I, IMECS 2009

[8] Farhad Hosseinzadeh Lotfi and Reza Fallahnejad (2010), "*Imprecise Shannon's Entropy and Multi Attribute Decision Making*" Entropy Journal 2010, Vol 12, pp 53-62

[9] Yuguo Qi, Fushuan Wen, Ke Wang, Li Li, S.N. Singh (2010). "*A Fuzzy Comprehensive Evaluation And Entropy Weight Decision-Making Based Method For Power Network Structure Assessment*" International Journal of Engineering, Science and Technology Vol. 2, No. 5, 2010, pp. 92-99

[10] Peiyue, L., Qian, H. and Jianhua, W. U. (2011) "*Hydrochemical formation mechanisms and quality assessment of groundwater with improved TOPSIS method in Pengyang county northwest China*", *E-Journal of Chemistry*, Vol. 8, No. 3, pp. 1164–1173.

[11] Kshitij Dashore, Shashank Singh Pawar, Nagendra Sohani, Devendra Singh Verma (2013). "*Product Evaluation Using Entropy and Multi Criteria Decision Making Methods*", International Journal of Engineering Trends and Technology (IJETT) - Volume4Issue5- May 2013

[12] Deepa Joshi and Sanjay Kumar (2014). "*Intuitionistic fuzzy entropy and distance measure based TOPSIS method for multi-criteria decision making*", Egyptian Informatics Journal (2014) 15, 97–104

[13] Anhai Li, Jun Zhao , Zhaochao Gong and Fenghua Lin (2015). "*Optimal Selection of Cutting Tool Materials Based on Multi-Criteria Decision-Making Methods in Machining Al-Si Piston Alloy*" International Journal of Manufacturing Technology

[14] Harish Garg, Nikunj Agarwal and Alka Choubey (2015). "*Entropy Based Multi-criteria Decision Making Method under Fuzzy Environment and Unknown Attribute Weights*" Global Journal of Technology & Optimization, 2015, Vol 6 No. 3

[15] Zhang-peng Tian , Hong-yu Zhang , Jing Wang , Jian-qiang Wang and

Xiao-hong Chen (2015). "*Multi-criteria decision-making method based on a cross-entropy with interval neutrosophic sets*", INTERNATIONAL JOURNAL OF SYSTEMS SCIENCE 2015

[16] Elham Ebrahimi, Mohammad Reza Fathi, Hamid Reza Irani (2016). "*A new hybrid method based on fuzzy Shannon's Entropy and fuzzy COPRAS for CRM performance evaluation (Case: Mellat Bank)*", Iranian Journal of Management Studies (IJMS) Vol. 9, No. 2, Spring 2016 pp. 333-358

[17] Harish Garg (2016). "*A New Generalized Improved Score Function of Interval-Valued Intuitionistic Fuzzy Sets and Applications in Expert Systems*" Applied Soft Computing 38 (2016) 988–999

[18] Javier Martínez-Gómez, Gonzalo Guerrón, Ricardo A. Narvaez C (2016). "*Cookware material selection by multi-criteria decision making (MCDM) methods*", International Journal of Engineering Trends and Technology (IJETT) – Volume 34, Number 8, pp 394-398

[19] Rao, R. V., & Patel, B. K. (2010). "*A subjective and objective integrated multiple attribute decision making method for material selection*". Materials and Design, 37(10), 4738-4747.

[20] Ashby MF, Brechet YJM, Cebon D, Salvo L. (2004) "*Selection Strategies For Materials And Processes*". Material & Design ; 25:51–67.

[21] A. S. Milani, A. Shanian, R. Madoliat, and J. A. Nemes (2005), "*The effect of normalization norms in multiple attribute decision making models: A case study in gear material selection,*" Structural and Multidisciplinary Optimization, vol. 29, no. 4, pp. 312-318

[22] R.V. Rao and J.P. Davim (2006). "*A decision-making framework model for material selection using a combined multiple attribute decision-making method*", International Journal Advanced Manufacturing Technology 35:751–760

[23] Shanian A, Savadogo O. (2006) "*Topsis Multiple-Criteria Decision Support Analysis for Material Selection of Metallic bipolar Plates for Polymer Electrolyte Fuel Cell*". J Power Sources; 159:1095–104.

[24] Shanian A, Savadogo O. (2006) "*ELECTRE I Decision Support Model for Material Selection of Bipolar Plates for Polymer Electrolyte Fuel Cells Applications*". Journal of New Materials for Electrochemical Systems 9, 191-199

[25] A. M. M. Sharif Ullah and K. H. Harib (2008), "*An intelligent method for selecting optimal materials and its application,*" *Advanced Engineering Information*, vol. 22, no. 4, pp. 473-483.

[26] Karande, P., & Chakraborty, S. (2012). "*Application of multi-objective optimization on the basis of ratio analysis (MOORA) method for materials selection*". Materials and Design, 37, 317-324.

[27] Shankar Chakraborty and Prasenjit Chatterjee (2013) "*Selection Of Materials Using Multi-Criteria Decision-Making Methods With Minimum Data*". Decision Science Letters 2 ;135–148

[28] Zavadskas, E.K., F. Peldschus and A. Kaklauskas (1994). "*Multiple Criteria Evaluation of Projects in Construction*". Technika, Vilnius.

[29] Janis, Irving L. and Mann, Leon (1977). "Decision making: A psychological analysis of conflict, choice, and commitment", New York: Free Press. ISBN 0029161606. OCLC 2542340

[30] *Guo and Kristina L. (June 2008). "DECIDE: A decision-making model for more effective decision making by health*

care managers". The Health Care Manager 27 (2): 118–127.

[31] Jahanshahloo GR, Lotfi FH, Izadikhah M. An algorithmic method to extend TOPSIS for decision-making problems with interval data. Applied Mathematics and Computation [Internet]. Elsevier BV; 2006 Apr;175 (2):1375–84. Available from: http://dx.doi.org/10.1016/j.amc.2005.08.048

[32] Pravin, G., Rajesh, K., Singhal, L. K., & Goyal, R. K. (2007). "Role of stainless steel to combat corrosion in the Indian sugar industry", International Sugar Journal, 109(1303), 449–453.

[33] Wesley, S. B., Goyal, H. S., & Mishra, S. C. (2012). "Corrosion behavior of ferritic steel, austenitic steel and low carbon steel grades in sugarcane juice", Journal of Materials & Metallurgical Engineering, 2(1), 9–22.

[34] Rajesh Kumar, S. (2011). "Corrosion protection of mild steel in sugar industry. International Journal of Food", Agriculture and Veterinary Sciences, 1 (1), 75–82.

[35] Prado, R. V., Uquilla, B., Aguilar, J., Aguilar, Y., & Casanova, F. (2010). "Abrasive wear effect of sugarcane juice on sugarcane rolls", Wear, 270, 83–87.

[36] Zumelzu, E., Cabezas, C., Opitz, O., Quiroz, E., Goyos, L., & Parada, A. (2003). "Microstructural characteristics and corrosion behaviour of high-chromium cast iron alloys in sugar media", Protection of Metals, 39(2), 183–188.

[37] Buchanan, V. E., Shipway, P. H., & McCartney, D. G. (2010). "Microstructure and abrasive wear behaviour of shielded metal arc welding hard facings used in the sugarcane industry", Wear, 263, 99–110.

[38] Casanova, F., & Aguilar, Y. (2008). "A study on the wear of sugar cane rolls", Wear, 265, 236–243.

[39] L. Anojkumar, M. Ilangkumaran, V. Sasirekha (2014) "Comparative analysis of MCDM methods for pipe material selection in sugar industry", Expert Systems with Applications 41, 2964–2980.

Chapter 6

Plithogenic SWARA-TOPSIS Decision Making on Food Processing Methods with Different Normalization Techniques

Nivetha Martin

Abstract

Decision making (DM) is a process of choosing the optimal alternative with the maximum extent of criteria satisfaction. The challenging aspect in making optimal decisions is the suitable choice of multi-criteria decision-making (MCDM) methods that consider the initial input as the expert's opinion on criteria satisfaction by the alternatives. This initial decision-making matrix representation discriminates MCDM as fuzzy, intuitionistic, neutrosophic to handle the decision-making environment that is characterized by uncertainty, impreciseness, and indeterminacy, respectively. A generalized kind of representation by plithogenic sets optimizes the decision-making risks. This chapter aims in developing SWARA-TOPSIS with plithogenic representations and discusses the efficiency of this integrated approach over the method of TOPSIS with equal criterion weight. A comparative analysis of four different normalization techniques is likewise made. The proposed plithogenic integrated MCDM model is validated with the decision making on four food processing methods. The final ranks of the alternatives are also compared under the proposed plithogenic SWARA-TOPSIS and TOPSIS models with different normalization techniques. The results witness the efficiency of the proposed model over the existing models.

Keywords: optimality, MCDM, SWARS-TOPSIS, plithogeny

1. Introduction

Multi-criteria decision-making (MCDM) methods are classified into multi-attribute decision-making and multi-objective decision-making in which the former determines the optimal alternatives and the latter finds the optimal alternatives that optimize the objective. The MCDM methods comprise a sequence of steps to derive the optimal solution to the decision-making problem. DM is the system of choosing the best alternative satisfying all the criteria to a great extent with the expert's assist, but the crucial thing is finding the criterion weight. At some circumstances, the criterion weights are assumed to be equal but it is not so in all the cases. The criterion weight states the significance of criteria and henceforth, the calculation of criterion weight is very essential. There are many methods to find the criterion weights such as analytic hierarchical process (AHP), analytic network process (ANP), best worst method (BWM), full consistency method (FUCOM), and stepwise weight assessment ratio analysis (SWARA). The method of SWARA appears to be simple and flexible in comparison with other methods of determining the criterion weight based on human expertise and it has several applications in prioritizing sustainability indicators of energy systems [1]. The method of TOPSIS (the technique for order of preference by similarity to ideal solution) is commonly used to rank the alternatives as it yields the best results in comparison with other methods and it has been discussed in a fuzzy environment by Neelima et al. [2] and Ansari et al. [3]. Babak et al. [4] and Houssine et al. [5] discussed TOPSIS under intuitionistic fuzzy and neutrosophic [6] environments.

The method of SWARA was used in combination with crisp COPRAS [7], fuzzy COPRAS [8], crisp VIKOR [9, 10], neutrosophic VIKOR [11], WASPAS [12], Delphi [13], ARAS, GRA [14], TOPSIS in different decision-making setting. The integrated approach of SWARA-TOPSIS was inferred to yield better results based on the study on its applications in supplier selection [15], reducing ecological risk factors [16], prioritizing the failures in a solar panel system. This integrated approach was discussed in the environments of fuzzy [17], intuitionistic, and neutrosophic [18, 19]. Ahmet et al. [20], Miranda et al. [21], and Nazanin et al. [22] discussed different data normalization techniques. To give a comprehensive picture of representing the expert's opinion, this integrated approach is discussed under plithogenic environment in this paper, which is not explored so far to the best of the knowledge. At recent times, researchers develop novel plithogenic MCDM methods. In these plithogenic decision-making models, the plithogenic operators together with the contradiction degree are used to find the aggregate opinion of the experts regarding the criterion satisfaction rate of the alternatives.

In this research work, plithogenic SWARA-TOPSIS is developed by applying plithogenic intersection operator to the expert's opinion on the initial decision-making matrix. The efficiency of different normalization techniques of the weighted matrices is determined by applying them to two different cases. The first case is plithogenic TOPSIS with equal criterion weight, and the second is plithogenic SWAR-TOPSIS. The comparison of both the cases will certainly unveil the efficiency of the proposed approach. The remaining content is segmented as follows, Section 2 presents the methodology; the section consists of the application of the proposed method to the decision-making of food processing technology; Section 4 discusses the result and the last section concludes the work (**Table 1**).

AHP	analytic hierarchical process
ANP	analytic network process
ARAS	additive ratio assessment method
BWM	best worst method
COPRAS	complex proportional assessment
FUCOM	full consistency method
GRA	gray relational analysis
SWARA	stepwise weight assessment ratio analysis
TOPSIS	technique for order of preference by similarity to ideal solution
VIKOR	VlseKriterijuska Optimizacija. I Komoromisno Resenje
WASPAS	weighted aggregated sum product assessment

Table 1.
List of acronyms.

2. Methodology

The method of plithogenic SWARA-TOPSIS is used to find the ranking of the alternatives. The steps involved are as follows:

Step 1: The initial decision-making matrix of order $u \times v$ with u alternatives and v criteria is constructed from the expert's perspective. This matrix consists of the criterion satisfaction by the alternatives, and the representation is made by using linguistic variables such as very high, high, moderate, low, and very low. The linguistic terms are not confined to these values alone. In general, a minimum of two expert's opinions is considered in framing the initial decision-making matrix. The aggregate expert's opinion is obtained using plithogenic intersection operators based on the representations (Fuzzy/intuitionistic/neutrosophic) of the linguistic variables.

Plithogenic Fuzzy Intersection $a \bigwedge_F b$.

Plithogenic Intuitionistic Intersection $(a_1, a_2) \wedge_{IFS} (b_1, b_2) = (a_1 \wedge_F b_1, a_2 \vee_F b_2)$

Plithogenic Neutrosophic Intersection $(a_1, a_2, a_3) \wedge_P (b_1, b_2, b_3) = (a_1 \vee_F b_1, \frac{1}{2}[(a_2 \wedge_F b_2) + (a_2 \vee_F b_2), a_3 \wedge_F b_3])$

$$a \bigwedge_F b = ab, a \vee_F b = a + b - ab$$

Step 2: The criterion weights are obtained by the method of SWARA, which are as follows:

i. The criteria are arranged in descending order by the experts based on their significance.

ii. The relative importance of the criterion placed in (h-1)th position over hth gives the comparative importance of the average value s_h

iii. The relative weights w_j of the evaluation criteria is determined

$$w_h = \frac{q_h}{\sum_{k=1}^{v} q_k}$$

where q_j, the recalculated weight

$$q_h = \begin{cases} 1 & h = 1 \\ \dfrac{q_{h-1}}{k_h} & h > 1 \end{cases} \text{ and } k_h = \begin{cases} 1 & h = 1 \\ s_{h+1} & h > 1 \end{cases}$$

Step 3: After finding the criterion weights by the method of SWARA, the aggregate normalized weighted matrix $D = (d_{ih})$ is determined by using any of the normalization techniques before which the criteria are classified as benefit criteria and cost criteria, where the former must be maximized and the latter to be minimized. The four normalization techniques are shown in **Table 2**.

Step 4: The positive ideal solution $D^+ = (d_1^+, d_2^+, d_3^+, \ldots d_v^+) = \max(d_{ih})$ for benefit criteria and $\min(d_{ih})$ for cost criteria. The negative ideal solution $D^- = (d_1^-, d_2^-, d_3^-, \ldots d_v^-) = \min(d_{ih})$ for benefit criteria and $\max(d_{ih})$ for cost criteria.

Normalization technique	Benefit criteria	Cost criteria
Linear scale transformation max method (NT1)	$\frac{x_{ih}}{x_{i\ max}}$	$\frac{x_{i\ min}}{x_{ih}}$
Linear scale transformation max-min method (NT2)	$\frac{x_{ih} - \min x_{ih}}{\max x_{ih} - \min x_{ih}}$	$\frac{\max x_{ih} - x_{ih}}{\max x_{ih} - \min x_{ih}}$
Linear scale transformation sum method (NT3)	$\frac{x_{ih}}{\sum_{i=1}^{u} x_i}$	$1 - \frac{x_{ih}}{\sum_{i=1}^{u} x_i}$
Vector-normalization method (NT4)	$\frac{x_{ih}}{\sqrt{\sum_{i=1}^{u} x_{ih}^2}}$	$1 - \frac{x_{ih}}{\sqrt{\sum_{i=1}^{u} x_{ih}^2}}$

Table 2.
Normalization techniques.

Step 5: F_i^+, the distance between the alternatives and the positive ideal solution F_i^- is the distance between the alternatives and the negative ideal solution is calculated as follows:

$$F_i^+ = \sqrt{\sum\nolimits_{h=1}^{v} \left(d_h^+ - d_{ih}\right)^2}; i = 1, 2, \ldots u$$

$$F_i^- = \sqrt{\sum\nolimits_{h=1}^{v} \left(d_h^- - d_{ih}\right)^2}; i = 1, 2, \ldots u$$

Step 6: The relative closeness to the ideal solution $R_i = \frac{F_i^-}{\left(F_i^+ - F_i^-\right)}$ is determined and the preferential ranking of the alternatives is made by the values of R_i. The alternatives with high scores are ranked from high to low.

3. Application to decision making on food processing methods

The proposed plithogenic SWARA-TOPSIS is illustrated with the decision making on the food processing technology. Food processing industries are the flourishing kind of industries in recent times. The lifestyle of the present generation has increased the consumption of processed food to a maximum extent. The consumers of processed food are quite steadily increasing as it is becoming inevitable. In general, these food industries employ various food processing technology for consumer acceptability and also introduce modern technology to meet the customer needs [23, 24].

The decision-making environment consists of four alternatives and five criteria that are stated as follows in **Table 3**.

The initial linguistic decision-making matrices given by two decision-makers are as follows:

Expert I

Methods Criteria	Z1	Z2	Z3	Z4	Z5
P1	M	H	M	H	M
P2	L	H	M	L	M
P3	M	H	VH	M	H
P4	VH	H	H	H	VH

Alternatives	Criteria
Chemical processing (P1)	Capital costs (Z1)
Biological processing (P2)	Microbial prevention (Z2)
Thermal processing (P3)	Time efficiency (Z3)
Non-thermal processing (P4)	Nutrients conservativeness (Z4)
	Longevity of shelf life (Z5)

Table 3.
Alternatives and criteria of the decision-making environment.

Linguistic terms	Neutrosophic representations
Very High (VH)	(0.95, 0.1, 0.1)
High (H)	(0.8, 0.2, 0.1)
Moderate (M)	(0.5, 0.5, 0.5)
Low (L)	(0.3, 0.7, 0.8)
Very Low (VL)	(0.1, 0.9, 0.9)

Table 4.
Quantification of linguistic terms.

Expert II

Methods Criteria	Z1	Z2	Z3	Z4	Z5
P1	H	VH	H	H	M
P2	VL	M	H	L	M
P3	H	VH	H	M	VH
P4	VH	VH	VH	H	H

Neutrosophic representations are used to quantify the linguistic values as given in **Table 4**.

The plithogenic aggregated expert decision matrix is

Methods Criteria	Z1	Z2	Z3	Z4	Z5
P1	0.397	0.5766	0.397	0.5678	0.3076
P2	0.073	0.397	0.397	0.167	0.3076
P3	0.397	0.5766	0.5766	0.3076	0.5766
P4	0.579	0.5766	0.5766	0.5678	0.5766

Case I: The criterion weights are assumed to be equal and the alternatives are ranked based on the scores of R_i obtained by using four different normalization techniques.

Normalization technique		Normalized weighted decision-making matrix					R_i	Rank
		Z1	Z2	Z3	Z4	Z5		
Linear scale transformation max method	P1	0.2	0.137704	0.196948	0.106694	0.2	0.664386	3
	P2	0.137704	0.137704	0.057926	0.106694	0.137704	0	4
	P3	0.2	0.2	0.106694	0.2	0.2	0.700953	2
	P4	0.2	0.2	0.196948	0.2	0.2	1	1
Linear scale transformation max-min method	P1	0.071937	0.2	0	0.2	0	0.51547	3
	P2	0.2	0	0	0	0	0	4
	P3	0.071937	0.2	0.2	0.07016	0.2	0.716921	2
	P4	0	0.2	0.2	0.2	0.2	1	1
Linear scale transformation sum method	P1	0.14509	0.054222	0.040776	0.070525	0.034789	0.613146	2
	P2	0.189903	0.037333	0.040776	0.020743	0.034789	0	4
	P3	0.14509	0.054222	0.059224	0.038206	0.065211	0.602772	3
	P4	0.119917	0.054222	0.059224	0.070525	0.065211	1	1
Vector-normalization method	P1	0.101952	0.107303	0.0802	0.129641	0.066565	0.605883	3
	P2	0.181971	0.07388	0.0802	0.03813	0.066565	0	4
	P3	0.101952	0.107303	0.116482	0.070232	0.124776	0.607144	2
	P4	0.057003	0.107303	0.116482	0.129641	0.124776	1	1

Case II: The criterion weights are obtained by using the method of SWARA: Expert I

Criteria	S_h	K_h	W_h	q_h
Z1	1	1	1	0.288
Z3	0.25	1.25	0.8	0.23
Z2	0.3	1.3	0.62	0.179
Z4	0.15	1.15	0.54	0.156
Z5	0.07	1.07	0.51	0.147

Expert II

Criteria	S_h	K_h	W_h	q_h
Z1	1	1	1	0.33
Z3	0.35	1.35	0.74	0.24
Z2	0.4	1.4	0.53	0.17
Z4	0.25	1.25	0.42	0.14
Z5	0.17	1.17	0.36	0.12

Criteria	Z1	Z2	Z3	Z4	Z5
Weight	0.31	0.24	0.17	0.15	0.13

Normalization technique		Normalized weighted decision-making matrix					R_i	Rank
		Z1	Z2	Z3	Z4	Z5		
Linear scale transformation max method	P1	0.057002	0.24	0.117048	0.147711	0.069351	0.922045	3
	P2	0.31	0.165245	0.117048	0.043444	0.069351	0	4
	P3	0.057002	0.24	0.17	0.080021	0.13	0.940439	2
	P4	0.039084	0.24	0.17	0.147711	0.13	1	1
Linear scale transformation max-min method	P1	0.111502	0.24	0	0.15	0	0.672361	3
	P2	0.31	0	0	0	0	0	4
	P3	0.111502	0.24	0.17	0.05262	0.13	0.869149	2
	P4	0	0.24	0.17	0.15	0.13	1	1
Linear scale transformation sum method	P1	0.22489	0.065067	0.03466	0.052894	0.022613	0.754312	1
	P2	0.29435	0.0448	0.03466	0.015557	0.022613	0	4
	P3	0.22489	0.065067	0.05034	0.028655	0.042387	0.105651	3
	P4	0.185871	0.065067	0.05034	0.052894	0.042387	0.291429	2
Vector-normalization method	P1	0.158026	0.128763	0.06817	0.097231	0.043267	0.749931	2
	P2	0.282055	0.088656	0.06817	0.028597	0.043267	0	4
	P3	0.158026	0.128763	0.099009	0.052674	0.081105	0.425359	3
	P4	0.088355	0.128763	0.099009	0.097231	0.081105	0.85551	1

4. Results

The results obtained in both the cases are summarized as follows in **Table 5**, and the relative closeness scores under both the cases are presented in **Figures 1** and **2**.

Based on the rankings of the alternatives obtained under both the cases, it clearly gives the preferential ranking of the alternatives. In almost all the cases, nonthermal

Normalization technique	Case I	Case II
Linear scale transformation max method	P4 > P3 > P1 > P2	P4 > P3 > P1 > P2
Linear scale transformation max-min method	P4 > P3 > P1 > P2	P4 > P3 > P1 > P2
Linear scale transformation sum method	P4 > P1 > P3 > P2	P1 > P4 > P3 > P2
Vector-normalization method	P4 > P3 > P1 > P2	P4 > P1 > P3 > P2

Table 5.
Ranking of the alternatives under cases I and II.

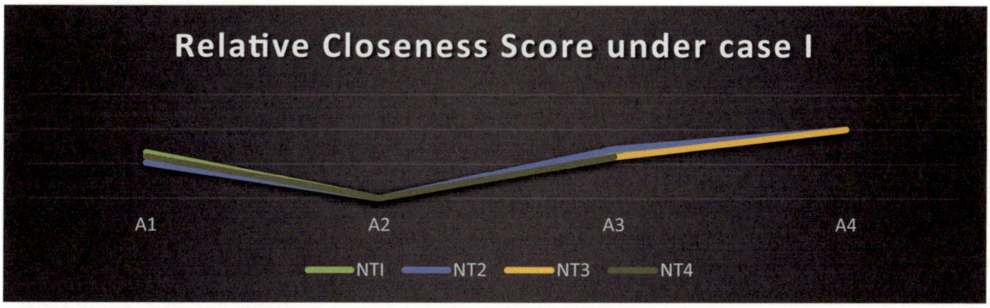

Figure 1.
Relative Closeness Score under case I.

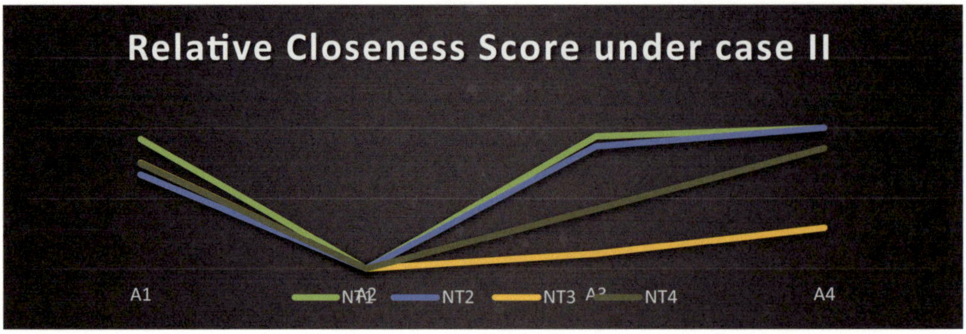

Figure 2.
Relative Closeness Score under case II.

processing technology acquires the first preference and chemical processing technology acquires the last preference. This ranking is validated under both the cases when various normalization techniques are used. The aggregate decision matrix obtained by using the plithogenic aggregate operators adds to the consistency of the proposed model. The ranking results differ only in both the cases under the normalization technique of the linear scale transformation sum method.

5. Conclusion

An integrated plithogenic SWARA-TOPSIS decision-making model is developed in this paper. A comparative analysis of various normalization techniques under two cases is made to determine the most preferred and least preferred food processing technology. The application of plithogenic to such a hybrid method is the novelty of this decision-making model. The proposed model shall be extended by using other plithogenic kinds of aggregate operators. This research work will certainly encourage the researchers to explore the applications of the proposed approach in various dimensions. The results obtained will also benefit the decision-makers in making an optimal selection on food processing technology.

Author details

Nivetha Martin
Department of Mathematics, Arul Anandar College (Autonomous), Madurai, Tamil Nadu, India

*Address all correspondence to: nivetha.martin710@gmail.com

References

[1] Zolfani SH, Šaparauskas J. New application of SWARA method in prioritizing sustainability assessment indicators of energy system. Engineering Economics. 2013;**24**:408-414

[2] Kore NB, Ravi K, Patil SB. A simplified description of FUZZY TOPSIS method for multi criteria decision making. International Research Journal of Engineering and Technology. 2017;**4**(5):1-4

[3] Jamal Ansari MT, Ahmed Al-Zahrani F, Pandey D, Agrawal A. A fuzzy TOPSIS based analysis toward selection of effective security requirements engineering approach for trustworthy healthcare software development. BMC Medical Informatics and Decision Making. 2020;**20**:1-13

[4] Rouyendegh BD, Yildizbasi A, Arikan UZB. Using intuitionistic fuzzy TOPSIS in site selection of wind power plants in Turkey. Adv. Fuzzy Syst. 2018; **2018**:1-14

[5] Tlig H, Rebi A. A TOPSIS method based on intuitionistic fuzzy values: A case study of North African airports. Management Science Letters. 2017;**7**:351-358

[6] Elhassouny A, Smarandache F. Neutrosophic-simplified-TOPSIS. Multi-criteria decision-making using combined simplified-TOPSIS method and neutrosophics. In: IEEE International Conference on Fuzzy Systems. 2016. Conference Proceedings; pp. 2468-2474

[7] Zavadskas EK, Hasan Aghdaie M, Hashemkhani Zolfani S. Decision making in machine tool selection: An integrated approach with SWARA and COPRAS-G methods. Engineering Economics. 2013;**24**(1):5-17

[8] Mishra AR, Rani P, Pandey K, Mardani A, Streimikis J, Streimikiene D, et al. Novel multi-criteria intuitionistic fuzzy SWARA–COPRAS approach for sustainability evaluation of the bioenergy production process. Sustainability. 2020;**12**(10):1-16

[9] Alimardani M, Hashemkhani Zolfani S, Hasan Aghdaie M, Tamosaitiene J. A novel hybrid SWARA and VIKOR methodology for economy. Technological and Economic Development of Economy. 2013;**19**(3): 533-548

[10] Geetha S, Narayanamoorthy S, Kang D. Extended hesitant fuzzy SWARA techniques to examine the criteria weights and VIKOR method for ranking alternatives. In: AIP Conference Proceedings. 2020. Conference Proceedings; p. 2261

[11] Salamai AA. An integrated neutrosophic SWARA and VIKOR method for ranking risks of green supply chain. Neutrosophic Sets and Systems. 2021;**41**:113-125

[12] Mardani A, Nilashi M, Zakuan N, Loganathan N, Soheilirad S, Mat Saman MZ, et al. A systematic review and meta-analysis of SWARA and WASPAS methods: Theory and applications with recent fuzzy developments. Applied Soft Computing. 2017;**57**:265-292

[13] Karabasevic D, Stanujkic D, Urosevic S, Popović H, Maksimovic M. An approach to criteria weights determination by integrating the DELPHI and the adapted SWARA methods. Management: Journal of Sustainable Business and Management Solutions in Emerging Economies. 2017; **22**(3):15-25

[14] Ghoushchi SJ, AbRahman MN, Raeisi D, Osgooei E, Ghoushji MJ. Integrated decision-making approach based on SWARA and GRA methods for

the prioritization of failures in solar panel systems under Z-information. Symmetry. 2020;**12**(2):1-21

[15] Narayanan AK, Jinesh N. Application of SWARA and TOPSIS methods for supplier selection in a casting unit. International Journal of Engineering Research & Technology. 2018;7(5):456-458

[16] Akcan S, Taş MA. Green supplier evaluation with SWARA-TOPSIS integrated method to reduce ecological risk factors. Environmental Monitoring and Assessment. 2019;**191**(12):1-22

[17] Percin S. An integrated fuzzy SWARA and fuzzy AD approach for outsourcing provider selection. Journal of Manufacturing Technology Management. 2019;**30**:531-552

[18] Ayca Supciller A, Toprak F. Selection of wind turbines with multi-criteria decision making techniques involving neutrosophic numbers: A case from Turkey. Energy. 2020;**207**:1-8

[19] Nada AN, Smarandache F, Abdel-Basset M, Haitham AE, Aboelfetouh A. An integrated neutrosophic-TOPSIS approach and its application to personnel selection: A new trend in brain processing and analysis. IEEE Access. 2019;7:29734-29744

[20] Aytekin A. Comparative analysis of the normalization techniques in the context of MCDM problems. Decision Making: Applications in Management and Engineering. 2021;**4**(2):1-27

[21] Miranda Lakshmi T, Vetriselvi K, Joshuva Anand A, Prasanna Venkatesan V. A study on different types of normalization methods in adaptive technique for order preference by similarity to ideal solution (TOPSIS). International Journal of Engineering Research & Technology. 2016;**4**(5):1-7

[22] Vafaei N, Ribeiro RA, Camarinha-Matos LM. Data normalisation techniques in decision making: Case study with TOPSIS method. International Journal of Information and Decision Sciences. 2018;**10**(1):19-38

[23] https://mastermilk.com/uploads/biblio/food_process_engineering_and_technology.pdf

[24] https://New_Food_Processing_Technologies_Development_and_Impact_on_Consumer_Acceptability

Chapter 7

Innovation Methodologies to Activate Inclusive Growth in the Organization

Garazi Carranza Ruiz de Loizaga and Begoña Sanchez Gonzalez

Abstract

Digitalization is transforming the way we move and produce, encouraging the industry to use the best available technologies focusing on people. Non technological innovations, especially, Workplace Innovation (WI) will play a key role in the digital revolution and acceleration of the technological advances, improving the competitiveness of the companies. This draws attention to the importance of the innovation culture and employee engagement focused on improving employee motivation and working conditions, thereby improving labor productivity, organizational efficiency, innovation capacity, market reactivity, and, as a result, business competitiveness. WI is a combination of structural and cultural practices that boosts employees' participation, improving the quality of work and organizational performance. These strategies aim to promote innovative work behavior to create, introduce and apply new ideas, processes and products. To address these issues this chapter analyses WI in rail sector and defines WI Scheme for rail sector. A theoretical background is presented based on a sample of 203 railway entities across European Union (EU). Then, data analysis and results are examined and the guide to implement WI scheme is defined. Finally, the results of the research, including limitations and concluding remarks are discussed.

Keywords: workplace innovation, business management, decision management, innovation, organizational innovation, open culture

1. Introduction

In recent years, the transformation of the organizational culture has become a disruptive way for companies to grow and innovate. Business practitioners, researchers and leaders are paying attention to innovation in the workplace to improve the organizational performance. Additionally, the COVID-19 crisis has highlighted the importance of digitalization and the need to fast-track the progress in technological innovations developed up to date. Consequently, the industry, no matters from which sector, needs to engage in the process of continuous improvement for being prepared to the new revolution in order to maintain their competitive advantage. In this situation, the role of Workplace Innovation (WI) is considered as an engine to improve organizations' ability to continuously generate innovations.

Rail is synonymous of technology, efficiency and sustainability. The railway industry is an important sector for Europe, with a turnover of 492 billion of euros. Since 2017, the industry's annual growth has been 3,6 and is expected to grow further at a rate of 2,3% until 2025 [1]. However, due to COVID-19 crisis the transport demand has been reduced by approximately 90% affecting the railway sector. The decrease of passenger and freight volumes results in postponements and cancelations of orders, as well as a lower services volume [1]. Although the railway sector has been affected by the consequences of the pandemic, there is a need to highlight rail transport plays a vital role in preserving the environment due to the low CO2 emissions, as well as supporting European society and its economy [2]. In this sense, the competitiveness and productivity growth of the railway industry depends, among other factors, on the company's ability to innovate, and rail research is a key driving force for Europe to maintain its competitiveness in technological development.

Social, economic and technological changes have driven the railway's sector migration towards the Open Innovation model. In spite of the great pressure from the business environment trends, stakeholders from the rail industry are still reluctant to open up their innovation strategy. WI has not been the sector's priority up to date, as it has been focused primarily on technological innovation to adapt to market demands. Therefore, the biggest challenge has been focused on providing innovative products offering quickness and flexibility to respond the changing customer's demands.

Technological innovation needs to be implemented together with non-technological innovation and WI presents an opportunity for this. This chapter develops and tests a research model based on WI concept on railway's companies by considering the literature and research related to the employees' personal innovation behavior, organizational practices, process practices as well as the impact on company performance. WI scheme developed for rail sector, is an overview of the results obtained by RailActivation project, which has received funding from the European Union's Horizon 2020 research and innovation program under grant agreement No 861887. The chapter analyses the key competences and skills that presently characterize the rail industry, and to draw a general picture of how these are developed, in which context, and through which particular mentoring process. Then, data analysis and results are examined to develop the WI scheme and a guide to implement it is defined. Finally, the research findings are discussed, including the limitations and concluding remarks.

2. Theoretical background

Workplace Innovation (WI) is a relatively new concept [3], being a combination of structural and cultural practices that enable employees to participate in the organizational change and renewal. Hence, improving the quality of working life and organizational performance [3]. According to the European Commission (EC) to stay at the competitive edge, companies need to invest not only in technological innovation but also in non-technological practices. Workplace Innovation can mean many things such as a change in business structure, human resources management, relationships with clients and suppliers, or in the work environment itself. It improves motivation and working conditions for employees, which leads to increased labor productivity, innovation capability, market resilience and overall business competitiveness. All enterprises, no matter their size, can benefit from WI.

The EC, by means of the European Workplace Innovation Network-EUWIN, launched in 2013, has also published a guide-to-guide companies on the implementation of WI. The network is quite active and connects nowadays more than 10,000 companies and other stakeholders. The guide refers to high performance jobs when:

1. Jobs are empowered and self-managed teams.

2. Flexible organizational structures, people-centered management practices and streamlined systems and procedures are based on trust.

3. Systematic opportunities for employee-driven improvement and innovation are available.

4. Leadership is co-created and distributed combined with 'employee voice' in strategic decision-making.

5. The enterprising behavior, the culture of innovation, the high levels of employee engagement, and the organizational and individual resilience, which flourish only when the other four combines to shape experience and practice across the whole organization.

WI focuses on work organization as a means of innovation and employee involvement, which aims to improve work quality and organizational performance. These techniques are designed to encourage employees to deliberately develop, implement and apply new ideas, process and products [4]. WI lies at the intersection of skills, technology and human resources management [5]. According to the literature, we can see the European workers percentage involved in improving work organization or processes is not really high (47%) [6].

The drivers for WI implementation are divided into two main groups [7]. On the one hand, the improvement of the organization economic goals and performance quality (e.g., increase of productivity, manufacturing quality, customer service, financial performance and profitability etc.). On the other hand, the quality of working life and employee engagement (e.g., increases employee motivation and well-being, playing a particularly important role in reducing stress, enhancing job satisfaction and mental health, and improving retention etc.).

The Employee Participation and Organizational Change (EPOC) analysis evidenced direct employee participation impacts on productivity, innovation and quality. The EPOC analyzed 6000 workplaces in Europe, and confirmed organizations with semi-autonomous groups had 68% reductions in costs, 87% of these entities reduced production times, 98% improved their products/services, and 85% increased their sales [8]. Furthermore, Swedish study evidences flexible organizations were more productive (+20–60%), had a lower rate of staff turnover (−21%) and had a lower rate of absence due to illness (−24%) [9]. The benefits of WI and the effect on entity efficiency and performance is as well evidenced by a review of sixte American articles, with improvements of between 15% and 30% in the performance of those companies [8].

Therefore, WI not only aims at promoting innovation capacities but also allows the companies to remain innovative and adapt to changes quickly and smoothly. WI strengthens an organizations' capacity to innovate by fostering both high-quality employment and good organizational performance [10]. Only the 25% of innovation is related to technological research, while the remaining 75% is related to management organization and work practices at the business level [8, 11, 12]. According to the literature, leaders are those in charge of building an innovative climate and motivate the team towards innovation [13]. This means, the innovative behaviors and attitudes that are conducive to innovative projects are boosted by leaders [14].

According to the research conducted among companies about WI, it can be seen there a positive relation between non-technological innovation and organizational performance, all resulting in more dynamism, innovation capacity and competitiveness. However, the influence of combined organizational factors and individual employee behavior adoption has not been thoroughly analyzed in the railway sector.

3. Analyzing workplace innovation in EU rail sector

3.1 Data and sample

The entities selected for this study belong to the European railway sector. The data used was collected randomly by an online survey drawn out based on the results of the benchmark and European WI concept and indicators [15]. The survey was divided into three sections: individual level, organizational level and process level. Furthermore, the effects of these three sections on the company's WI is also considered, in a results level.

The typology of questions used has been varied, using open answers, multiple-section, one-choice questions and Likert scale to measure the degree/disagree level.

Data was collected over 54-day period (between 02/12/2019 and 24/01/2020) and the final sample included 203 respondents from 16 European countries. This variety of countries enriches the sample of respondents shown in **Figure 1**.

Regarding the quantitative analysis, considering that European Rail Industry employs nearly 400,000 people [1] the study has a confidence level of 95% and a margin of error of 7%.

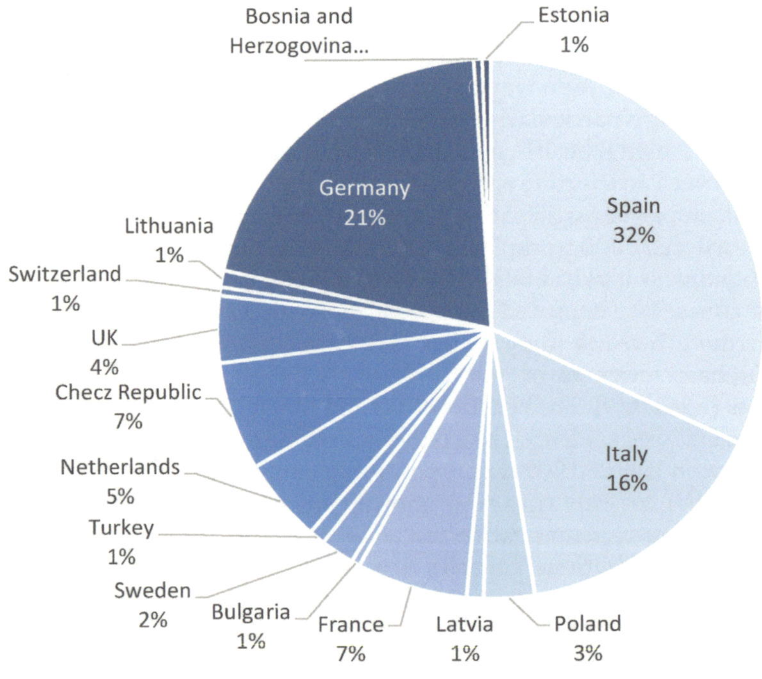

Figure 1.
Sample description (countries).

3.2 Definition of the general trends of WI in the European railway sector

The analysis aimed to examine which organizational, process and individual factors play a role in innovation adoption at the employee's level.

3.2.1 Organizational level

Organizational variables concern the context in which work is carried out. As long as WI is lacking, technological innovation is regarded a necessary but not sufficient prerequisite for change and improvement. As a result, WI refers to the essential organizational adjustments that will enable employees to properly incorporate and apply technological innovation. Most of the respondents (79,5%) indicated that during the last three years their companies had introduced new product or new process to the market. Furthermore, 60,2% of the respondents confirmed that additionally, their entities introduced organizational and marketing innovation strategies as shown in **Figure 2**.

The majority of the product and process innovations were developed by the companies' themselves, and these innovations resulted from collaborative work with other entities and institutions. Companies should go beyond their internal processes and develop cooperation with external organizations or professionals. This means combining their internal knowledge with external knowledge to move forward in their strategy. In this sense, it should be highlighted that not many rail entities focus their innovation on modifying other entities innovative solutions and this is shown in **Figure 3**.

Figure 4 shows how each company has its own approach to organize their innovations. Based on the results, most of the entities involve different departments in

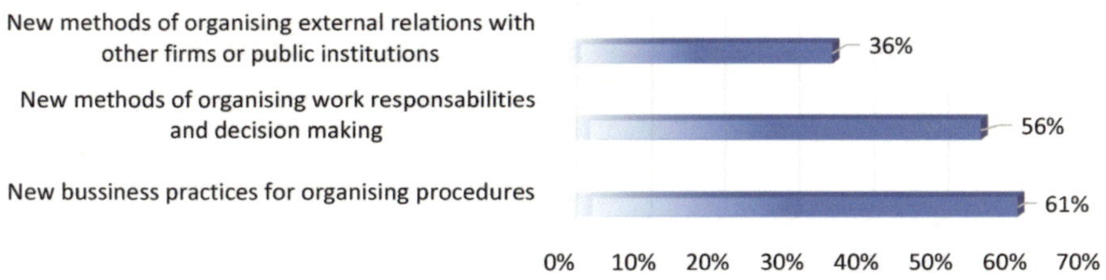

Figure 2.
Innovations introduced during the last three years in EU entities.

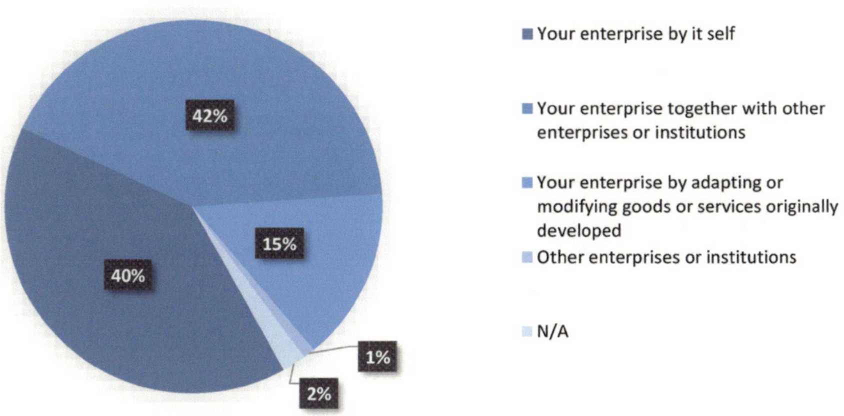

Figure 3.
Innovation's development in EU rail entities.

their innovation processes. However, in most of the cases, the engineering department is the one that leads the innovations.

Among organizational innovation, entities mostly implement new business practices for organizing procedures (62,3%). More than half of the respondents confirmed their organization had used new methods for organizing work assignment and decision making in their enterprises. These improvements were focused on the use of a new system of employee responsibilities, teamwork, decentralization, integration or de-integration of departments, as well as education/training systems. The remaining 40,7% introduced new methods of organizing external relations with other firms or public institutions. These changes were mostly focused on the use of alliances, partnerships, outsourcing or subcontracting.

The improvement of quality goods or services (60%), the reduction of time to respond to customer or supplier needs (57,5%), and the improvement of the ability to develop new products or processes were assigned the highest priority among the objectives for firms addressing organizational innovations over the previous three years (47%). An open culture will allow to face the challenge of launching innovative products, offering quickness and flexibility to respond to changing demands from their customers, as shown in **Figure 5**.

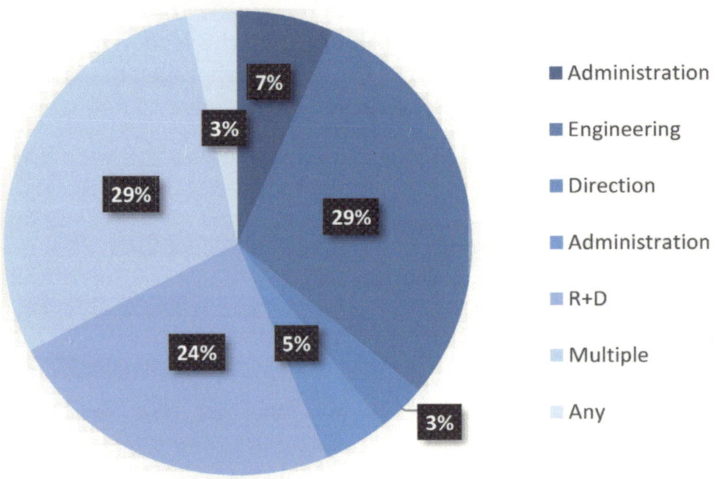

Figure 4.
Departments in charge of the product and process innovations development.

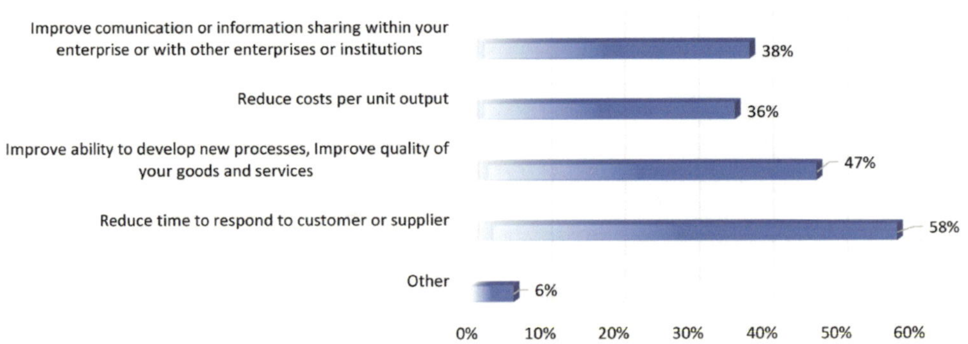

Figure 5.
Objectives for organizational innovations introduced in EU railway enterprises during the last three years.

Companies that work in the railway sector are prompt to introduce changes in their internal processes. In particular, great changes in relation to the use of technology, the way to coordinate and allocate the work to employees, the remuneration system, recruitment policies and in the working time arrangements have been confirmed (**Figure 6**).

As mentioned in Section 2, WI is a complex process which depends on various organizational and management factors. With regards the changes in the external processes, these seem to be less important than the internal ones. More than half of the respondents have confirmed their organizations had adopted new strategies for organizing job responsibilities and decision making. The most used information methods are internal sources and public sector sources. Both of them are used by more than a half of the respondents. Market sources (e.g. suppliers of equipment, materials, components, or software) and opinion of clients or customers from the public sector are very frequent also (both have more than 40% of positive answers). Nevertheless, information provided by consultants and commercial labs were not considered relevant source of the information for innovation projects, as shown in **Figure 7**.

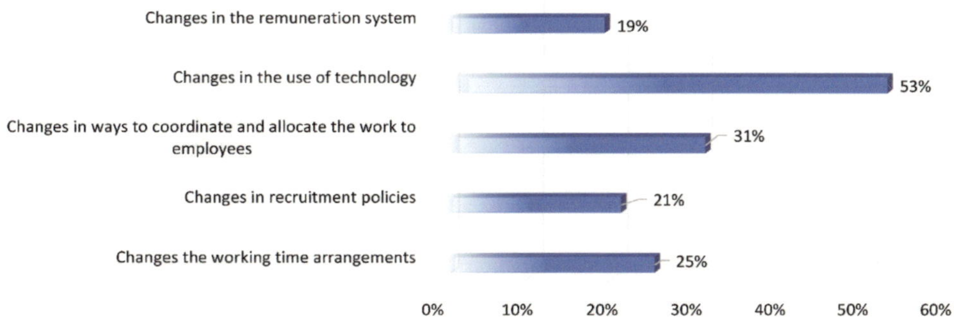

Figure 6.
Internal changes introduced in EU railway enterprises during the last three years.

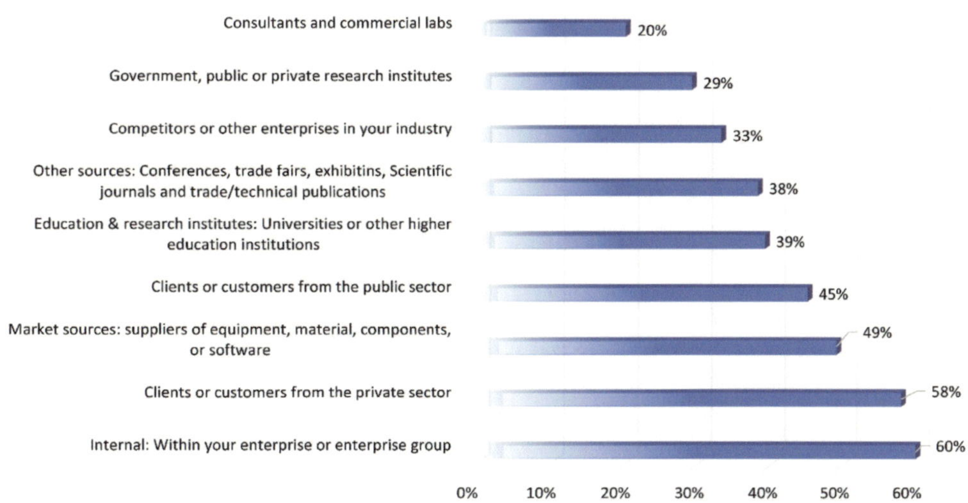

Figure 7.
Information sources used for new innovation projects or contributed to the completion of existing projects during the last three years.

According to the achieved results, brainstorming sessions are the most common tools the entities implement in their innovation practices (61,9%), followed by multidisciplinary or cross functional work teams (56,7%). These methods are based on staff rotation through different departments, financial and non-financial incentives, and public recognition, among others (**Figure 8**).

The most common method to involve the employees are regular meetings between employees and immediate managers (73%). The Committees or task forces are less common, as well as the communication methods such as internal newsletters, notice boards and email. Additionally, open meetings to all employees, suggestions schemes for collection of ideas and employee surveys are the most used ones by big entities (**Figure 9**).

3.2.2 Process level

At process level is measured the development of new approaches/practices as a result of the implementation of various WI instruments, analyzing the effect of methods on the staff's ability to generate new ideas. Autonomy and participation concern the degree to which employees can decide the way their work is carried out.

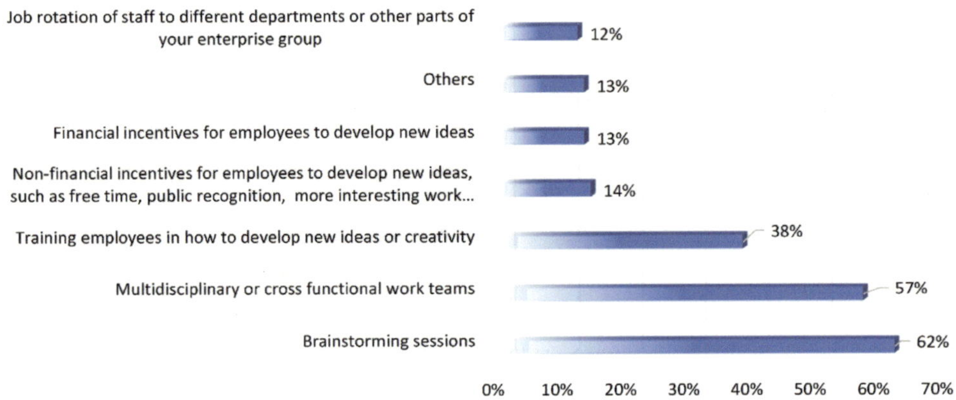

Figure 8.
Methods of staff stimulation in order to develop new ideas or creativity.

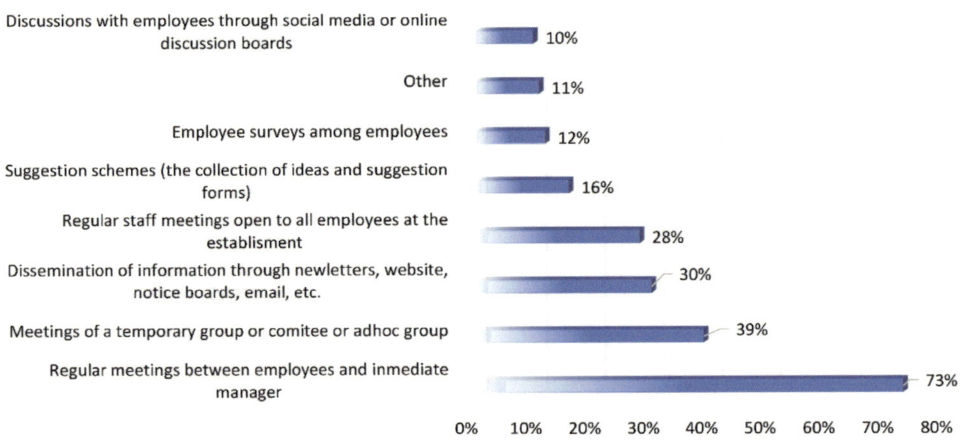

Figure 9.
Methods of involving employees into enterprises' innovation activities.

Almost half of respondents indicated that daily work decisions are taken in collaboration between employees and managers. However, the number of employees involved in the follow up is not really relevant. Normally, it is the manager the responsible of monitoring the tasks, as it is shown in **Figure 10**:

Innovation behavior concerns the extent to which employees feel they are involved in the development of innovation. For all job levels, highest percentage of employee's involvement was in the development of process innovation (58,45%), as well as for product innovation (57,67%). However, the study reveals that employees do not feel really engaged in organizational innovation. **Table 1** shows the obtained results.

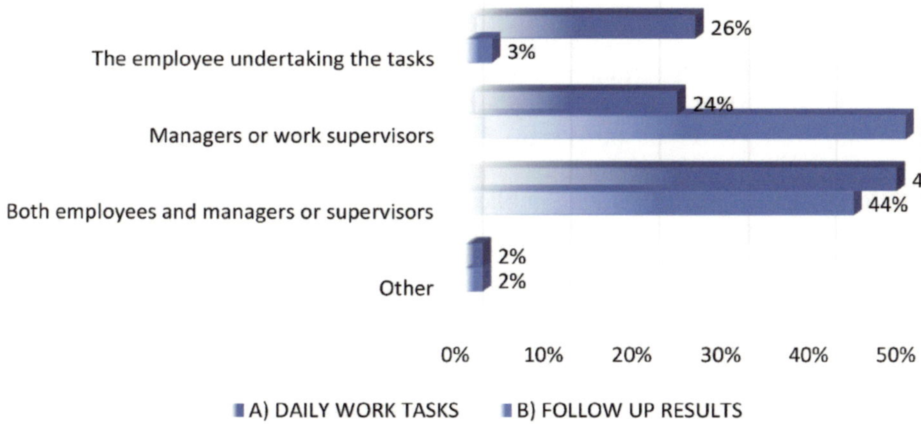

Figure 10.
Difference between decision taking for daily work tasks and follow up results.

Developed innovation	Position						Total (row)
	Assistant		Director		Manager		
	f	%	*f**	%	*f**	%	*f*
Product innovation							
No	13	56,5%	13	32,5%	30	38,0%	56
Yes	10	43,5%	27	67,5%	49	62,0%	86
Total	**23**	**100,0%**	**40**	**100,0%**	**79**	**100,0%**	**142**
Process Innovation							
No	9	39,1%	15	37,5%	35	44,3%	59
Yes	14	60,9%	25	62,5%	44	55,7%	83
Total	**23**	**100,0%**	**40**	**100,0%**	**79**	**100,0%**	**142**
Marketing Innovation							
No	8	34,8%	23	57,5%	46	58,2%	77
Yes	15	65,2%	17	42,5%	33	41,8%	65
Total	**23**	**100,0%**	**40**	**100,0%**	**79**	**100,0%**	**142**
Organizational Innovation							
No	17	73,9%	20	50,0%	53	67,1%	90
Yes	6	26,1%	20	50,0%	26	32,9%	52
Total	**23**	**100,0%**	**40**	**100,0%**	**79**	**100,0%**	**142**

**f =frequency.*

Table 1.
Type of developed innovation/role in entity income crosstabulation.

Figure 11 show the position perspective on involvement of employees into development of different types of innovations.

Existing approaches to the organizations' Knowledge and Information Management (KIM) were also evaluated. These aspects are focused on keeping and sharing best practices among the entity. In most of the cases (66,8%), there is an established procedure for keeping records of the good practices or lessons learned. Additionally, 56,7% of the entities that implemented these documenting procedures for monitoring external ideas or technological developments are doing it as a part of the responsibilities of general staff and 28,4% are using staff assigned specifically to this task, as shown in **Figure 12**.

Organizations have the need for new models of relationships based on sharing and making information accessible, the exchange of ideas and open collaboration. Most of the respondents had their own technology surveillance systems (69,9%) for monitoring market trends and technological developments. Among the methods used for monitoring external sources, the following are highlighted: Internet (58,6%), seminars and trade fairs (57,1%) and personnel training (49%). Other methods such as visits to other workplaces, reading publications in both professionals' journals and research and scientific magazines are not relevant for rail industry (**Figure 13**).

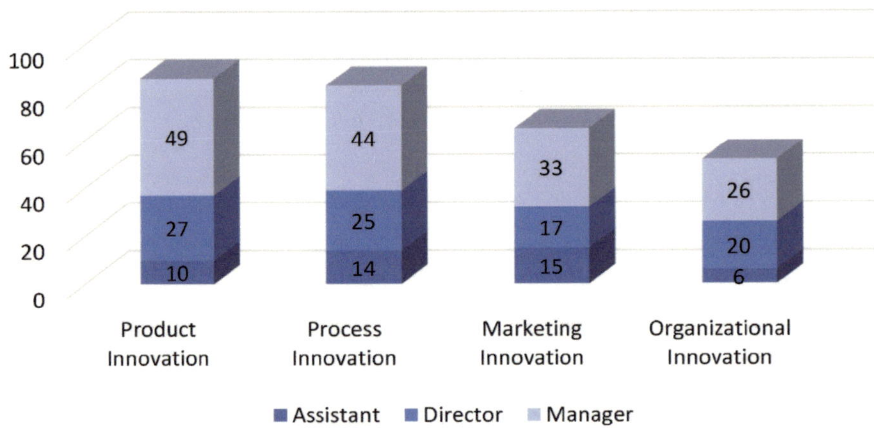

Figure 11.
Position perspective on involvement of employees into development of different types of innovations (in frequency of participation).

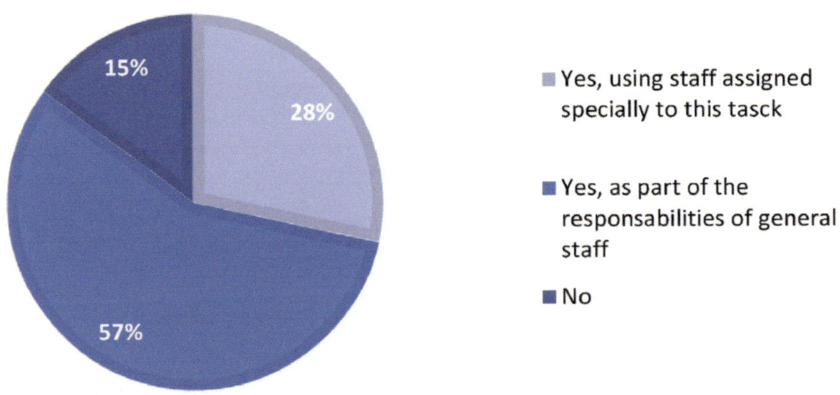

Figure 12.
Particularities of KIM in EU railway enterprises (organization of work of employees who document and keep records of their good work practices.

3.2.3 Individual level

The individual level refers to the attitudes of the employees towards innovation, as well as their individual characteristics, such as age and gender. The only type of innovation in which women have a higher chance than men of being involved is management innovation, which accounts for around 19% of the difference. The drawn-up cross-tabulation (**Table 1**) allows us to see that all age groups are participating in the development of all four types of innovation.

Table 2 shows that the middle-aged employees (36–55 years old) have the highest frequency of participation in innovation development. However, if we

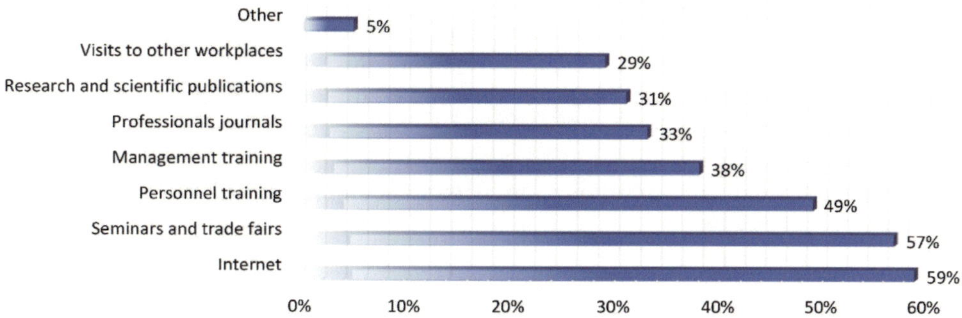

Figure 13.
Methods and instruments used for monitoring of external ideas or technological developments for new or changed products, processes or services.

Developed innovation	**Age**						**Total (row)**
	18–35		36–55		56–65		
	f	%	*f**	%	*f**	%	*f*
Product Innovation							
No	13	65,0%	42	36,5%	15	46,9%	70
Yes	7	35,0%	73	63,5%	17	53,1%	97
Total	**20**	**100,0%**	**115**	**100,0%**	**32**	**100,0%**	**167**
Process Innovation							
No	13	65,0%	55	47,8%	9	28,1%	77
Yes	7	35,0%	60	52,2%	23	71,9%	90
Total	**20**	**100,0%**	**115**	**100,0%**	**32**	**100,0%**	**167**
Management Innovation							
No	9	45,0%	66	57,4%	19	59,4%	94
Yes	11	55,0%	49	42,6%	13	40,6%	73
Total	**20**	**100,0%**	**115**	**100,0%**	**32**	**100,0%**	**167**
Organizational Innovation							
No	12	60,0%	75	65,2%	21	65,6%	108
Yes	8	40,0%	40	34,8%	11	34,4%	59
Total	**20**	**100,0%**	**115**	**100,0%**	**32**	**100,0%**	**167**

Table 2.
Type of developed innovation/age crosstabulation.

look at the average probability of participation in the innovation development for different age groups, the 56–65 years old participants are those who have the highest probability of being involved in innovation development (50%). The second highest involvement in innovation development is among young employees (41,25%), and the lowest (37,63%) is among middle-aged employees (36–55 years).

4. Workplace innovation scheme for rail industry

The Scheme pretends to be a flexible itinerary that will drive the company to better competitiveness using WI. The analysis in Section 3 evidences that companies must pay attention to the environment to identify the barriers that prevent teams to be more productive. Therefore, managers must believe in the WI and commit the team, as they will be the responsible of implementing the new tools and measure results to progressively move towards a full open culture that promotes digital transformation.

The driver for Workplace Innovation includes economic as well as social and human aspects, such as:

- Strategic orientation: to be innovative and competitive, organizations need to react to in their environment such as client and competitor behavior, new technological developments, and legislation, etc. this requires purchasing of new knowledge from outside, networking and cooperation with external partners.

- Organizing smarter: the ability of the company to invent new combination of organization, staff deployment and technical applications with a clear focus on the renewal or improvement of work processes.

- Flexible work: increasing flexibility of work through increasing the employability of the staff, facilitating flexible working time and/or contracts, self-rostering, etc. with attention to individual arrangement on working time, work performance, personal development and flexible employment.

- Product-market improvement: innovation by searching for new markets and clients, and the improvement of products and services.

These elements were already part of the questionnaire used in the consultation analysis and are also the basis of the WI Pilot Scheme. The Scheme will drive the company through an itinerary to understand where they stand on WI focusing on the following three interrelated aspects shown in the **Figure 14**:

- The Organization as such

- The employee

- The approach to technological and market developments

The company can select the blocks based on their specific needs, some companies will go for all the blocks, while others will select and implement only those they

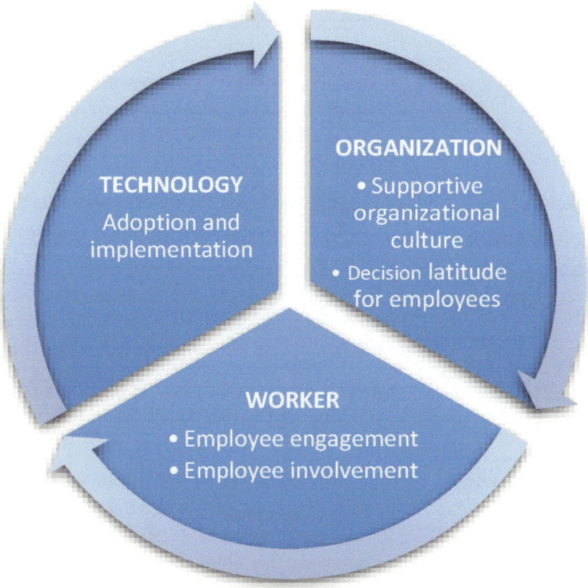

Figure 14.
Workplace innovation scheme.

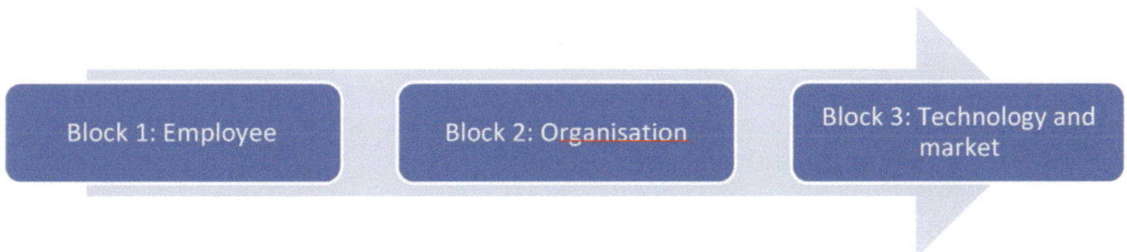

Figure 15.
WI scheme for rail sector.

want to improve. The blocks and the itinerary suggested to improve the Workplace Innovation within a company are the following ones shown in **Figure 15**:

4.1 Block 1: employees

In this block or step, the company will analyze, and address aspects directly related to employees within a company. The main purpose is to check how the employees feel within a company and focus on a better engagement and involvement. **Table 3**, shows the structure suggested for the Block on Employees, based on the previous research. Seven relevant aspects are suggested to be considered in a company to check the status of WI under the Block Employees:

4.2 Block 2: organization

Following the same logic as for the Block on Employees, the following results have been raised by the people participating in the survey and, on this basis, these are the eleven key factors suggested to review and consider for improving WI oriented to the organization (**Table 4**):

Block 1. Employees. Aspects to consider	Block 1. Employees. Some ideas to do it
• Innovation culture among employees	• Encourage innovation culture: Be honest and open, share ideas, explore initiatives without fear of retribution, allocate time for the employees to break from routine roles to inspire new thoughts.
• Cross functional teams	• Promote the development of cross actions among different teams: employees from different parts of the business; brainstorming sessions, improvements to processes together, etc.
• Encourage different perspectives	• Look for employees who understand business vision, align with its culture – which is not necessarily the same one, may have different perspectives, come from diverse backgrounds, etc.
• Gender issues	• Take it into consideration. Average of women in the railway sector. Identify their responsibilities, their positions in the company, etc.
• Training / Professional career	• To know the level of education of employees. Contrast it with the needs of the company and detect gaps. Identify training needs and support individual training and individual training plans for employees. Trainings about creativity, innovation, etc.
• Employees from different positions work together	• Employees from different positions and responsibilities get together to improve the work organization and processes of different departments.
• Clear responsibilities	• The responsibilities of the employees should be clear, defined and shared, aiming to avoid the lack of motivation among the staff.

Table 3.
Workplace innovation under the block employees.

4.3 Block 3: technology and market

Based also in our research, these are the eleven topics that are suggested as key topics to assed WI under Block 3 (**Table 5**):

4.4 How to implement WI scheme for rail sector?

The Pilot Scheme can be implemented by each company on an individual basis, the recommendation would be for each company to create a small team devoted to WI (including employees from different profiles and responsibilities) that follows up the situation of the company (**Figure 16**). The time devoted to the implementation of the Scheme should be decided by each company. The following three steps are suggested:

More in detail, the following is suggested:

Step 1. Workplace Innovation Kick off. The idea is to check the initial situation of the company regarding Workplace Innovation. An internal analysis including a Strengths, Weaknesses, Opportunities and Threats (SWOT) matrix as a result could be very useful. This will help to better contextualize and decide a further approach. The SWOT matrix allows a strategic analysis useful for a further planning to achieve the objectives or expected results. The Strengths and Weaknesses are related to internal factors while the Opportunities and Threats depend on external factors, as shown in the table.

Based on the initial SWOT produced, a meeting where the results are shared with the rest of employees is suggested. On this basis, an updated matrix can be proposed and at the same time, decide where the weaknesses and strengths regarding Workplace Innovation are. Following this, the company will decide if they go for the three blocks of the Pilot Scheme or for any of them.

Block 2. Organization. Aspects to consider	Block 2. Organization. Some ideas to do it?
• Provide support for sharing ideas	• Many large companies already have methods to allocate time and means to their employees to break from routine roles, to inspire new thoughts, etc. by means of meetings, suggestion boxes, suggestion area on the internal intranet.
• Generational change	• Employees' age and their position, what are the reasons behind, when it is necessary to transfer knowledge from the most experienced personnel to other workers, etc.
• Procedure to assess new ideas from employees.	• Ensure there is a specific process which everyone understands for assessing each new idea. This must be supported by acknowledgement and feedback in a timely manner. Introduce a new idea or *what if*? section to regular meetings, brainstorming sessions.
• Implement employees' ideas and suggestions in a fast and regular way.	• When employees see that they are influencing the direction of the business, they will be extremely motivated to continue sharing ideas, working towards the success of the idea and encouraging productivity of other employees.
• Suggest rewards to employees	• Rewards can be for individuals or even for teams or for the whole workforce. The important thing is that employees see that their efforts to improve the business are appreciated. They could be non-financial incentives such as free time, recognition, more interesting work, etc. Or financial with a specified in advance remuneration system.
• Establish a collaboration space	• Provide a dedicated area that will promote interaction with employees.
• Improve communication or information sharing	• Dissemination of information can be done through newsletters, website, notice boards, email, etc. depending on the type of information that is shared. Discussions with employees through social media or in online discussion boards, employee surveys among employees, etc.
• Establish a feedback culture at all organization levels	• This fact provides company members with feedback on their work. It also encourages them to participate in relevant decisions of the company.
• Promote and Share Good Practices/ lessons learnt	• Keep records of their good work practices or lessons learned and share it with other employees.
• Clarify which are the departments or areas in charge of innovation	• There are different options: to have a department where the innovations are centralized, to make innovations in for each department, to coordinate all actions, etc.
• Work Teams	• See if the work is done individually or in teamwork. Design the best protocols, carry out the work in the most efficient and satisfactory way, choose their own members, choose their own leaders, decide on their day-to-day and weekly tasks themselves, know who is the responsible for the quality of their work, members that perform several different tasks in the team etc.

Table 4.
Workplace innovation under the block organization.

Results:

- Create a Workplace Innovation team in the company.
- Produce a SWOT analysis regarding the WI.

Block 3. Technology and market. Aspects to consider	Block 3. Technology and market. Some ideas to do it?
• New product/services identification	• Which new product/services have been introduced in the market by the company and when, not only by the company itself, but also by competitors, stakeholders, etc.
• Marketing innovation	• Study the marketing situation in the company. Know the new trends, see how they can be adapted. Innovating in the way of communicating internally is also a key activity.
• Communication or information sharing with other enterprises or institutions	• Improve communication or information sharing with other enterprises or institutions. Both at the marketing level and at the relational level.
• Co-Development product/processes	• Co-Development with other enterprises or institutions, sharing of objectives, possible cooperation or alliances, participation in innovation projects, etc.
• Proactive approach to business	• Maintain the business model of the company continually updated and matching with changing conditions.
• Benchmarking in a systematic way	• Establishment of a methodology to monitor external ideas, technological developments, new or modified processes or services.
• Use more collaborative information sources	• Active participation in conferences, trade fairs, exhibitions scientific journals and trade/technical publications, professional and industry associations, etc.
• New business practices to organize internal procedures	• New practices such as: supply chain management, business reengineering, knowledge management, lean production, quality management, etc.
• Review and reformed if necessary	• Review for instance: the logistics, delivery or distribution methods for your inputs, goods or services.
• Review the production costs strategy	• It should be continuously adapted, agile to the changes that are made in the production process.
• Changes in the use of Technology	• Invest in having the latest technology that could allow companies to stay competitive and provide the best quality of services or products as possible. Also, apply new technologies at communication level to improve the communication and connection with employees, leaders, and co-workers anytime and anywhere. Systems like Project Management Software, CRM, etc., that can help and improve internal processes.

Table 5.
Workplace innovation under the block 3, technology and market.

- Workshop with employees to share the SWOT and results.
- Update SWOT and decide for the block of the Pilot Scheme to implement.

Step 2. The company will implement the Pilot Scheme and provides recommendations for action. Based on the results gathered under Step 1, the company will implement the Pilot Scheme. The Company can select one of the blocks, two or all. The company should easily check their strong the strong and weak points for the blocks suggested and decide how to implement reinforcement and corrective actions respectively.

Results:

- Implement the pilot scheme, all Blocks or the ones they consider based on the results from Step 1.

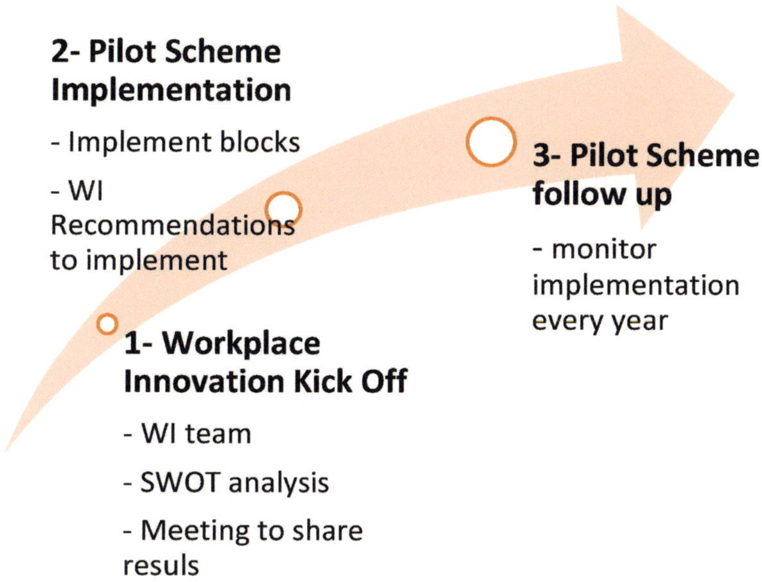

Figure 16.
WI scheme for rail sector, steps for implementation.

Step 3. A follow up is suggested every year. This monitoring is very important to ensure implementation of results and potential updates to include.

Results:

- Follow up every year if possible.

5. Conclusions

At the heart of all transitions are teams and leaders who have the courage to think openly to create a long-term perspective. The literature confirms the digital transformation is influenced by the culture of innovation, the high levels of employee commitment and the capacity for organizational and individual transformation. Digital transformation is the key to business competitiveness in a changing and increasingly demanding market [16]. However, a culture that encourages innovation and creativity is needed to succeed in the railway technological transformation. While the technological investment increases, the digital revolution raises new requirements for completing the transition successfully. In this sense, one of the challenges in the digital age is the adaptation of values, procedures and experiences that characterize the entity through its employees.

A tentative conclusion from the analysis is that employee engagement is an essential driver of WI [17]. The analysis has shown that four elements are relevant for a successful innovation adoption: participatory implementation, innovation behaviors, usefulness of innovation and results demonstrability.

At the organizational level, the results revealed that organizational factors have different impacts on innovation climate. Employee-driven creativity influences the daily evolution of WI practices and gradual improvements, most railway organizations do not use their autonomy to improve WI practices [16]. These findings depart from the WI existing studies that suggest job autonomy can be relevant to guide one's behavioral intentions and has influence positively the company performance [16, 18]. However, within the process level, the result suggests that participatory implementation plays a key role in WI Implementation. This result is in line with previous research, which confirm teamwork, internal cooperation and dialog will facilitate react more quickly to new ideas and challenges. In the correlation analysis it can be seen that the priority of the railway industry is to ensure the future by responding to business dynamics, rather than building an organizational model based on efficiency or quality or working life [16]. However, considering the change is unavoidable, railway organizations must to changes in order to be prepared for the future. There is evidence that participatory work environments and mechanisms for employee voice are associated with higher levels of innovative behavior [6]. Participatory implementation at the process level is positively related to results demonstrability and usefulness of innovation [16].

As a result, the railway industry's management practices should involve autonomous coordination. This means that instead of only suggesting ideas, the management should engage, stimulate and support the team. Then, based on their experience and point of view, employees would be able to recommend how the ideas should be developed [6, 17]. WI's current challenge thus, is to bridge the gap between employees and management.

As expected, there is a positive relation between innovation behavior and usefulness of innovation. But what's more important is that participatory implementation has an effect on all aspects of employees' perceptions of innovation (results demonstrability and usefulness of innovation). These results are aligned with previous research that evidences individual creativity has positive and significant effect on innovative behavior [19]. Finally, it can be seen there is no significant influence between the perception of innovation or innovation adoption among employees, not having a relevant role in WI autonomy and participation.

The main conclusions reached after the intensive consultation and test of the WI Scheme for rail sector is that the defined scheme is appropriate for Rail sector and it is suitable for other sectors. It is simple and flexible enough to be implemented in companies, that at the same time, can select and implement following an easy process the block or blocks they consider more relevant to better implement WI. The WI Scheme reached a great number of stakeholders and companies from different sectors. The follow up actions on the impact reached showed that the companies had a very positive reaction on the Pilot Scheme. Some observations can be made from these cases and confirm the railway industry is closely involved in the transformation towards WI practices at the process level. Within the scheme, the Block on Employees are the most relevant when implementing Workplace Innovation within an organization, followed by the organizational one and by far, the technology focused one.

However, in order to have a good implementation of the WI Scheme employees of each function should participate regardless of their role, and age, and involving several business functions as innovation goes beyond boundaries. The Scheme and Methodology is easy to use in other contexts too, when a need arises. Main obstacles that could arise are; if in the Scheme, only of technical profiles focused on product innovation are involved; if there is not enough recognition of the value of communication & management and the focus on tasks and less on getting as complete an overview as possible.

Therefore, a tentative conclusion of the analysis is that the change in the working system must be combined with a greater participation of the employees. Employees can commit to an innovative culture through the development of personal competences, but above all, it is important that employees have enough information to know where the company wants to evolve.

Future research would be necessary to analyze the preconditions for participatory structures within work teams. This is an essential factor in the WI since it is also related to the innovative behavior of employees and their commitment to the company. Companies in the sector need committed workers who are willing to face the industrial revolution of the sector. The European railway industry has the potential to be highly competitive, but it will not be so in a few decades if the transformation of workplaces is not promoted in order to attract engage and retain young talents [16]. As previously stated, the railway industry is traditional sector and in order to adapt to the changing environment it has capacities to implement innovative culture that allow continuous change in response to consumer demands. Furthermore, further research on the factors that could influence railway efficiency in the future as a result of COVID-19 should be made in order to facilitate the acceleration of railway strategies ensuring long term sustainability of the sector.

Acknowledgements

We thank respondents who provided insight through the online survey and give us the opportunity to analyze the results offering conclusions.

Funding

This Project has received funding from the European Union's Horizon 2020 research and innovation program under grant agreement No 861887.

Availability of data and material

The datasets generated during and/or analyzed during the current study are available from the corresponding author on reasonable request.

List of acronyms

WI	Workplace Innovation
OI	Open Innovation
SMEs	Small and medium entities
SWOT	Strengths, Weaknesses, Opportunities and Threats
EUWIN	European Workplace Innovation Network

Author details

Garazi Carranza Ruiz de Loizaga[1*] and Begoña Sanchez Gonzalez[2]

1 MAFEX-Spanish Railway Association, Bilbao, Spain

2 TECNALIA Research and Innovation, Bilbao, Spain

*Address all correspondence to: garazi@mafex.es

References

[1] Berger, R., 2020. World Rail Market Study–Forecast 2020 to 2025. UNIFE, the European Rail Industry Association.

[2] ERRAC(2017). Rail 2050 Vision. Rail the backbone of Europe's mobility.

[3] European Commission, 2014. Workplace innovation. Concept and indicators.

[4] Bos-Nehles, A., Renkema, M., Janssen, M., 2017. HRM and innovative work behavior: a systematic literature review. Personnel Review, Vol 46, Issue 7, 1228-1253.

[5] Beblavý, M., Maselli, I., & Martellucci, E., 2012. Workplace Innovation and Technological Change. CEPS Special Reports, No 65.

[6] Totterdill, P., & Exton, R., 2017. Creating the bottom-up organization from the top: Leaders as enablers of Workplace Innovation. Workplace Innovation: Theory, Research and Practice, 189-207.

[7] Oeij P. R.A., Dhondt S., Žiauberytė-Jakštienė R., Corral A., Totterdill P., 2016, Implementing workplace innovation across Europe: Why, How and What? Economic and Social Changes: Facts, Trends, Forecast, Vol. 5, 195-218.

[8] Totterdill, P., Dhondt, S., & Boermans, S., 2014. Your Guide to Workplace Innovation. European Workplace Innovation Network.

[9] Kroupa, A., 2007. European Foundation for the Improvement of Living and Working Conditions.

[10] Oeij, P., Rus, D., Dhondt, S., & Van Hootegem, G. (2019). Workplace innovation in the era of disruptive technologies. International Journal of Technology transfer and commercialization. Vol. 16, pp 208-309.

[11] Volberda, H. and van den Bosch, F., 2004, Rethinking the Dutch innovation agenda: Management and organization matter most, ERIM Report Series Research in Management, ERS-2004-009-STR, Erasmus Research Institute of Management, (ERIM).

[12] Pot, F., Koningsveld, E., Erg, E., 2009a. Quality of working life and organizational performance-two sides of the same coin? Scandinavian Journal of oek, Environment& Health.

[13] Wipulanusat, W., Panuwatwanich, K., & Stewart, R., 2017. Exploring leadership styles for innovation: an exploratory factor analysis. Ekonomia i Zarzadzanie, Vol. 9, 7-17.

[14] Oke, A., Munshi, N., & Walumbwa, F., 2009. The influence of leadership on innovation processes and activities. Oragnizational Dynamics, Vol. 28, Issue 1, 64-72.

[15] Kesselring A., Cosima B., and Scoppetta, A., 2014. Workplace innovation: Concepts and indicators. Brussels: European Commission, DG for Enterprise and Industry.

[16] Carranza G., Garcia M, Sánchez B., 2020. Activating inclusive growth in railway SMEs by workplace innovation, Transportation Research Interdisciplinary perspectives.

[17] Oeij, P., Gaspersz, J., Van Vuuren, T., & Dhondt, S., 2017. Leadership in innovation projects: an illustration of the reflective practitioner and the relation to organisational learning model. Journal of Innovation and Entrepreneurship, Vol. 6, Issue 2, 1-20.

[18] Preenen, P., Oeij, P., Dhondt, S., Kraan, K., & Jansen, E, 2016. Job autonomy matters for young companies' performance growth. World Review of

Entrepreneurship Management and Sustainable Development, Vol. 12, Issue 1, 74-100.

[19] Asbari, M., Purba, J., Hariandja, E., & Sudibjo, N., 2021. From Leadership to Innovation: Managing Employee Creativity. Jurnal Manajemen Strategi Dan Aplikasi Bisnis, 4(1), 143-154.

Chapter 8

Improved Probabilistic Frequent Itemset Analysis Strategy of Learning Behaviors Based on Eclat Framework

Xiaona Xia

Abstract

Interactive learning environment is the key support for education decision making, the corresponding analytics and methodology are the important part of educational technology research and development. As an important part and the research challenge, learning behaviors are uncertain and produce complex data relationships, which makes the learning analysis process more difficult. This chapter studies the feasibility of Eclat framework applying in educational decision making and get the corresponding the data analysis results. We take probabilistic frequent itemsets and association rules as research objectives, extract and standardize multiple data subsets; Based on Eclat framework, using data vertical format, we design and improve the models and algorithms in the process of data management and processing. The results show that the improved models and algorithms are effective and feasible. On the premise of ensuring robustness and stability, the mining quality of probabilistic frequent itemsets and association rules is guaranteed, which is conducive to the construction of key execution topology of learning behaviors, and improves the accuracy and reliability of data association analysis and decision prediction. The whole analysis methods and demonstration processes can provide references for the study of interactive learning environment, as well as decision suggestions and predictive feedback.

Keywords: Learning Analytics, Decision Making, Eclat Framework, Probabilistic Frequent Itemsets, Association Rules, Decision Prediction, Interactive Learning Environment

1. Introduction

Content resources, interaction patterns, collaborative models, organizational planning and influencing factors related to learning processes constitute learning behaviors, which are also key elements to describe learning behaviors [1, 2]. The learning processes supported by online technology and data technology ensure the completeness and continuity of learning behavior data. Massive learning behaviors is an important part of education big data, which provides the possibility for the full development of learning analytics [3, 4]. Learning behavior data can be divided into two categories: horizontal format and vertical format from the perspective of data structure and feature attributes. These two categories are inseparable about the components of learning behaviors, which are the atomic units to describe learning behaviors, such as url, forumng, questionnaire, etc. The horizontal format of learning behaviors is a vector set composed of multi-dimensional attributes, and the vertical format is a vector set composed of multi-level learners. From the perspective of horizontal format, the researches define learning behaviors as the collection of learners, appropriate learning analytics and tools are used to carry out data statistics and rule exploration. However, it is difficult to calculate and compare the influences of components of learning behaviors, which is not conducive to the construction of a new education mode, and it is relatively difficult to implement the calculation and comparison of the influences of learning behaviors more passive.

Learning behaviors represent continuous learning processes, and there are associated needs and execution results [5]. The analysis of learning behavior based on vertical format can provide more intuitive and accurate characteristics for the study of the groupness and individuality of the learning behavior components. However, the analysis process based on the vertical format is a complex problem with multiple factors. It is impossible to find a suitable decision making and prediction framework. Through sampling, the breadth and depth of data processing are limited, and it is difficult to achieve a feasible decision. Due to the shortcomings and gaps in technology and model, learning behaviors constitute data and potential relationships cannot be gotten fully mining and complete analysis. In terms of research methods and application practices of learning behaviors, there are still many problems to solve [6, 7].

In this chapter, vertical data is analyzed for an online learning behavior big data set. The vertical data analysis of learning behaviors is carried out from the data structure and characteristics. Based on Eclat framework, a probabilistic frequent itemset learning algorithm is designed, and its feasibility and reliability are demonstrated and compared. Within the effective performance indicators, the probabilistic frequent itemsets and association rules are calculated and mined from the learning behavior components, and the correlation is demonstrated. Then we explore the rules and characteristics of learning behaviors, and provide decision feedback and suggestions for the design improvement and relationship of learning behaviors.

2. Related work

Mining probabilistic frequent itemsets is a branch of data analytics. There are explicit or implicit association data, which is the key basis for prediction, decision making and recommendation of other learning behavior components. On the current big data platform, the decision algorithm and recommendation algorithm based on frequent itemsets mining are used to track data. However, due to the particularity and complexity of learning behaviors, as well as the autonomy and randomness of learning processes, there is no general technical means to ensure the integrity and sufficiency to implement the analysis and calculation with the goal of decision making and prediction. In this regard, it is necessary to participate in benign learning behavior component construction and recommendation. The research on frequent itemsets has shown an urgent technical demand in the field of education big data. There have been relevant results to demonstrate the urgency and reality of empirical methods and technical means.

The research on probabilistic frequent itemsets of learning behavior components, after combing the relevant theoretical and application results, mainly focuses on the data statistics and association rules of horizontal format, which is reflected in the following aspects:

2.1 Frequent itemset mining based on apriori

Frequent itemset mining based on Apriori takes the construction of itemset association rules as the premise. The mining process is based on the horizontal format and completes the extraction of rules through iterative search strategy. After data connection and pruning, the itemsets satisfying the association rules are formed [8–11]. If one itemset satisfies the minimum support and a certain confidence, it is defined as a frequent itemset. Apriori algorithm is used to analyze the relevance of learning behaviors, the main idea is to select the learning platform, locate the components of learning behaviors, realize the association between learning behaviors and learning effects, define learning behavior as “cause”, and define learning effect as “result”. The traditional Apriori algorithm is improved flexibly. With the help of clustering, weighted balance, decision tree evaluation and other means, the data tracking are realized. The research target is to optimize learning behaviors and improve learning efficiency. However, the frequent itemset mining process of Apriori needs to scan the original data many times. When the original data is large, the number of times of iterative scanning is too much, which seriously affects the efficiency of the algorithms.

2.2 Frequent itemsets mining based on FP-growth

Frequent itemset mining based on FP-growth also uses horizontal data format, but the data structure is essentially different. The process of data analysis is mainly divided into two steps: constructing FP tree and mining frequent itemsets. Through the construction of FP tree, the expression of itemsets associated transaction is realized, that is, one path of FP tree corresponds to a transaction, and the transaction is composed of items. Different transactions may have the same items, which makes the path of FP tree overlap. The more overlapped, the greater the path compression space, the higher the access efficiency of FP [12–15]. FP-growth is used to mine frequent itemsets of learning behaviors. Its main idea is similar to Apriori. According to the research target of learning behaviors, users require to select the data set of learning behaviors, define the itemsets and research target, put forward hypothesis test, explore the rules by means of classification, clustering and decision making, draw a conclusion, and verify the existing education and teaching according to the data analysis results, but there are some problems. Due to the diversity, randomness and complexity of learning behaviors, FP-growth algorithm has obvious limitations in the study of learning behaviors. When the itemsets of learning behavior are too many or the relationships are complex, it will lead to too many sub nodes of FP tree, which will greatly reduce the efficiency of the algorithms, and can not get accurate and complete frequent itemsets. FP-growth algorithm is very difficult to learn.

2.3 Frequent itemsets mining based on Eclat framework

Compared with Apriori and FP(Frequent Pattern)-growth, The fundamental difference of Eclat is that the algorithm analysis of Eclat uses vertical data format, and is essentially a deep optimization search mechanism. The rule search space is effectively divided into subspace sets through concept lattice and equivalence relationships. The support calculation of each itemset does not require repeated retrieval of the entire dataset [16–19]. The main idea of using Eclat framework to study learning behaviors need the support of big data set of learning behaviors, through data transposition and standardization processing, we can get the itemsets and the transaction set. On this basis, the relevant models and algorithms of Eclat framework are improved and redesigned. On the premise of support, confidence and promotion, frequent itemsets and association rules are mined. Taking the final frequent itemsets and association rules as the references. Vertical data analysis and research based on Eclat framework can improve the speed of data search, association and analysis, and also improve the reliability of data validation results to a certain extent.

However, the Eclat framework is rarely used in the data processing of learning behaviors. Therefore, the improvement of algorithms and models has no effective results, which is directly related to the difficulty of technology caused by the complexity of learning behaviors. If Eclat is used to transpose and intersect all items and transactions, or if the number of items and transactions is too large, the efficiency of the algorithms will be affected. Therefore, the mining of frequent itemsets in Eclat framework should be assisted by other algorithms and tools, which is more practical. This chapter will integrate the advantages and feasible attempts in the application of Eclat framework, such as technical improvement, model design, tool application, etc., so as to provide more effective methods for the follow-up study of big data of learning behaviors and others.

3. Elements of learning behaviors and research problems

We select a big data set of learning behaviors of UK open university in four periods in recent two years, and the data scale reaches hundreds of millions. From the perspective of course category, we realize the tracking and comparison of learning behaviors of the same category and different categories, and make adaptive decision. The courses are divided into two categories: Literature and Technology. For each category, two courses are selected, namely L1 and L2, T1 and T2. Different courses have different periods of learning behaviors, with the help of assessment, the learning effects are achieved. There is correlation between learning behaviors and learning effects, and there is mutual restrictive and driving relationships between the components of learning behaviors. The empirical problems and testing strategies are established between learning behaviors and learning effects, the research conclusions and decision making reflection are the basis for the improvement and optimization of data-driven learning behaviors.

Tables 1–4 show the components and indicators of learning behaviors corresponding to the four courses of L1, L2, T1 and T2. The four tables involve four learning periods: P1, P2, P3 and P4. The data distribution of the tables indicates that not all courses have learning behavior in each period. The indicators involve two statistics: the median and the mode, which are used to investigate the population trend. Different indicators are selected according to different types of components. "assessment" represents the assessment method of courses, that is composed of enumeration components, mainly including CT (Computer Test), TT (Teacher

P2		P4	
forumng	668	content	1080
homepage	369	resource	8
content	147	subpage	16
resource	1	url	0
assessment	TT	assessment	TT
final_result	pass	final_result	pass

Table 1.
Components and indicators of L1.

P3		P4	
forumng	23	forumng	26
homepage	106	homepage	112
collaborate	0	collaborate	0
content	17	content	24
page	0	page	0
quiz	276	quiz	312
resource	32	resource	34
subpage	56	subpage	54.5
url	4	url	4
assessment	TT	assessment	TT
final_result	With-drawn	final_result	With-drawn

Table 2.
Components and indicators of L2.

P2		P3		P4	
dualpane	3	dualpane	0	dualpane	0
forumng	112.5	forumng	73.5	forumng	126
homepage	195	homepage	160.5	homepage	189
collaborate	0	collaborate	1	collaborate	1
content	506	content	447.5	content	466
wiki	117	wiki	86.5	wiki	126
page	0	page	0	page	0
quiz	137	quiz	113	quiz	108
resource	7	resource	11	resource	9
subpage	22	subpage	17	subpage	19
url	27	url	27.5	url	22
assessment	TT	assessment	TT	assessment	TT
final_result	withdrawn	final_result	withdrawn	final_result	pass

Table 3.
Components and indicators of T1.

Test) and exam (computer and Teacher joint test); "final_result" represents the result of the course assessment and is also an enumeration type, including four components: excellent, pass, fail and withdrawn. "assessment" and "final_result" measure the group tendency of courses. Other components are the main parts of the interaction processes. They all describe the interaction frequency, which has the autonomy and randomness of learners. The strength of interaction frequency is assessed by the median to investigate the distribution range.

From **Tables 1–4**, we can see that the concentration of group selection of "assessment" is very obvious. Most of the learners have completed the course assessment by teachers, but the assessment results are quite different, and the assessment results of the same course in different learning periods are also different. About P4 of L2, as same as P2 and P3 of T1, learners tend to give up the assessment.

P1		P2		P3		P4	
dataplus	0	dataplus	0	dataplus	0	dataplus	0
dualpane	2	dualpane	0	dualpane	0	dualpane	0
forumng	229.5	folder	1	folder	1	forumng	150
glossary	0	forumng	183	forumng	143	glossary	0
homepage	282	glossary	0	glossary	0	homepage	229
content	795	homepage	234	homepage	201	htmlactivity	4
elluminate	8	collaborate	1	oucollaborate	1	collaborate	1
wiki	13	content	566	oucontent	482	content	638
page	9	wiki	11	ouwiki	8	wiki	9
questionnaire	3.5	page	7	page	7	page	2
quiz	581.5	questionnaire	3	questionnaire	0	questionnaire	2
resource	32	quiz	543	quiz	521	quiz	557
subpage	219.5	repeatactivity	0	resource	22	repeatactivity	0
url	23	resource	26	subpage	162	resource	25
assessment	TT	subpage	180	url	12	subpage	184
final_result	Pass	url	13	assessment	TT	url	14
		assessment	TT	final_result	pass	assessment	TT
		final_result	pass			final_result	excellent

Table 4.
Components and indicators of T2.

In P4 of T2, most of the learners obtain excellent assessment results, and most of them pass the course. From "assessment" and "final_result", the group indicators of Literature courses and Technology courses are similar.

As for other components of learning behaviors, it can be found from the data that the category of components and the participation of isomorphic components show strong discrete characteristics. The results show that the types of interaction components in two learning periods of L2 and three learning periods of T1 are consistent, and the median is relatively close, which indicates that the distribution of learners' participation in these interactive components is basically consistent. The two learning periods of L2 have the same "final_result" mode, and the assessment results of T1 have obvious differences. The comparison of the types or numbers of interaction components related to the same course in different learning periods directly shows the differences. The interactions are significantly different, and there is a gap in the median of the same interaction component, such as "content" of two learning periods of L1. At the same time, the types of interaction components that belong to Literature or Technology courses are subject to the courses. The learners of L1 and L2 have their own interactive components, and T1 and T2 are the same.

Therefore, their interaction components of L1, L2, T1 and T2 reflect the autonomous learning characteristics, and the component constraints of assessment methods and results realize the differentiation of learners. The problems and relationships are shown in **Figure 1**, which is divided into the following four steps:

1. The mining of frequent itemsets will take different interaction components as reference items, and realize the analysis and mining of frequent itemsets based on reference items according to certain probability;

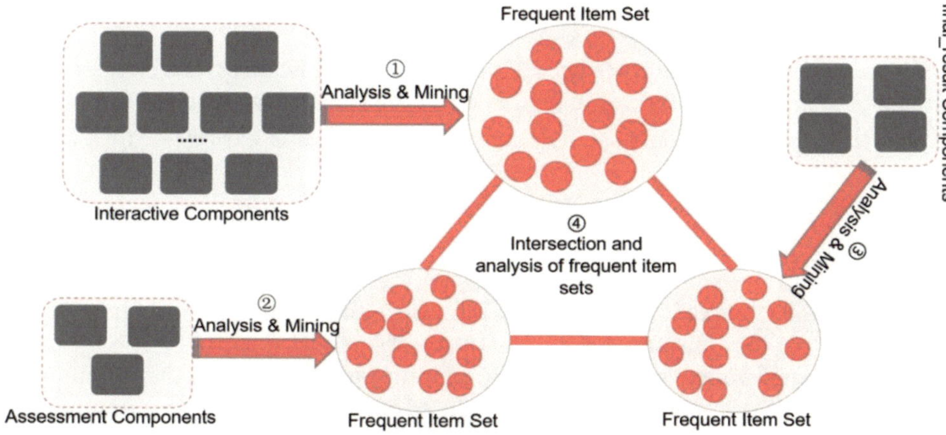

Figure 1.
The research problems and logical relationships.

2. Taking three enumeration methods of "assessment" as component reference items, according to certain probability, the frequent itemsets analysis and mining based on reference items are realized;

3. The four enumeration methods of "final_result" are component reference items. Based on a certain probability, the analysis and mining of frequent itemsets based on reference items are realized;

4. Based on a certain probability, the intersection of the three groups of frequent itemsets obtained from (1), (2) and (3) is solved and analyzed, and the inherent association logic and restrictive conditions are evaluated. On this basis, the rule of data-driven learning behaviors, prediction direction and decision making are explored.

The certain probability in the four steps depends on the selected algorithm requirements and measurement support. Based on the improved Eclat framework, we complete the four steps of the research problems, uses the three indicators "Support", "Confidence" and "Lift" to realize constraints, analyzes threshold and test criteria, and mines probabilistic frequent itemsets and association rules.

4. Improved Eclat framework

For the four learning behavior datasets corresponding to L1, L2, T1 and T2, the execution results of the reference items can be described in the form of probability, but not the "Support" calculation mode. The expected "Support" of reference items should be used to describe the execution frequency of uncertain components [20], that is a feasible and target analysis strategy, which is the model basis for improving the Eclat framework.

4.1 Related models

The Related Models for the improvement of Eclat framework are as follows.

4.1.1 Expected "Support" of reference items

Given a probabilistic data set with N reference item instances, the expected "Support" of a reference term X is expressed as the cumulative value of the probability in the probabilistic data set. The calculation formula is $\exp ect - \sup(X) = \sum_{i=1}^{N} p_i(X)$.

4.1.2 Frequent itemsets

Based on the expected "Support" of a reference item, a probabilistic data set with Nreference item instances is given, if it meets $\exp ect - \sup(X) \geq N \times \min\_RST$, the reference item X is a frequent item set. $\min\_RST$ is the minimum relative "Support" threshold, which is calculated by the ratio of the minimum absolute "Support" threshold to the reference item instance. Generally, this value can be specified according to the data distribution.

4.1.3 Probability frequency

Combined with the conditions of frequent itemsets, given a probabilistic data set with N reference item instances, the probability frequency of the reference term is defined as: $proF(X) = proF\{\exp ect - \sup(X) \geq N \times \min\_RST\}$.

4.1.4 Probabilistic frequent itemsets

Given a probabilistic data set with N reference item instances, if meeting $proF(X) \geq \min\_proF$, the reference item X is a probabilistic frequent itemset, $\min\_proF$ is the minimum frequent probability threshold, which can also be specified according to the data distribution.

4.2 Algorithm design

Many algorithms for mining frequent itemsets mostly use horizontal data format with transaction as vector [5, 21]. The uncertainty of learning behavior data makes the analysis of learning behavior need vertical data format. One complete learning behavior of learners constitutes a transaction. Based on Eclat framework, it is suitable to adopt *tidlist* data structure, and add a probability parameter to each item of learning behaviors to indicate the possibility of a specific transaction.

The vertical data format of learning behavior data is a binary tuple $(x, tidlist(x))$, which represents the item set of learning behaviors, and x is the identifier of each item, that is, the number of each learning behavior, $tidlist(x)$ is the list of items of x. If each item contains an identifier i_i and an existence probability $p_X(i_i)$, $tidlist(x)$ is expressed as a tuple $\{(i_1, p_x(i_1)), (i_2, p_x(i_2)), \cdots, (i_i, p_x(i_i))\}$. In the algorithm design of vertical data format, it is necessary to complete the calculation of probability frequency. Here we use two-dimensional array $P_x[i,j]$ to represent the probability quality function, which means the X probability of the i occurrence in the previous j reference items. Therefore, the calculation process of probability frequency is described as PFC(Frequent Pattern Calculation) program.

PFC program

Input: Item set $X(i_i, p_X(i_i))//1 \leq i \leq |I|$, I represents the maximum number of transactions.

Output: $P_x[i,j]$
Process

1. PFC()

2. For j=0 to $|I|$

3. $P_x[0,j]$=1

4. EndFor //Initialize the first row units of $P_x[i,j]$ of a to 1

5. For j=0 to $|I|$

6. For i=0 to $\min\_Value(j, \min\_RST)$// $\min\_Value(j, \min\_RST)$ is used to compare j and min_RST, then return the minimum value.

7. If $i > j$ then $P_x[i,j]=0$

8. Else if $i > j$ then $P_x[i,j] = \prod_{i=1}^{j} p_x(i_i)$

9. Else if $i < j$

10. Then $P_X[i,j] = P_X[i-1, j-1] \cdot p_X(i_j) + \max(P_X[i, j-1], P_X[i-1, j]) \cdot (1 - p_X(i_j))$

/*This formula is a kind of dynamic decision programming, and the maximum probability frequency is obtained by the adjacent units.*/

11. End If

12. End If

13. End If

14. End For

15. End For

16. Output: $P_x[i,j]$

Based on the calculation results of probability frequency, Eclat algorithm is designed. There are three main steps:

Firstly, according to the vertical data format, the transactions and corresponding items are extracted from the learning behavior data set, with the help of bi-directional sorting strategy, transactions are initialized. The items are stored according to *tidlist*. Then, it analyzes the "Support" of the transactions stored in *tidlist*, and discards the transactions with lower "Support" (support $< min\_RST$).

Secondly, the items of learning behaviors are pruned and optimized, and the $k-$item set from *tidlist* is extracted by intersection, and the probability frequency of $k-$item set is realized by multiplication operation.

Thirdly, mining probabilistic frequent itemsets recursively in candidate itemsets. In the mining process, pruning strategy based on *tidlist* is implemented to reduce the search time complexity. Furthermore, based on the projection of $k-$frequent itemsets, the probability data composed of frequent itemsets are obtained.

These three steps constitute a recursive process, and the whole algorithm process is described as LB(Learning Behavior)-Eclat program.

LB-Eclat Program

Input: $T//T$is the data set for storing vertical data formats.
Process:

LB-Eclat(T)

While all $X_i \in T$

  $I_i = \varphi$

  While $X_j \in T\&\&\ expect - rup(X_i) > expect - rup(X_j)$

    $X_{ij} = X_i \cup X_j$

    $tidlist(X_{ij}) = tidlist(X_i) \cap tidlist(X_j)$

    Call PFC(X_{ij})//call PFC program

    If $P_X[i,j] \geq min\_proF$

    Then $T = T \cup \{X_{ij}\};\ I_i = I_i \cup \{X_{ij}\}$

  End While

End While

While $I_i \neq \varphi$

  LB-Eclat(I_i)

End Whille

Output: all probabilistic frequent itemsets.

---

5. Experiments

The learning behavior components shown in **Tables 1**-4 are different in scale and sparsity. Combined with the density of learning behavior components, the specific situation is shown in **Table 5**. In order to realize the comparison and test of the algorithms, the traditional Eclat algorithm and the Eclat algorithm based on descending "Support" (DES Eclat) are selected to carry out the experiments.

L1-P2	sparse density	L1-P4	sparse density	L2-P3	moderate density	L2-P4	dense density
T1-P2	sparse density		T1-P3	sparse density	T1-P4	moderate density	
T2-P1	moderate density	T2-P2	dense density	T2-P3	moderate density	T2-P4	dense density

Table 5.
Density of data sets.

5.1 Performance Indicators

Based on the Eclat framework, the traditional Eclat algorithm, des-Eclat algorithm and LB-Eclat algorithm are written into Python 3.7 and run in the same experimental configuration. In the whole experiment process, we set different $\min\_RST$ to mine frequent itemsets, and record the indicators generated in the whole processes, which are mainly reflected in the running time of the algorithm, the proportion of memory and the number of probabilistic frequent itemsets.

The test of each indicator is divided into three series according to the sparsity of the data set. The comparative statistical results of corresponding time are shown in **Figures 2**–**4**. The larger the $\min\_RST$, the smaller the time curve distribution of each subgraph. It can be seen from **Figure 2** that the algorithm execution results of sparse density dataset based on the same value show that the traditional Eclat algorithm has advantages. The special sorting of data of DES-Eclat and LB-Eclat increases the time complexity, and the analysis process increases the data time. The execution time of LB-Eclat algorithm is the lowest in **Figures 3** and **4**, which

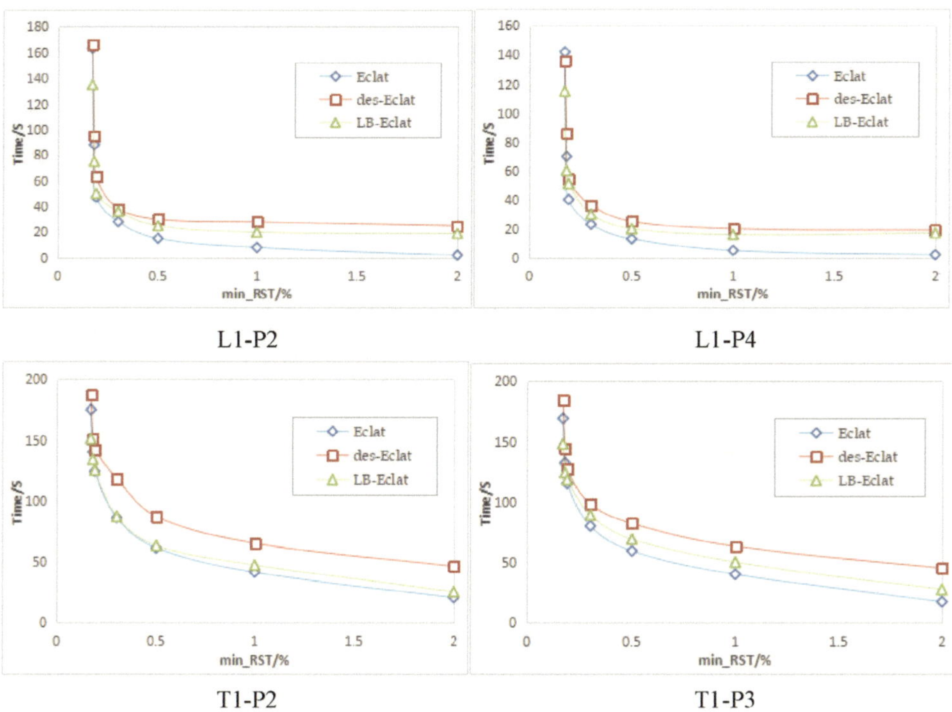

Figure 2.
Comparison of running time of three algorithms on sparse density datasets.

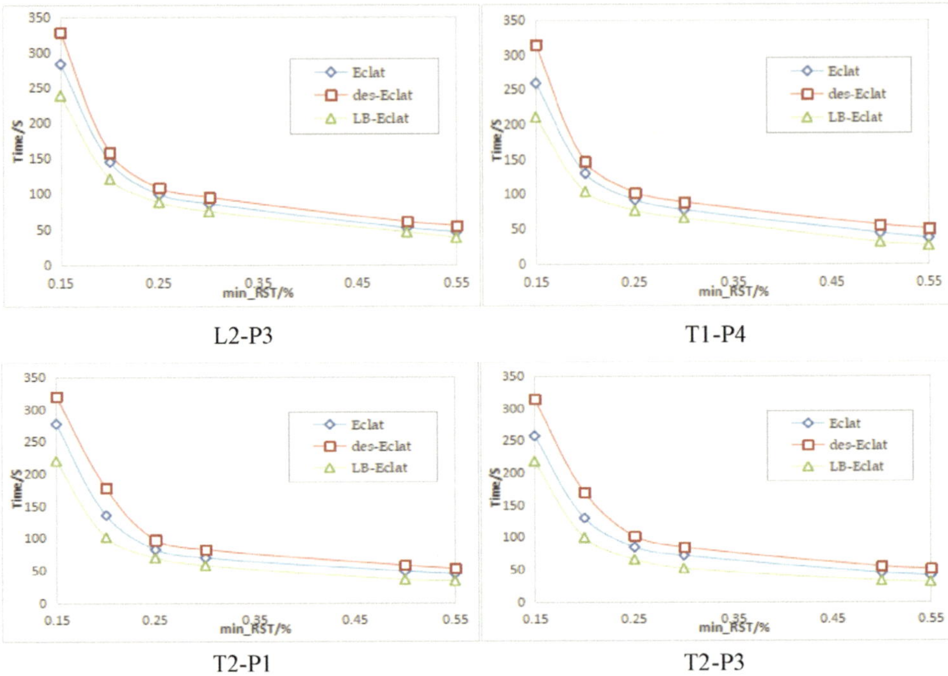

Figure 3.
Comparison of running time of three algorithms on moderate density datasets.

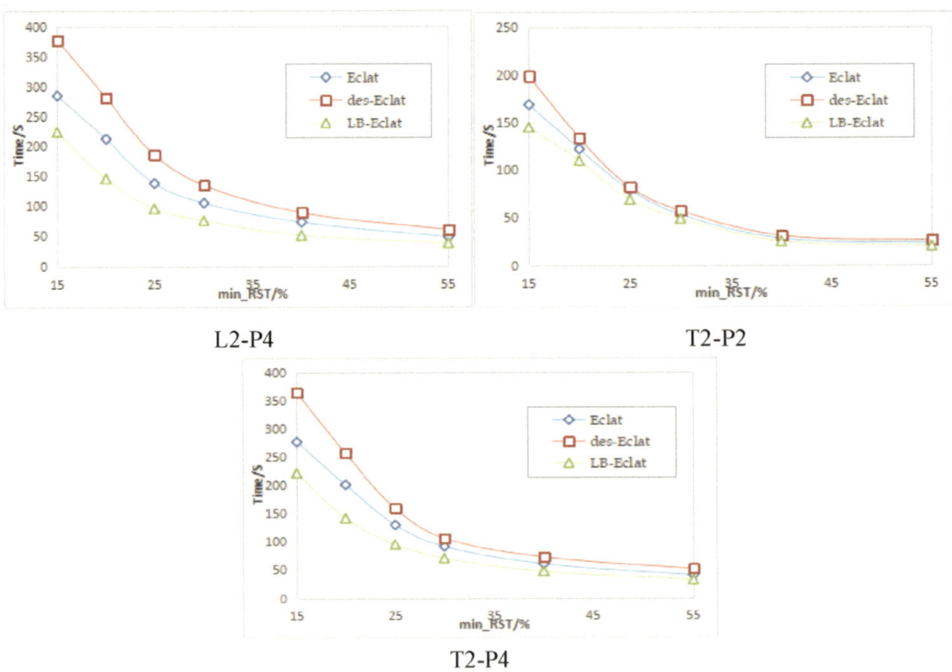

Figure 4.
Comparison of running time of three algorithms on dense density datasets.

indicates that the improvement of the algorithm is more conducive to the analysis of data sets with higher density, and is more effective for mining and processing frequent itemsets of learning behaviors. It can not be found from the time that the DES-Elat algorithm based on the reverse order strategy has a long running time.

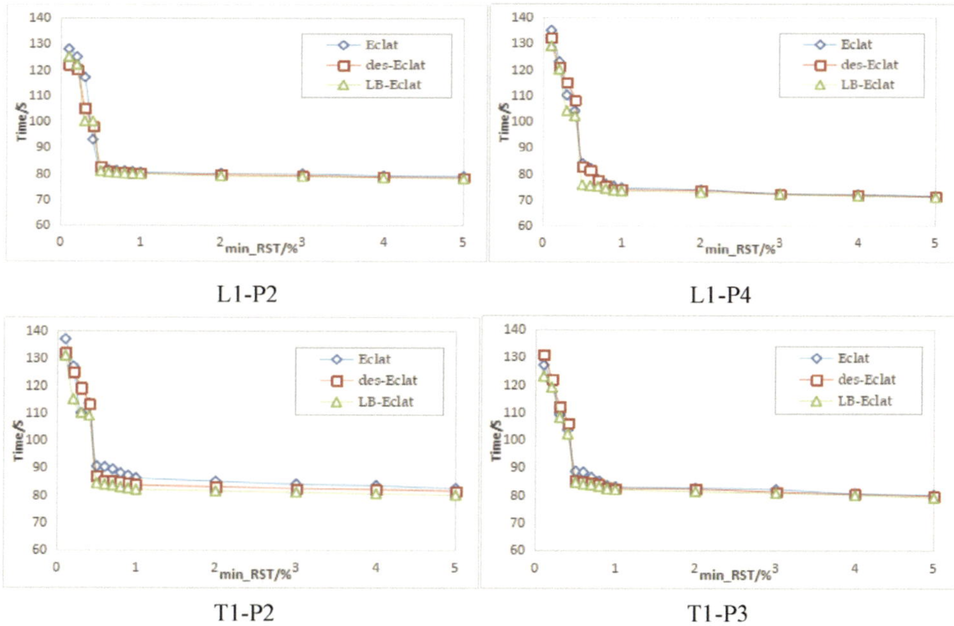

Figure 5.
Comparison of memory space of three algorithms on sparse density datasets.

The comparative results of memory space of the three algorithms are shown in **Figures 5–7**. No matter what the density of data set, the three algorithms occupy the same memory space distribution, the value change trend is the same, LB-Eclat algorithm is slightly smaller than other algorithms, the larger the data set density,

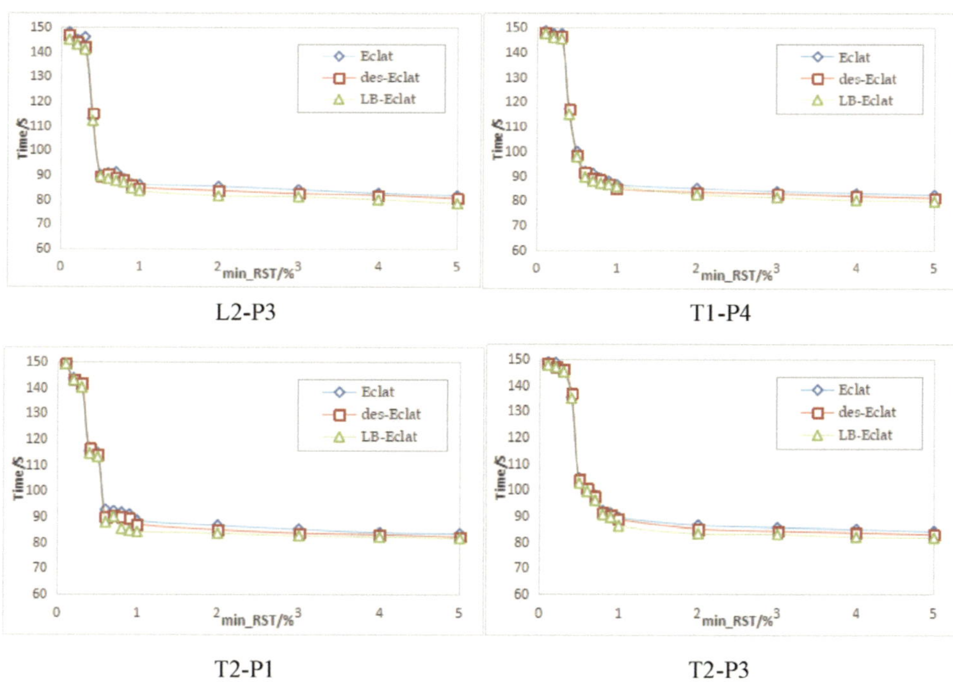

Figure 6.
Comparison of memory space of three algorithms on moderate density datasets.

compared with the traditional Eclat algorithm and des-Eclat algorithm, the smaller the space complexity, that improve the utilization of memory.

The comparison results of probabilistic frequent itemsets mined by the algorithms are shown in **Figures 8–10**. With different min _*RST*, the number of

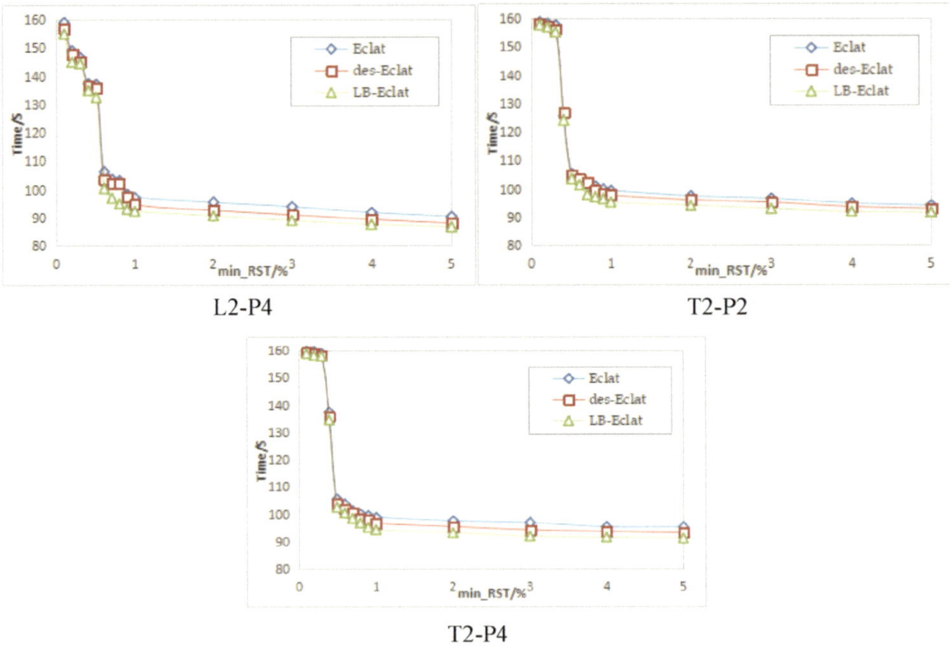

Figure 7.
Comparison of memory space of three algorithms on dense density datasets.

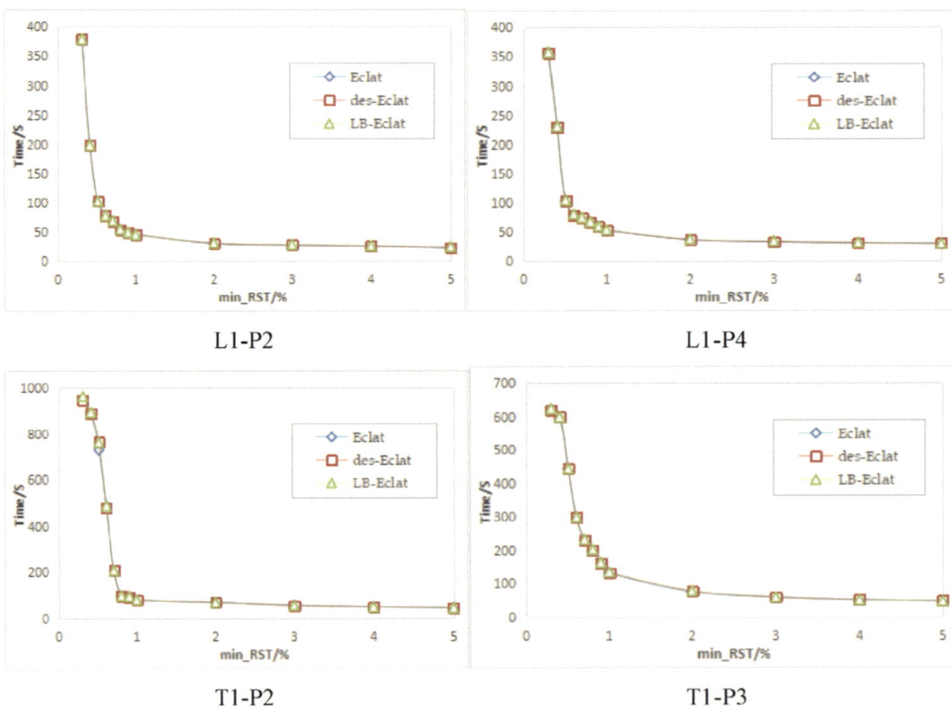

Figure 8.
Comparison of probabilistic frequent Itemsets of three algorithms on sparse density datasets.

probabilistic frequent itemsets depends on the items of learning behaviors and the density of transactions. Although the running time and memory space of the three algorithms are different on the same dataset, the number of probabilistic frequent

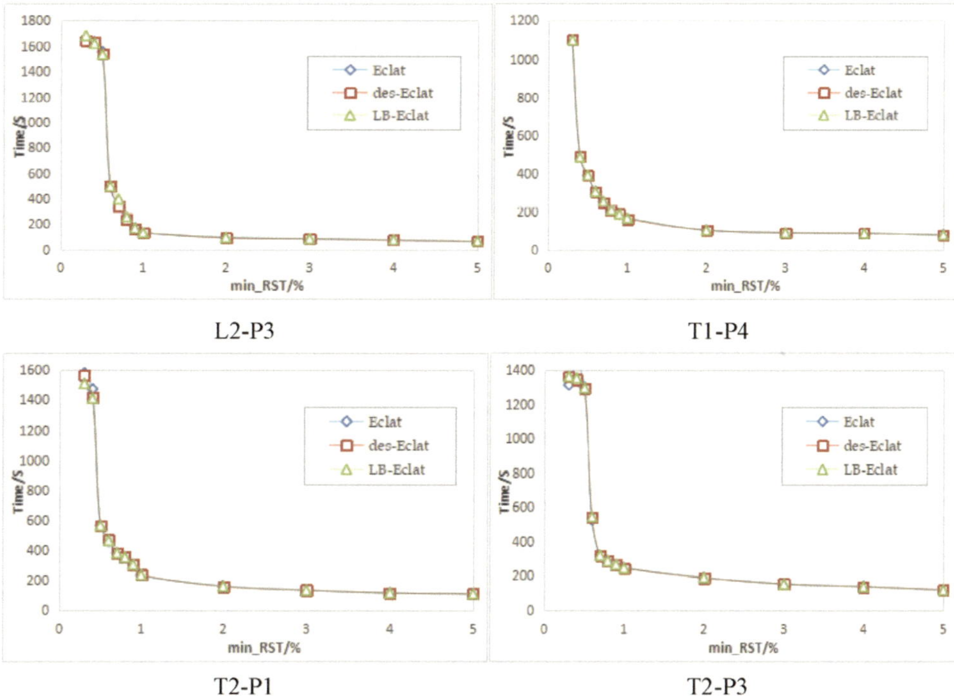

Figure 9.
Comparison of probabilistic frequent Itemsets of three algorithms on moderate density datasets.

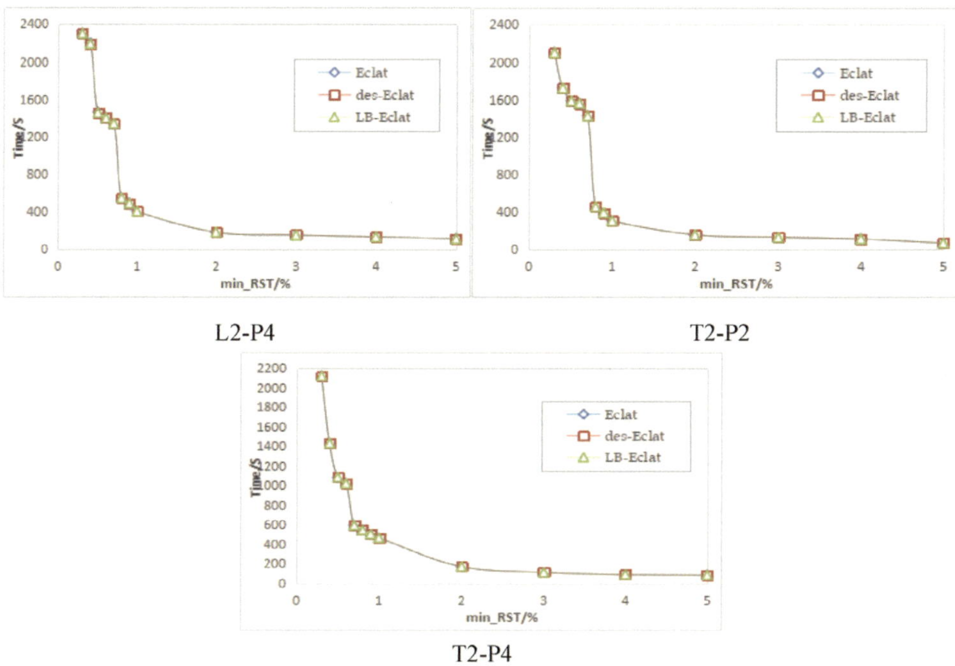

Figure 10.
Comparison of probabilistic frequent Itemsets of three algorithms on dense density datasets.

itemsets obtained is basically the same. With the increase of $\min\_RST$, the fewer the number, the smaller the value, The larger the number, the more transactions and items need to be analyzed and calculated, which will inevitably increase the time complexity and space complexity.

The experimental results show that the LB-Eclat algorithm is effective in the study of uncertain learning behavior probabilistic frequent itemsets. About the running time and memory space, LB-Eclat is better than the other two approximate algorithms in mining and analyzing the probabilistic frequent itemsets of sparse density data sets, moderate density data sets and dense density data sets. Since there are 11 learning behavior data sets, the data are all from the real learning processes, and the comparison test process is fully complete. The indicators show that LB-Eclat algorithm are robust and realistic.

6. Probabilistic frequent itemsets analysis of learning behaviors

Based on LB-Eclat algorithm, the probabilistic frequent itemsets of 11 data sets of learning behaviors are mined, and the itemsets with high probability are found. On the basis of “Support” (>0.3) and “Conference” (>0.7), the probability frequent itemsets of each dataset are mined, and then the association degree of rules generated by itemsets is verified by “Lift”. If “Lift” > 1, the association degree of relevant rules is high. In the mining results of probabilistic frequent itemsets, 2-itemsets are the most, as shown in **Tables 6–8**, the other 3-itemsets and 4-itemsets are mainly based on the intersection and combination of 2-itemsets. The higher the density of data sets, the more frequent itemsets are mined. Based on the constraints of “Support” and “Confidence”, some data sets are limited to 2-itemsets, such as L1-p2 and L1-p4.

From the distribution of frequent 2-itemsets in **Tables 6–8**, they have the following characteristics:

1. There is a strong correlation between the components of learning behaviors, and even has a more obvious impact on the components of learning results. In the data set of approximate density, the frequent itemsets of Technology courses are significantly more than that of Literature courses. It shows that the learning behavior components of Technology courses have a strong diversity, and there is a continuous and serial interaction between the components, which makes learners form the approximate frequency participation. Compared with Literature courses, the components of Technology courses are more conducive to the formation of frequent itemsets of learning behaviors.

L1-P2	**T1-P2**		**T1-P3**
forumng, homepage	forumng, homepage	content, url	forumng, homepage
forumng, content	homepage, content	wiki, url	forumng, wiki
content, final_result	homepage, wiki	subpage, url	forumng, url
forumng,final_result	homepage, subpage	homepage, final_result	homepage, content
L1-P4	homepage, url	content, final_result	homepage, wiki
	content, wiki	wiki, final_result	homepage, url
content, subpage	content, quiz	url, final_result	content, wiki
content,final_result			
T1-P3	content, url	homepage, final_result	wiki, final_result
	wiki, url	content, final_result	url, final_result

Table 6.
Probabilistic frequent 2-itemsets of sparse density data sets.

L2-P3	T1-P4	T2-P1	
forumng, homepage forumng, subpage forumng, url homepage, quiz homepage, subpage homepage, url quiz, subpage resource, subpage subpage, url homepage, final_result page, final_result quiz, final_result resource, final_result subpage, final_result	forumng, homepage forumng, wiki forumng, url homepage, content homepage, wiki homepage, url content, wiki wiki, url forumng,final_result homepage,final_result content, final_result wiki, final_result quiz, final_result subpage,final_result url, final_result	dataplus, content dataplus,questionnaire dataplus, url dualpane, content dualpane,questionnaire dualpane, subpage dualpane, url forumng, homepage homepage, content homepage, questionnaire homepage, subpage homepage, url content, page content, questionnaire content, quiz content, resource content, subpage	content, url wiki, subpage page, questionnaire page, subpage page, url questionnaire,subpage questionnaire, url quiz, subpage resource, subpage subpage, url dataplus, final_result dualpane, final_result forumng, final_result homepage, final_result content, final_result page,final_result questionnaire, final_result
quiz, final_result resource, final_result	subpage, final_result url, final_result		
T2-P3			
dataplus, content dataplus, questionnaire dataplus, url dataplus, subpage folder, quiz folder, subpage	forumng, homepage forumng, subpage homepage, content homepage, wiki homepage, questionnaire homepage, subpage homepage, url content, wiki content, questionnaire	content, subpage content, url wiki, questionnaire wiki, subpage wiki, url questionnaire, subpage questionnaire, url quiz, subpage subpage, url	dataplus, final_result folder, final_result forumng, final_result homepage, final_result content, final_result questionnaire, final_result quiz, final_result subpage, final_result url, final_result

Table 7.
Mining results of probabilistic frequent 2-itemsets of moderate density data sets.

2. For sparse density data sets, "forumng", "homepage" and "content" are beneficial to form frequent 2-itemsets with other components, which is obviously reflected in different data sets of Literature and Technology courses. "wiki" also has frequent interaction with other components in Technology courses; For moderate density and dense density data sets, frequent 2-itemsets are similar, "forumng", "homepage", "content", "url", "quiz" and "subpage" all have strong component correlation. For Technology courses, frequent itemsets formed by "dataplus", "dualpane", "wiki" and "questionnaire" are used widely and frequently.

For the frequent itemset association rules of learning behavior components, three indicators are used to measure, which are "Support", "Confidence" and "Lift". "Support" determines the correlation between the components. "Lift" > 1 indicates that there is association and has positive correlation. The higher "Lift" is, the more valuable the association rules are; if "Lift" < 1 and smaller, there is negative correlation; if Lift = 1, the components are independent and have no correlation. The association rules with "Lift" > 1 and high confidence are listed and shown in **Table 9**, these association rules are the basis for tracking, adjusting and optimizing learning behaviors.

On the whole, the association rules corresponding to the probabilistic frequent itemsets of sparse density data sets are less, and the association rules of Literature courses are less in the same density data sets [22]. For the moderate density and dense density data sets of Technology courses, rules are formed among the

L2-P4	T2-P2		
forumng, homepage	dataplus, questionnaire	content, wiki	subpage, url
homepage, subpage	dataplus, dualpane	content, page	dataplus, final_result
quiz, subpage	dataplus, content	content, questionnaire	dualpane, final_result
forumng, final_result	dataplus, page	content, quiz	folder, final_result
homepage, final_result	dataplus, url	content, subpage	forumng, final_result
page, final_result	dualpane, content	content, url	content, final_result
quiz, final_result	dualpane, page	wiki, questionnaire	homepage, final_result
subpage, final_result	dualpane, questionnaire	wiki, subpage	content, final_result
	dualpane, subpage	wiki, url	wiki, final_result
	dualpane, url	page, questionnaire	page, final_result
	folder, subpage	page, subpage	questionnaire, final_result
	forumng, homepage	page, url	quiz, final_result
	homepage, content	questionnaire, subpage	subpage, final_result
	homepage, wiki	questionnaire,	url, final_result
	homepage, subpage	urlquiz, subpage	
	homepage, url		
T2-P4			
dataplus, dualpane	dualpane, questionnaire	content, subpage	page, subpage
dataplus, content	homepage, content	content, url	page, url
dataplus, wiki	homepage, subpage	wiki, page	questionnaire, subpage
dataplus, page	homepage, url	wiki, questionnaire	questionnaire, url
dataplus, questionnaire	content, wiki	wiki, subpage	quiz, subpage
dataplus, subpage	content, page	wiki, url	resource, subpage
dataplus, url	content, questionnaire	page, questionnaire	subpage, url
dualpane, page			

Table 8.
Probabilistic frequent 2-itemsets of dense density data sets.

	Support	Conference	Lift	Rules
L1-P2	0.2301	0.8127	1.2832	{homepage, content} → {forumng}
L1-P4			None	
T1-P2	0.2152	0.7836	1.5241	{homepage} → {forumng}
T1-P3	0.2701	0.7435	1.7195	{content, wiki, subpage, url} → {homepage}
	0.2558	0.8281	1.6399	{content, wiki, subpage} → {url}
L2-P3	0.3291	0.8536	1.8408	{homepage, subpage, url} → {forumng}
	0.2453	0.7166	1.6807	{quiz, subpage, url} → {homepage}
	0.2132	0.5369	1.3577	{subpage, quiz} → {final_result}
T1-P4	0.1731	0.8467	1.7063	{homepage, wiki, url} → {forumng}
	0.2229	0.8757	1.7530	{content, wiki, url} → {homepage}
	0.3681	0.5355	1.2122	{content, wiki} → {final_result}
T2-P1	0.3522	0.7739	1.4773	{content,questionnaire,url} → {dataplus}
	0.4119	0.7049	1.6980	{content, questionnaire, subpage, url} → {datapane}
	0.3859	0.7978	1.5795	{homepage} → {forumng}
	0.4619	0.7953	2.0856	{content, questionnaire, subpage, url} → {homepage}
	0.4207	0.8682	1.7532	{page, questionnaire, quiz, resource, subpage, url} → {content}
	0.3361	0.7452	1.6985	{questionnaire, subpage, url} → {page}
	0.4747	0.7210	1.4747	{subpage, url} → {questionnaire}

	Support	Conference	Lift	Rules
	0.5151	0.8386	2.0553	{resource, url} → {subpage}
	0.3361	0.5548	1.2858	{content, subpage, quiz} → {final_result}
T2-P3	0.2023	0.7734	1.6246	{content, questionnaire, url, subpage} → {dataplus}
	0.1285	0.8243	1.6447	{homepage, subpage} → {forumng}
	0.2704	0.8609	1.7790	{content, wiki, questionnaire, subpage, url} → {homepage}
	0.3022	0.8631	1.7404	{wiki, questionnaire, subpage, url} → {content}
	0.3253	0.8098	1.5003	{url} → {subpage}
	0.2521	0.5250	1.5236	{folder, content, quiz, subpage} → {final_result}
L2-P4	0.1781	0.8473	1.4871	{homepage} → {forumng}
	0.3934	0.5563	1.0403	{subpage} → {final_result}
T2-P2	0.1989	0.7732	1.6777	{questionnaire, dualpane, content, page, url} → {dataplus}
	0.2486	0.7531	1.6984	{content, page, questionnaire, subpage, url} → {dualpane}
	0.2019	0.8072	1.5534	{homepage} → {forumng}
	0.3947	0.7515	1.7227	{content, wiki, subpage, url} → {homepage}
	0.3025	0.8761	1.7971	{wiki, page, questionnaire, quiz, subpage, url} → {content}
	0.3342	0.7527	1.6687	{questionnaire, subpage, url} → {page}
	0.2624	0.7085	1.2884	{subpage, url} → {quiz}
	0.3128	0.8552	1.6777	{url} → {subpage}
	0.3760	0.5452	1.4449	{folder, content, quiz, subpage} → {final_result}
T2-P4	0.2763	0.8002	1.7168	{dualpane, content, wiki, page, questionnaire, subpage, url} → {dataplus}
	0.2262	0.7934	1.7061	{content, subpage, url} → {homepage}
	0.2756	0.8858	1.7399	{wiki, page, questionnaire, subpage, url} → {content}
	0.3966	0.7606	1.7510	{questionnaire, subpage, url} → {page}
	0.3149	0.8222	1.9056	{url} → {subpage}

Table 9.
Association rules generated by probabilistic frequent Itemsets.

components of learning behaviors, and some of the components can produce rules with high credibility and strong relevance with the final assessment results.

It can be seen from **Table 9** that there are common association rules of components among different data sets, which indicates that these rules have strong generality; for Literature courses or Technology courses, there are some similarities in association rules, but there are also obvious differences; For the same course, in different periods, the results show that the association rules of probabilistic frequent itemsets have both intersection and differences. About {content, questionnaire, subpage, url} → {homepage}, {resource, url} → {subpage} and {resource, url} → {subpage}, the "Lift" values are higher, indicating that the association degree is very high. From the table, it is easy to form strong association rules around "questionnaire", "quiz", "forumng", "homepage", "resource", "subpage", "url" and so on. "dataplus", "dualpane", "folder", "wiki" and so on have strong relevance in Technology courses. Some of components have an obvious impact on the learning results. The extraction of these association rules can greatly simplify the categories of components in **Tables 1**–4.

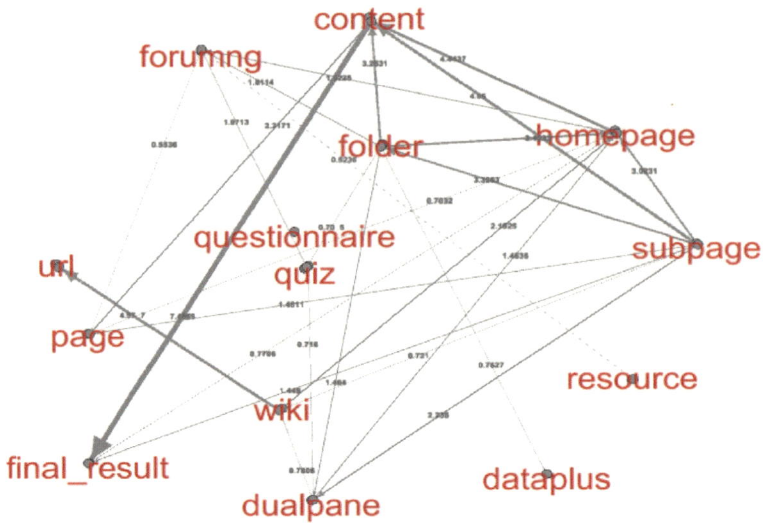

Figure 11.
The key topology of learning behaviors based on probabilistic frequent Itemsets and association rules.

The mining of probabilistic frequent itemsets and the learning of association rules are conducive to the evaluation and recommendation of components in the construction of learning behaviors [22–24]. At the same time, the formation process of learning behaviors can realize the aggregation of effective components according to these association rules. For the components related to association rules, we can build elastic proximity relationships or timely guidance strategies and recommendation mechanisms. This can effectively guide the learning processes, on the other hand, according to the needs of learning objectives, we can design association rules of probabilistic frequent itemsets according to the historical data, which is conducive to analyze and predict feasible participation components.

Based on the data in **Tables 6–9**, the nodes and edges of component interaction processes are constructed, and the key constituent units of learning behavior data sets are generated by Gephi. **Figure 11** shows the topological structure and relationship weight of probabilistic frequent itemsets. There are 14 participation components involved and the weight of each relationship (edge) is calculated automatically. The thickness of the line indicates the strength of the relationship, and the dotted lines represent the potential relationships. The construction and extraction of the key topology of learning behaviors supported by probabilistic frequent itemsets are completed, which is a referential result of data-driven learning behavior prediction and decision making.

7. Decision-making scheme for improving learning behaviors

Studying learning behavior through big data can promote learners to improve their learning processes and learning effects [25]. Aiming at the mining and association analysis of probability frequent itemsets, we realize 11 data subsets of learning behaviors with components as the basic structure characteristics. On the basis of Eclat framework, the vertical data format is adopted to design and improve the data structure and analysis algorithm for learning behavior components. Through the indicator comparison of approximate algorithms, the improved algorithm is effective and feasible for the analysis processes of data subsets, especially in the application of moderate density and dense density data set. Based on the data analysis results, "Support", "Confidence" and "Lift" are the measurement indicators, and the corresponding thresholds are set. The probabilistic frequent itemsets and association rules are mined, and the key topology of learning behaviors supported by the probabilistic frequent itemsets are constructed. The whole processes of mining and analyzing probabilistic frequent itemsets are based on the vertical data format, which ensures the depth and breadth of data research results for decision prediction.

The research of learning behaviors is a specific branch of big data. It is different from other types of data characteristics. Because of the periodicity, continuity, collectivity and individuality of learning behaviors, there may be greater instability and discreteness between the generated data and the expected data. It is very difficult in data analysis and decision making, so it is necessary to design appropriate data structures and algorithms [26, 27] to carry out multi-dimensional empirical study on learning behaviors. Through a series of work and research results of probabilistic frequent itemsets analysis, the following decision schemes are obtained.

7.1 Learning content will affect the frequent itemsets of learning behaviors

Learning content determines learners' tendency. The data of learning behaviors focuses on two Literature courses and two Technology courses, which correspond to multiple learning periods respectively. On the whole, the learning process of Technology courses more complicated, the learning behavior components are more diverse, and the online learning process description is also quite complete and comprehensive, that forms larger scale datasets. Learning content will affect the data density, components and the actual learning processes of learners, which determines the frequent itemsets mining results. For example, from the probabilistic frequent itemsets of the two learning periods of L1 course, the online learning processes corresponding to the learning contents do not have advantages, there is no effective correlation between the components and the learning assessment results, and the advantages of online learning mode are not obvious, which may be more suitable for the teaching mode.

Therefore, the construction of learning behaviors depends on the learning content. According to the mining results of frequent itemsets of historical data and the analysis of association rules, the learning mode of the course is optimized in the new learning period. Based on the learning content, we guide or expand the components of learning behaviors, so as to enhance the learning interest.

7.2 Teaching goals will affect the frequent itemsets of learning behaviors

The same learning content in different learning period, can produce different learning behavior data density, so as to get different frequent itemsets. In different learning periods, the frequent itemsets and association rules obtained by the algorithm are similar, but there are also obvious differences. The components are not the same, and some data sets are quite different. Learners in different periods have different teaching needs, and then correspond to different teaching objectives; On the other hand, the participation and traction in the learning process make the different participation components, and the stickiness of different components are different, which determines the frequent items, and thus produces different association rules, it even affects learners' assessment methods and learning results.

Therefore, the construction of learning behaviors should consider the learning periods and the actual learners, flexibly construct teaching objectives, and design adaptive learning behavior components. In the learning processes, we should also timely analyze the learning behaviors, mine the existing problems and learners' preferences, adjust the components in time, and optimize the learning methods appropriately. We should build a real-time and effective data tracking and analysis mechanisms.

7.3 The frequent itemsets of learning behavior have the characteristics of explicit and implicit association

There are differences in interaction mode of learning behavior components in different platforms, but the demands of serving learning behaviors are the same, that is to realize the continuity of learning behaviors and achieve the learning effects through the interaction of components. Through the mining of probabilistic frequent itemsets and the analysis of association rules, the components of frequent itemsets have explicit association features, and different frequent itemsets may also have implicit association features. It has a strong recommendation value for the prediction and feedback of latent learning behaviors. The key topological relationships of learning behaviors are shown in **Figure 11**, that can provide references for the follow-up learning processes of similar or the same courses, and expand learning methods.

Therefore, the construction of learning behaviors should not only consider the learning content and teaching objectives, but also refer to the historical effective learning behaviors, and also need to carry out effective learning process reform and learning strategy change based on data analysis, gradually promote learners to develop effective learning habits and methods, and construct new learning behavior components. According to the learning situation, stage learning feedback, potential behavior recommendation and implicit interest mining are achieved in order to improve the learning quality.

7.4 Learning behavior needs the adaptive support of specific algorithm and data structure

The generation of learning behaviors is a multi-dimensional process. The research strength of these data determines the cognitive strength of learning behaviors. There are different perspectives on the composition of learning behaviors, which determines different research methods. How to carry out relatively sufficient modeling description and business processing of learning behaviors presents challenges to learning analytics. Some existing software tools and analysis methods can not guarantee the appropriate quantification, standardization and initialization, the analysis process and experimental conclusion may not be thorough and comprehensive. Compared with the statistics and test of learning behaviors carried out by sampling, the effective and comprehensive analysis of learning behaviors is more convincing.

Therefore, the empirical analysis of learning behaviors should be the comprehensive application process of data-driven technologies and methods. Combined with the data characteristics, the technical requirements are demonstrated, and the structures and algorithms suitable for data attributes and process characteristics are designed. This aspect has huge research space and prospect in the field of education big data, which poses challenges for researchers. Learning analytics of educational big data is essentially data analysis, and it is a comprehensive application of computer science and technology, statistics, engineering, etc., and the design and development of general tools in this respect still need time [28]. For a specific data set, it is feasible and more realistic to design suitable data structures and algorithms for decision making.

8. Conclusion

The learning analysis of learning behaviors is a complex process. The data structure, attribute characteristics and relationship categories bring more difficulties. Moreover, the data has strong uncertainty and instability, so it is difficult to achieve technical unity and generality [29]. The development of online learning model gives new definitions and norms to learning behaviors, and also requires new data structure, attribute characteristics, relationship categories, etc. many technologies and methods that can be used in the research of learning behaviors may be inefficient for new data, or do nothing for the new research branches. This research is about the design and application of intelligent data mining technology on a big data set of learning behaviors. Based on Eclat framework, the data structure and algorithms are improved. Starting from the vertical data format, mining probabilistic frequent itemsets, analyzing association rules, and realizing data-driven decision making. In the subsequent research of learning behaviors, for uncertain data, we continue to conduct in-depth research and demonstration of methods and technologies, improve the quality of data analysis and relationship perspective, and provide more valuable conclusions for decision making and prediction feedback of learning behaviors.

Compliance with ethical standards

The authors certify that there is no conflict of interest with any individual/organization for the present work.

A list of acronyms

FP	Frequent Pattern
PFC	Frequent Pattern Calculation
LB-Eclat	Learning Behavior Eclat
Descending Eclat	Descending “Support”

Author details

Xiaona Xia[1,2,3]

1 Faculty of Education, Qufu Normal University, Qufu, Shandong, China

2 Chinese Academy of Education Big Data, Qufu Normal University, Qufu, Shandong, China

3 School of Computer Science, Qufu Normal University, Rizhao, Shandong, China

*Address all correspondence to: xiaxn@sina.com

References

[1] Kusemererwa, C., Munene, J. C., Laura, O. A., & Balunywa, J. W. (2020). Individual learning behavior: do all its dimensions matter for self-employment practice among youths in uganda?. Journal of Enterprising Communities: People and Places in the Global Economy, Vol. 14 No. 3, pp. 373-396. DOI: 10.1108/JEC-02-2020-0012

[2] Wang, X., Guchait, P., & Paamehmetolu, A. (2020). Tolerating errors in hospitality organizations: relationships with learning behavior, error reporting and service recovery performance. International Journal of Contemporary Hospitality Management, Vol. 32 No. 8, 2635-2655 DOI: 10.1108/IJCHM-01-2020-0001

[3] B, Z. Y. A., C, G. Z. A. B., C, D. L. A. B., & B, H. L. A. (2020). Learning crowd behavior from real data: a residual network method for crowd simulation. *Neurocomputing*, 404(3), 173-185, DOI: 10.1016/j.neucom.2020.04.141.

[4] Schmerse, D. (2020). Preschool quality effects on learning behavior and later achievement in germany: moderation by socioeconomic status. *Child Development*, Volume 00, Number 0, 1-18, DOI: 10.1111/cdev.13357.

[5] Lai, S., Sun, B., Wu, F., & Xiao, R. (2020). Automatic personality identification using students' online learning behavior. IEEE Transactions on Learning Technologies, 13(1), 26-37, DOI:10.1109/TLT.2019.2924223

[6] Ines Šarić-Grgić, Ani Grubišić, Ljiljana Šerić, & Robinson, T. J. (2020). Student clustering based on learning behavior data in the intelligent tutoring system. International Journal of Distance Education Technologies, 18 (2), 73-89, DOI:10.4018/IJDET.2020040105.

[7] Yokoyama, M., & Miwa, K. (2020). STUDENTS' CONCEPTION OF LEARNING AND LEARNING BEHAVIOR FROM MULTIPLE-GOALS PERSPECTIVE. *7th International Conference on Educational Technologies 2020*, 33-40, DOI: 10.33965/icedutech2020_202002L005.

[8] Silva, J., Varela, N., Luz Adriana Borrero López, & Rafael Humberto Rojas Millán. (2019). Association rules extraction for customer segmentation in the smes sector using the apriori algorithm. Procedia Computer ence, 151, 1207-1212, DOI: 10.1016/j.procs.2019.04.173.

[9] Hossain, T. M., Watada, J., Jian, Z., Sakai, H., & Aziz, I. A. (2020). Missing well log data handling in complex lithology prediction: an nis apriori algorithm approach. International journal of innovative computing, information & control: IJICIC, 16(3), 1077-1091, DOI: 10.24507/ijicic.16.03.1077

[10] Hong, J., Tamakloe, R., & Park, D. (2020). Discovering insightful rules among truck crash characteristics using apriori algorithm. Journal of advanced transportation, 2020(2), 1-16, DOI: 10.1088/1742-6596/1477/2/022032

[11] Bashkari, S., Sami, A., & Rastegar, M. (2020). Outage cause detection in power distribution systems based on data mining. *IEEE Transactions on Industrial Informatics*, PP(99), 1-1, DOI: 10.1109/TII.2020.2966505

[12] Abdullah, S. S., Sedig, K., & Rostamzadeh, N. (2020). Multiple regression analysis and frequent itemset mining of electronic medical records: a visual analytics approach using visa_m3r3. Data, 5(2), 1-26, DOI: 10.3390/data5020033.

[13] Chaghari, A., Mohammad-Reza Feizi-Derakhshi, & Mohammad-Ali

Balafar. (2020). The combination of term relations analysis and weighted frequent itemset model for multidocument summarization. Computational Intelligence, 36(2), 783-812, DOI: 10.1111/coin.12270

[14] Raj, S., Ramesh, D., Sreenu, M., & Sethi, K. K. (2020). Eafim: efficient apriori-based frequent itemset mining algorithm on spark for big transactional data. Knowledge and Information Systems, 62(4), 3565–3583, DOI: 10.1007/s10115-020-01464-1

[15] Rahman, A., Mutiarawan, R. A., Darmawan, A., Rianto, Y., & Syafrullah, M. (2020). Prediction Of Students Academic Success Using Case Based Reasoning. *2019 6th International Conference on Electrical Engineering, Computer Science and Informatics (EECSI)*. IEEE, 171-176, DOI:10.23919/EECSI48112.2019.8977104

[16] Singh, P., Singh, S., Mishra, P. K., & Garg, R. (2020). RDD-Eclat: Approaches to Parallelize Eclat Algorithm on Spark RDD Framework. *Second International Conference on Computer Networks and Communication Technologies*, 755-768, DOI: 10.1007/978-3-030-37051-0_85

[17] Zhang, C., Tian, P., Zhang, X., Jiang, Z. L., Yao, L., & Wang, X. (2019). Fast eclat algorithms based on minwise hashing for large scale transactions. IEEE Internet of Things Journal, 6(2), 3948-3961, DOI: 10.1109/JIOT.2018.2885851

[18] Robu, V., & Santos, V. D. D. (2019). Mining Frequent Patterns in Data Using Apriori and Eclat: A Comparison of the Algorithm Performance and Association Rule Generation. 2019 6th International Conference on Systems and Informatics (ICSAI), 1478-1481, DOI: 10.1109/ICSAI48974.2019.9010367

[19] Man, M., Jusoh, J. A., Saany, S. I. A., Bakar, W. A. W. A., & Ibrahim, M. H. (2019). Analysis study on r-eclat algorithm in infrequent itemsets mining. International Journal of Electrical and Computer Engineering, 9 (6), 5446-5453, DOI: 10.11591/ijece.v9i6.pp5446-5453

[20] Atis KAPENIEKS, Iveta DAUGULE, Kristaps KAPENIEKS, Viktors ZAGORSKIS, Janis KAPENIEKS Jr, Zanis TIMSANS, & Ieva VITOLINA. (2020) TELECI Approach for e-Learning User Behavior Data Visualization and Learning Support Algorithm. Baltic Journal of Modern Computing, Vol. 8, No. 1, 129-142, DOI: 10.22364/bjmc.2020.8.1.06.

[21] Lin Tan, Yali Chen, Runhan Yang, Li Lai. (2020) Empirical Research on the Effect of Collaborative Learning in Blended Learning Mode Based on KNN Algorithm. ICIET 2020: *Proceedings of the 2020 8th International Conference on Information and Education Technology*, March 2020, 48-52, DOI: 10.1145/3395245.3395251

[22] Chebi, H., Tabet-Derraz, H., Sayah, R., Meroufel, A., & Meraihi, Y. (2020). Intelligence and adaptive global algorithm detection of crowd behavior. International Journal of Computer Vision and Image Processing, Volume 10, Issue 1, 2020, 24-40, DOI: 10.4018/IJCVIP.2020010102

[23] Xia, X. (2021). Interaction recognition and intervention based on context feature fusion of learning behaviors in interactive learning environments. Interactive Learning Environments, Advance online publication 17 Jan 2021. 1-19. DOI: 10.1080/10494820.2021.1871632

[24] Yuniarti, T., Widhianningrum, P., & Sulistyowati, N. W. (2020). A study of accounting learning achievements using emotional intelligence and learning behavior, ASSETS Jurnal Akuntansi dan Pendidikan, 9(1):52-60, DOI: 10.25273/jap.v9i1.4179

[25] Xia, X. (2020). Random field design and collaborative inference strategies for learning interaction activities. *Interactive Learning Environments*, Advance online publication 30 Dec 2020. 1–25. DOI: 10.1080/10494820.2020.1863236

[26] Smiderle, R., Sandro José Rigo, Marques, L. B., Coelho, J. A. P. D. M., & Jaques, P. A. (2020). The impact of gamification on students' learning, engagement and behavior based on their personality traits. Smart Learning Environments, 7(1), 1-11, DOI: 10.1186/s40561-019-0098-x.

[27] Xia, X. (2020). Learning behavior mining and decision recommendation based on association rules in interactive learning environment. *Interactive Learning Environments*. Advance online publication 4 Aug 2020. 1–16. DOI: 10.1080/10494820.2020.1799028

[28] John, C., & Meinel, C. (2020). Learning Behavior of Men and Women in MOOC Discussion Forums – A Case Study. 2020 IEEE Global Engineering Education Conference (EDUCON). IEEE, 300-307, DOI:10.1109/EDUCON45650.2020.9125322

[29] Jiang, L., & Dong, K. (2020). Artificial intelligence-based learning behavior data mining and network teaching quality monitoring mechanism. Journal of Physics Conference Series, 1533, 032058, DOI: 10.1088/1742-6596/1533/3/032058

Chapter 9

The Application of Simple Additive Bayesian Allocation Network Process in System Obsolescence

Oluwatomi Adetunji

Abstract

In designing a system, multi-dimensional obsolescence design criteria such as Scheduling; Reliability, Availability, Maintainability; Performance and Functionality; and Costs affect its overall lifespan. This work examines the impacts of these factors on systems during the design phase using a new application called the Simple Additive Bayesian Allocation Network Process (SABANP). The application uses a combination of Multi-Criteria Decision Making (MCDM) methodology and a Bayesian Belief Network to address the impact of obsolescence on a system. Unlike the requirement of weights that are prevalent in the analysis of MCDM, this application does not require weights. Moreover, this application accounts for functional dependencies of criteria, which is not possible with the MCDM methodologies. A case study was conducted using military and civilian experts. Data were collected on systems' obsolescence criteria and analyzed using the application to make trade-off decisions. The results show that the application can address complex obsolescence decisions that are both quantitative and qualitative. Expert validation showed that SABANP successfully identified the best system for mitigating obsolescence.

Keywords: Obsolescence, Multi-Criteria Decision Making, Bayesian Belief Network, Simple Additive Bayesian Allocation Network Process, Diminishing Manufacturing Sources and Material Shortages (DMSMS)

1. Introduction

Obsolescence is an event bound to happen. It occurs when a component or system (hardware and software) cannot carry out required functions or continue to be useful. Reasons include the component not being available for purchase in its original form from the original manufacturer or producer; not being maintainable, affordable to repair, or reliable; technology evolution; and anything else that causes a component or system to no longer be viable [1–3]. Obsolescence also encompasses discontinuance. However, Pecht and Das [4] made a distinction between the "obsolescence" and "discontinuance" concepts. Discontinuance takes place when the manufacturer stops the production of a component, which occurs at a part-number or manufacturer-specific level, while obsolescence occurs at a technology

 IntechOpen

level [4, 5]. Obsolescence can happen to products, systems, processes, software, policy, standards and organizations.

Many solutions have been proposed for managing obsolescence. However, over the past decade, it is estimated that over $9 billion has been wasted on this problem [6]. The problem is often a result of the rate of technological advancement in systems rendering them obsolete. Managing obsolescence has traditionally been done with a reactive approach. This means that the action taken to resolve the issue occurs after the obsolescence is found. Today, with the rapid growth of digital technology, digital systems and software are reaching their end-of-life sooner rather than later.

Moreover, the contractual agreement between Original Equipment Manufacturer (OEM) and the government is often limited in scope and reactive in nature. This chapter proposes a new application model — a proactive approach that takes into account obsolescence factors that affect systems during the design phase.

The proposed model uses a combination of a Bayesian Belief Network and an MCDM for identifying systems that are more susceptible to obsolescence, which can provide an alert to the system owners to take action before the obsolescence occurs. The combined application of Bayesian Belief Network and MCDM to manage obsolescence in this work serves as the addition to the body of knowledge. This chapter refers to the extension of this methodology as the Simple Additive Bayesian Allocation Network Process (SABANP). The SABANP enables the analyst to define the complex model by connecting a particular Bayesian Believe Network process to the system components (i.e., the leaf nodes), whereby obsolescence characteristics are modeled as an event. When modeling the dynamic characteristics as events, the following set of processes is developed to model the variety of obsolescence criteria:

1. The time when the event occurs or the time to obsolescence,

2. The order by which the events will likely occur, and

3. The event occurrence dependence on time and costs.

The costs that include procurement are required because of their ramifications on the obsolescence problem. The end result of obsolescence in a system is the significant costs it incurs for the organization. The DoD estimated costs upward of $750 M annually for managing obsolescence [7]. Obsolescence is time-dependent; therefore, the model assumed a 95% confidence that systems would be obsolete within two years.

2. Background

In managing system obsolescence, three approaches are used: reactive, proactive and strategic. The reactive approach addresses the obsolescence after the component or part is obsolete, while the proactive one addresses the obsolescence before it occurs [8]. The strategic approach often uses a combination of reactive and proactive approaches to manage the risk of obsolescence; however, the decision models that address obsolescence are underdeveloped [6]. The most agreed upon approach to managing obsolescence is the proactive strategy since it ensures that systems with long life spans are continuously and effectively maintained [9, 10].

Originally, the work began from the need to find better and more effective ways to deal with obsolescence in a proactive manner. To do so, the following obsolescence criteria were chosen from the literature [2, 11, 12]:

(1) Performance and Functionality (P&F); (2) Cost, which includes Acquisition, Licensing and Support; (3) Personnel Training (PT); (4) Reliability, Availability, and Maintainability (RAM); (5) Procurement (PR), which includes Vendor Assembly and Installation Support; (6) Configuration Management (CM); (7) Data Rights and Technical Documentation (DR&TD); and (8) Open Architecture and Standards (OA&S). We also added (9) Technology Readiness Level (TRL), which was adapted from the DoD Technology Readiness Assessment Guidance [13], and (10) Obsolescence Schedule Risk (O&SR).

Each criterion was assessed as either "higher is better" (HG) in the case of a criterion that has a benefit to the stakeholder, or "lower is better" (LW) in the case of non-benefit to the stakeholder to determine the criterion's weight factor. For example, Cost is defined as LW because high ownership and acquisition costs are a non-benefit to the stakeholder. The same can be said of O&SR. This convention is accounted for within the model construct as shown in **Table 1**.

Experts were asked to assess each system's P&F; Costs; required level of PT; RAM; whether they are easily Procurable (PR); installation support and vendor assembly in the design phase. These systems run on software programs, and experts were also asked via a survey to assess each system's CM, the availability of DR&TD, the OA&S, and the TRL by assigning grades on a scale ranging from 0 to 9. These criteria were agreed upon by the experts and are based on the literature review.

Experts rated the O&SR on a scale of 1–5, where 5 represents the highest score and 1 the lowest score. While the rest of the criteria scales are from 0–9, a scale of 1–5 was used for the O&SR because a risk matrix that goes from 1–5 is easily conceptualized by expert practitioners.

2.1 Criteria weights

Weights (w_j) were required to sum to one, and all criteria weights met this requirement. The ratings represent the weights of the ten criteria as provided by the decision maker based on experience and expertise. The weight data served as the inputs to the Technique for Order of Preference by Similarity to Ideal Solution (TOPSIS) model. This decision making method, that is, TOPSIS was used to validate the Simple Additive Bayesian Allocation Network Process. **Table 2** shows the decision maker-weighted values for each criterion, which total to 1 or 100%.

Criteria (x_j)	**(1) P&F**	**(2) Cost**	**(3) PT**	**(4) RAM**	**(5) PR**	**(6) CM**	**(7) DR&TD**	**(8) OA&S**	**(9) TRL**	**(10) O&SR**
Weight Factors	HG	LW	HG	HG	HG	HG	HG	HG	HG	LW

Table 1.
Criteria benefit and non-benefit weight factors.

Criteria (x_j)	**(1) P&F**	**(2) Cost**	**(3) PT**	**(4) RAM**	**(5) PR**	**(6) CM**	**(7) DR&TD**	**(8) OA&S**	**(9) TRL**	**(10) O&SR**
Weights (w_j)	0.19	0.12	0.06	0.15	0.11	0.07	0.09	0.07	0.06	0.08

Table 2.
Decision maker-assigned weight values.

2.2 The time-discrete Bayesian belief network modeling

The Bayesian Networks are composed of nodes and arcs [14, 15]. Bayesian Networks have the capability to perform diagnostic analysis because of its rich graphical and embedded mathematical capability of modeling and analyzing dynamic behavior of systems [16]. Nodes, in this case, represent Random Variables and arcs between nodes represent the dependencies between the random variables [14]. It uniquely defines joint probability distribution of the random variables. Once the joint probability distribution is known, any random variable query can be solved. Furthermore, random variables can be either infinite (continuous random variable) or finite (discrete random variable) [14]. This chapter only considers discrete random variable since the data that are gathered are from experts and the distribution is discrete. There are three types of nodes: root nodes, sequential root nodes, and leaf nodes. Root nodes are nodes without incoming arcs or without parents, and sequential root nodes are nodes that have incoming arcs and outgoing arcs or are both parents and children. Leaf nodes are nodes without outgoing arcs or without children. Root nodes will have marginal prior probability tables that are associated with them, and sequential root nodes and leaf nodes have conditional probability tables that are associated with them [14]. A conditional probability table provides the probability of each random variable state conditional on the values of its parent nodes. To determine the joint probability distribution, the Chain Rule is used and assumes that the conditional independence is encoded in the designed Bayesian Believe Network structure between the variables.

The joint probability distribution of the variables set $\{X_1, X_2, \dots, X_M\}$ is given as follows [4]:

$$P\left[X_1, X_2, \dots, X_m\right] = \prod_{i=1}^{m} P[X_i | parents(X_i)], i = 1, 2, 3 \dots, m \tag{1}$$

Recent research works have resulted in better and more efficient algorithms for computing and inferring probabilities in Bayesian Networks. The inference has become easier to the point that algorithms can utilize the independence assumptions between variables and its powerful computations make the command execution quicker for the user. Bayesian Networks have been used extensively in areas such as medical diagnosis, troubleshooting systems, manufacturing control, etc. Nevertheless, it has not been used to mitigate or predict obsolescence in systems with Subject Matter Experts' (SMEs) input or qualitative analysis.

To develop the model, a discrete-time Bayesian Believe Network is formulated to model the system obsolescence. The leaf node or random variable represents the system component. The system component herein is categorized as a component, sub-system or system that interacts between collections of components. These leaf nodes that are used in the experiment are the Integrated Bridge System that are found on Naval Vessels, as described in Section 2.4.

By using this model, one can analyze the interactions among the criteria and find the critical criteria that could have the most adverse effects on a system's operations. This model is used to develop simulation test scenarios, such as what if the costs were not a significant factor in the tradeoff analysis or what if the configuration management does not have any effect on the system's lifecycle. This analysis can also gather information on which obsolescence-related attributes should be prioritized with respect to the design, development, testing, and maintenance.

2.3 Expert judgment

The expert judgments were used to gather the required input data for this experiment. The expert-assigned scores were documented and aggregated for each leaf node based on the agreed upon obsolescence criteria, after normalization of the scores. Though the systems that were employed for the experiment were fielded on Navy ships, the experts were asked to initiate a scenario in which system development was being planned on a new ship class in order to determine the best system against obsolescence through which it can be mitigated.

The system of reference Integrated Bridge System was established after iterative discussions with experts. The research participants were recruited by e-mail with nineteen obsolescence experts completing and returning responses. The minimum requirement for expert judgment participation was set at fifteen returned surveys. Therefore, this number of responses is acceptable for expert judgment. The demographic data also reflected the experts' diverse experiences. All participants had at least four years of experience in managing obsolescence and DMSMSs with some exceeding 35 years of experience. Approximately 10% had a Ph.D., 58% had a master's degree, and 32% had a bachelor's degree. The analysis also revealed that 70% were employed by organizations with 500 or more employees, and these organization sizes ranged from 500 to 100,000 employees.

Participants were asked to complete the study that consisted of approximately 90 data fields. The survey data responses were documented, and the ranking of each alternative on each criterion across the experts was aggregated, normalized and transposed into the model. Exceptions were made for the Cost criterion data scale where the actual cost range data were used. The criteria agreed upon by the experts were used to formulate the survey questions.

2.4 An integrated bridge system (IBS)

An IBS serves as the context of the survey instrument. The IBS on the Naval vessels of the USS Arleigh (DDG-51), the USS Ticonderoga (CG-47) and the USS Nimitz (CVN-68) were examined in this work. The IBS serves as the system-under-test. An IBS is designed to assist the vessel navigator in selecting information that is relevant to the operational context by collecting, processing, and presenting relevant data without cluttering displays with other information that may not be needed at that point. It takes a systems approach to the automated collection, processing, control, and display of ship-control and vital navigational sensor data to maximize the bridge watch efficiency and safety. An IBS is based on human-machine interaction, which integrates all navigational functions and provides accurate navigational information to operators or users with no human error. Its capabilities include multifunction workstations, multiple layers of redundancy, Commercial Off-the-Shelf (COTS) hardware, ease of maintenance, and open system design (i.e., intersystem links to other systems). These systems fall under the purview of being mission essential. Mission essential systems are systems that can have an adverse impact on the mission if they are not operational due to obsolescence.

2.5 Research process

The following steps were used in the research process. One must first determine the current deterministic MCDM methods that are applicable for use in nonlinear (multidimensional) decision analysis. Then, currently available mission-ready systems that serve as points of reference for the study was identified. Finally, an analysis was conducted using the Simple Additive Bayesian Allocation Network Process model with expert judgments in the analysis of alternatives in order to select the best system against obsolescence.

3. Methodology

Simple Additive Bayesian Allocation Network Process (SABANP) utilized the components of the Simple Additive Weighing (SAW) method as the input variables to the Bayesian Belief Network. SAW is an MCDM. To better understand SABANP, it is necessary to provide details of what SAW is and how it is used in the model. The SAW model, which is also known as the WSM or the "weighted average," is a common approach used for multicriteria analysis [17].

One must first calculate the normalized decision matrix for the benefit criteria (higher is better), where n_{ij} is the normalized score of the ith alternative with respect to j^{th} criterion, and r_{ij} are the values in the decision matrix provided by the experts [17, 18]:

$$n_{ij} = {}^{r_{ij}}/_{r_{ij}^{max}}, i = 1, 2, 3, \dots m, j = 1, 2, 3 \dots, n \tag{2}$$

r_{ij}^{max} is the maximum value of the ith alternative with respect to each jth criterion in the decision matrix.

For the non-benefit criteria (lower is better), r_{ij}^{min} is the minimum value of the ith alternative with respect to each jth criterion in the decision matrix [6]:

$$n_{ij} = {}^{r_{ij}^{min}}/_{r_{ij}}, i = 1, 2, 3, \dots m, j = 1, 2, 3 \dots, n \tag{3}$$

The normalized Matrix for IBS is found in **Table 3**.

The best alternative is the one that maximizes A_i in Eq. (4) below. The weights (w_j) are the weighted criteria values, and they sum to 1 as shown in **Table 2**.

Criteria	IBS DDG-51 Class	IBS CG-47 Class	IBS CVN-68 Class
(1) P&F	1	0.920	1
(2) Cost	0.984	1	0.815
(3) PT	0.9717	0.937	1
(4) RAM	1	0.889	0.959
(5) PR	1	0.896	0.976
(6) CM	1	0.896	0.976
(7) DR&TD	0.947	0.895	1
(8) OA&S	0.987	1	0.939
(9) TRL	1	1	0.979
(10) O&SR	1	0.938	0.978

The time for the system to reach obsolescence was modeled with a 95% confidence interval, i.e., the software and hardware would be obsolete within two years.

Table 3.
SAW normalized matrix.

$$A_i = \sum_{j=1}^{n} w_j n_{ij}, i = 1, 2, 3 \dots, m \tag{4}$$

The SAW model is governed by additive utility theory [19]. As shown in the equation above, each alternative aggregate value is equivalent to the summation of its multiplication. In a one-dimensional case in which the units are similar—for example, seconds, feet, and dollars—the WSM is easy to use [17, 20]. The approach becomes difficult when applied to decision-making problems that are multidimensional [21]. The weights were assessed during the data collection using the direct weighting method. The direct weighting method allows the decision maker to rank the criteria and provide subjective values to the criteria weights based on the defined rank. However, the weights were not needed in the SABANP model to calculate the best alternative. Eqs. (2) and (3) were used since SABANP requires only the normalization of the experts' inputs. The normalized scores ranging from 0 to 1, as shown in **Table 3**, were transposed into the SABANP model for the analysis.

3.1 Simple additive Bayesian allocation network process (SABANP)

The SABANP process begins by populating the survey's raw data into the decision matrix. As shown in **Table 4**, the score of criterion C_j with regard to alternative A_i is r_{ij} and the weight of the C_j *is* W_j. The weights are not required for the analysis.
The following steps are required to conduct SABANP analysis:

1. The normalized decision matrix is first determined (Eqs. (2) and (3)). The normalized score (r_{ij}) is computed to turn the different attribute dimensions r_{ij} into nondimensional attributes, allowing for comparison throughout the attributes.

2. After the normalized decision matrix is determined, the true and false functions are utilized to establish the initial probabilities:

$$\text{The true function is given as } T(n_{ij}), \text{where } T(n_{ij}) = n_{ij}; \tag{5}$$

$$\text{And the false function is given as } F(n_{ij}), \text{ where } F(n_{ij}) = 1 - T(n_{ij}) = n_{ij}^*$$

	C1	C2	...	Cn
A 1	r_{11}	r_{12}	...	r_{1n}
A 2	r_{21}	r_{22}	...	r_{2n}
A 3	r_{31}	r_{32}	...	r_{3n}
.	.	.	.	.
.	.	.	.	.
.	.	.	.	.
Am	r_{m1}	r_{m2}	...	r_{mn}
	W_1	W_2	...	W_n

Table 4.
Raw data decision matrix.

	C1	C2	...	Cn			C1	C2	...	Cn
A 1	X_{11}	X_{12}	...	X_{1n}	⇒	A 1	n_{11}, n_{11}^*	...	...	n_{1n}, n_{1n}^*
A 2	X_{21}	X_{22}	...	X_{2n}		A 2	n_{21}, n_{21}^*	...	...	n_{2n}, n_{2n}^*
A 3	X_{31}	X_{32}	...	X_{3n}	⇒	A 3	n_{31}, n_{31}^*	...	...	n_{3n}, n_{3n}^*
.	.	.	.	.		.	.	.	.	.
.	.	.	.	.		.	.	.	.	.
.	.	.	.	.	⇒	.	.	.	.	.
Am	X_{m1}	X_{m2}	...	X_{in}		Am	n_{m1}, n_{31}^*	...	...	n_{in}, n_{in}^*

Table 5.
Data decision matrix.

3. Initial probabilities, n_{ij} and n_{ij}^* are assigned to each variable set $\{X_{ij}\}$ in the joint distribution function (Eq. (6)) as shown in **Table 5**.

The joint probability distribution (JPD) of the variables set $\{X_{11}, X_{21}, \ldots, X_{mn}\}$ is given as follows:

$$P[X_{11}, X_{21}, \ldots, X_{mn}] = \prod_{i=1}^{m} \prod_{j=1}^{n} P[X_{ij} | parents(X_{ij})], i = 1, 2, 3 \ldots, m; j = 1, 2, 3 \ldots, n \quad (6)$$

In modeling the system, the IBS system data collected from experts with respect to the systems alternatives and criteria were analyzed using the SABANP. NETICA™ software was used to develop the model. NETICA™ is a powerful, easy-to-use, complete program for developing belief networks and influence diagrams. It provides an interface for drawing networks, and creating relationships between variables which can be probabilities, equations, or data files.

The systems were modeled using RAM, P&F, PR, CM, DR&TD availability, OA&S, TRL, PT, and O&SR as inherent factors that affect the system's design with effects on the costs and time to obsolescence. The NETICAL™ software model shows the captured image when the model was simulated twice or when N = 2 as displayed in **Figure 1**, where N represents the number of times the model and simulation were run. A graphical representation of it is shown in **Figure 2** for the IBS 1 on DDG-51. **Figures 3** and **4** show the graphical representations of the SABANP models of the IBSs (2 and 3) on CG-47 and CVN-68, respectively.

The research question was centered on the following: Does using the newly derived methodology (SABANP) to evaluate multiple obsolescence characteristics in a System enable one to predict which system is less susceptible to obsolescence?

The null hypothesis is that SABANP cannot predict which System is less susceptible to obsolescence, and the alternative hypothesis is that SABANP can predict which system is less susceptible to obsolescence. Additionally, statistical analysis was not conducted. Rather, the model was ran one hundred times (100x,) and the results were aggregated for accepting or rejecting the null hypothesis. A sensitivity analysis was also performed on the results.

Three questions were used within the survey to validate the SME inputs. These questions were used to cross-examine the survey data received from the experts. The data were analyzed to check for inconsistencies. Individual responses to system rankings and criteria weights were plotted to ensure that there were no outliers, and that the data are attributed to a credible sample of expert practitioners.

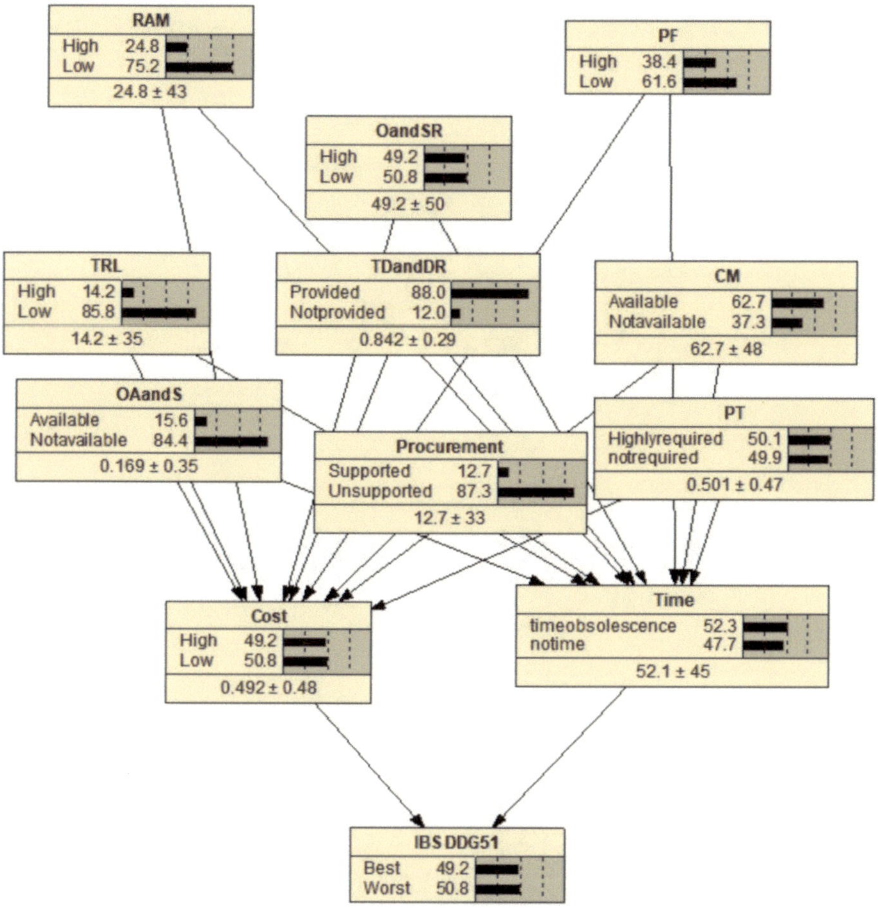

Figure 1.
System design characteristics of the SABANP model (N = 2) with netica software.

Each criterion was modeled on two functions. The function was based on a true or false table. To construct the table, the true table was given an arbitrary phrase like high, provided, available, supported, highly required, time to obsolescence and best. For example, for RAM, the true table states the following: what is the probability that the system has a high RAM? For P&F, the true table states the following: what is the probability that the system's P&F is high? This logic of the true table for these examples is applied to the remaining criteria.

The same logic was applied to the false table. To construct the false table, an arbitrary phrase like low, not provided, not available, unsupported, not required, no time and worst was used. For example, for PT, the false table states the following: what is the probability that Personnel Training is not required for the system? In addition, for time, what is the probability that the system will not be obsolete in two (2) years? **Table 6** represents the true and false table probabilities. The true table probabilities are the normalized values of the expert judgments that are displayed in **Table 3**. The false table is the difference between the probability of each event as described in Eq. (5). The criteria are modeled as events. For example, when one event's true table value is 0.9, the false table value is 0.1. The JPD of the model is given as Eq. (6) and modeled using NETICA™ respectively for IBS 1, IBS 2 and IBS 3 system. Each system is modeled based on the probabilities of each criterion (RAM; P&F; PR; CM; DR&TD availability; OA&S; TRL; PT; and O&SR) given Cost and Time to obsolescence.

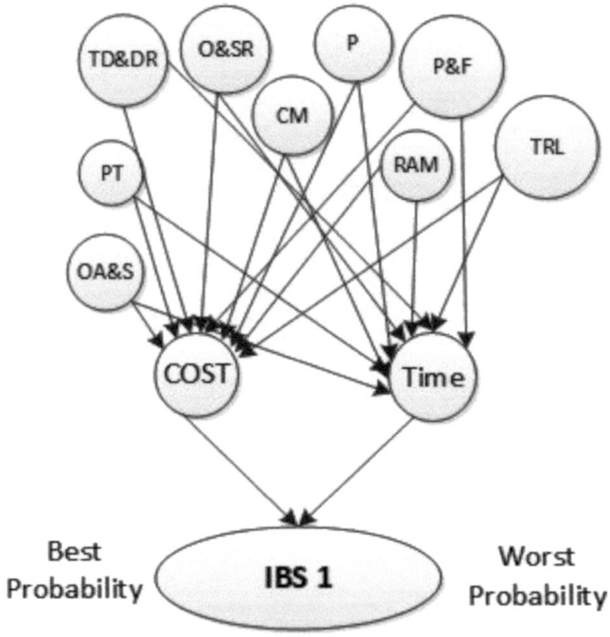

Figure 2.
The IBS for DDG-51 and its equivalent SABANP model.

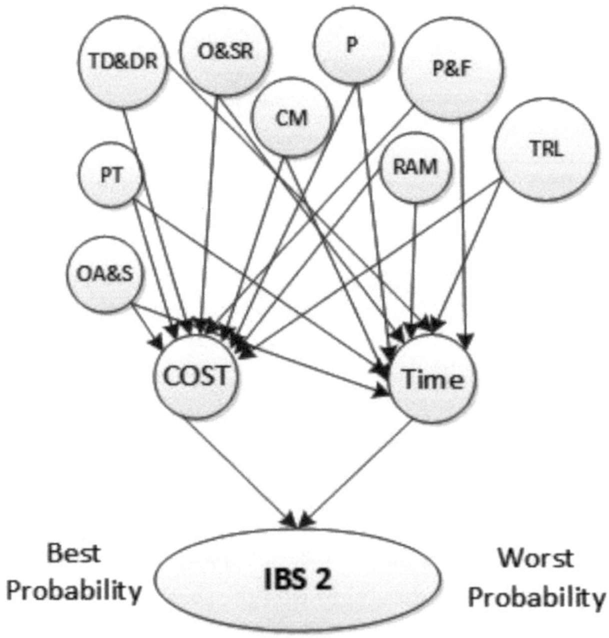

Figure 3.
The IBS for CG-47 and its equivalent SABANP model.

3.2 Multi criteria decision making (MCDM)

What is MCDM? MCDM methods provide a way to combine qualitative data (such as expert opinions) and quantitative data in order to analyze various

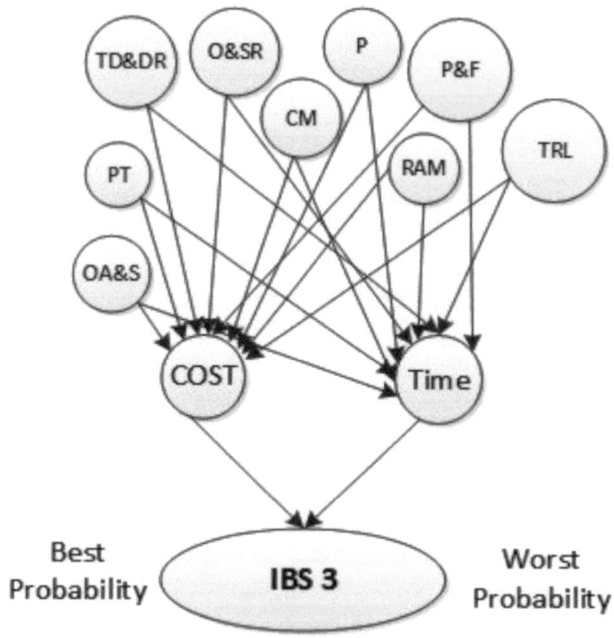

Figure 4.
The IBS for CVN-68 and its equivalent SABANP model.

Criteria	TRUE IBS DDG-51 Class	FALSE IBS DDG-51 Class	TRUE IBS CG-47 Class	FALSE IBS CG-47 Class	TRUE IBS CVN-68 Class	FALSE IBS CVN-68 Class
(1) P&F	1	0	0.920	0.08	1	0
(2) Cost	0.984	0.016	1	0	0.815	0.185
(3) PT	0.9717	0.028	0.937	0.063	1	0
(4) RAM	1	0	0.889	0.111	0.959	0.041
(5) PR	1	0	0.896	0.104	0.976	0.024
(6) CM	1	0	0.896	0.104	0.976	0.024
(7) DR&TD	0.947	0.053	0.895	0.105	1	0
(8) OA&S	0.987	0.013	1	0	0.939	0.061
(9) TRL	1	0	1	0	0.979	0.021
(10) O&SR	1	0	0.938	0.062	0.978	0.022

Table 6.
True and false table.

alternatives [17]. When nonlinear factors are present, MCDM techniques are beneficial for discriminating among alternatives. Nonlinear factors are cases where the units of measurement (e.g., feet, seconds, Fahrenheit, and miles/hr.) are not the same. In the case of linear factors, the units of measurement are the same across the attributes or criteria. MCDM techniques can be categorized as fuzzy, stochastic or deterministic [20]. Additionally, a popular MCDM was examined for validation and or comparison to the SABANP result. The MCDM is TOPSIS. TOPSIS was chosen because of its popular usage in the literature and because it is capable of providing a deterministic data approach that accounts for the expert judgment participation, the dimensional criteria space, the methodical representation, and the explanation.

Four steps are required in any decision-making approach that relies on numerical analyses of alternatives to assess system factors' nonlinearity when selecting an MCDM methodology:

1. establish the relevant alternatives and criteria,

2. allocate numerical values to the criteria weights and the alternatives' impacts on the criteria,

3. assess the nonlinearity related to the system in consideration when choosing an MCDM method, and.

4. process numerical values to rank each alternative [17, 21].

There are several methods used to determine criteria weights, such as weight-assessment models [22, 23]. Certain authors have stated that standards are not available for defining which technique yields the most accurate criteria weight because whether the technique is biased is uncertain [24]. Others have suggested pairwise assessment matrices to calculate the significance or weights of criteria [18, 25]. A weighting method can be categorized as subjective or objective, algebraic or statistical, decomposed or holistic, and indirect or direct [17, 26]. In this study, the direct weighting method is selected because this method allows the decision maker to rank the criteria and provide subjective values to the criteria weight based on the defined rank. The direct weighting method was utilized in the analysis of TOPSIS, however, SABANP requires no weight inputs. Often weights are difficult to quantify when there are many experts. The benefit of having no weights is that it simplifies the decision matrix and provides for optimal decision making.

3.2.1 TOPSIS analysis

Established by Yoon [27] and Hwang & Yoon [28], the basic principle underlying TOPSIS is that the selected alternative should have the shortest distance from the positive ideal solution and the farthest distance from the negative ideal solution [29]. **Figure 5**, which is adapted from Adetunji's [6] graphic, depicts an assumption

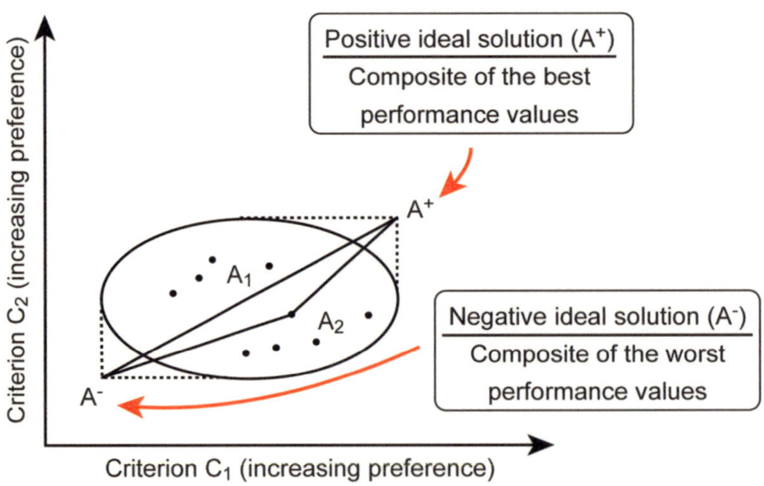

Figure 5.
Technique for order of preference by similarity to ideal Sslution (TOPIS) graphical representation.

for two criteria, where (A^-) is the negative ideal solution and (A^+) is the positive ideal solution [17, 28]. The negative ideal solution is made up of the worst performance value of all the alternatives. The positive ideal solution is made up of the best performance value of all the alternatives.

Justifying the selection of A_1 is difficult [17, 29] as shown in the visual example in **Figure 5**; therefore, the proximity (relative closeness) to each of these performance poles (A^-) and (A^+) is measured in the Euclidean sense [17, 28, 30], for which the square root of the sum of the squared distances along each axis is in the 'attribute space' [30].

The following steps are required to conduct a TOPSIS analysis:

1. The normalized decision matrix is first determined using Eq. (7). The normalized score (r_{ij}) is calculated to transform the various attribute dimensions X_{ij} from the raw data into non-dimensional attributes, thus allowing for comparisons among the attributes [17, 28, 29]:

$$r_{ij} = X_{ij}/\sqrt{\sum_{i=1}^{m} X_{ij}^2}, \text{where } i = 1, 2, 3, 4 \dots, m; j = 1, 2, 3, 4 \dots, n \tag{7}$$

   Table 7 shows the normalized decision matrix.

2. Calculate the weighted normalized values (v_{ij}) by multiplying r_{ij} by the criterion weights (w_j) [17, 28, 29] (see **Table 8** and Eq. (8)):

$$v_{ij} = w_j r_{ij}, \text{where } j = 1, 2, 3, 4 \dots, n; i = 1, 2, 3, 4 \dots, m \tag{8}$$

   The weighted normalized values are shown in the weight normalized matrix in **Table 8**.

3. Evaluate the positive (A^+) and negative (A^-) ideal solution using Eq. (9) [17, 28, 29]:

Criteria	IBS DDG-51 Class:	IBS CG-47 Class:	IBS CVN-68 Class:
(1) P&F	0.386	0.355	0.386
(2) Cost	0.332	0.327	0.401
(3) PT	0.362	0.355	0.392
(4) RAM	0.377	0.364	0.388
(5) PR	0.399	0.354	0.382
(6) CM	0.397	0.356	0.387
(7) DR&TD	0.371	0.351	0.392
(8) OA&S	0.382	0.387	0.363
(9) TRL	0.373	0.373	0.366
(10) O&SR	0.374	0.398	0.382

Table 7.
TOPSIS normalized decision matrix for IBS.

Criteria	IBS DDG-51 Class:	IBS CG-47 Class:	IBS CVN-68 Class:
(1) P&F	0.073	0.067	0.073
(2) Cost	0.040	0.039	0.048
(3) PT	0.022	0.021	0.024
(4) RAM	0.057	0.055	0.058
(5) PR	0.044	0.039	0.042
(6) CM	0.028	0.025	0.027
(7) DR&TD	0.033	0.032	0.035
(8) OA&S	0.027	0.027	0.025
(9) TRL	0.022	0.022	0.022
(10) O&SR	0.030	0.032	0.031

Table 8.
TOPSIS weighted normalized decision matrix for IBS.

$$A^{+} = \left\{ \left(\underset{i}{max} \; v_{ij} \,|\, j \in J \right), \left(\underset{i}{min} \; v_{ij} | j \in J^{+} \right) | \, where \; i = 1, 2, 3, 4 \ldots, m \right\} \tag{9}$$

$$= \left\{ v_1^{+}, v_2^{+}, v_3^{+} \ldots, v_j^{+}, \ldots, v_n^{+} \right\},$$

$$A^{-} = \left\{ \left(\underset{i}{min} \; v_{ij} \,|\, j \in J \right), \left(\underset{i}{max} \; v_{ij} | j \in J^{-} \right) | \, where \; i = 1, 2, 3, 4 \ldots, m. \right\}$$

$$= \left\{ v_1^{-}, v_2^{-}, v_3^{-} \ldots, v_j^{-}, \ldots, v_n^{-} \right\},$$

$$\mathrm{J}^{+} = \{\mathrm{j} = 1, 2, 3, 4 \ldots, \mathrm{n} |\, \mathrm{j \; relates \; to \; the \; benefit \; criteria}\}.$$

$$J^{-} = \{ \, j = 1, 2, 3, 4 \ldots, n | \, j \; relates \; to \; the \; non - benefit \; criteria \}$$

The A^{+} and A^{-} solutions are shown in **Tables 9** and **10** respectively.

V1-V10	Positive Ideal
V1+ =	0.073
V2+ =	0.039
V3+ =	0.024
V4+ =	0.058
V5+ =	0.044
V6+ =	0.028
V7+ =	0.035
V8+ =	0.027
V9+ =	0.022
V10+ =	0.030

Table 9.
TOPSIS positive ideal solutions for IBS.

V1-V10	Negative Ideal
V1- =	0.067
V2- =	0.048
V3- =	0.021
V4- =	0.055
V5- =	0.039
V6- =	0.025
V7- =	0.032
V8- =	0.025
V9- =	0.022
V10- =	0.032

Table 10.
TOPSIS negative ideal solutions for IBS.

4. Calculate each alternative separation from the positive (s_i^+) and negative (s_i^-) ideal solutions (use the n-dimensional Euclidean distance) using Eq. (10) [17, 28, 29]:

$$S_i^+ = \sqrt{\sum_{j=1}^{n} (v_{ij} - v^+{}_j)^2} \text{ where } i = 1, 2, 3, 4 \dots m, \tag{10}$$

$$S_i^- = \sqrt{\sum_{j=1}^{n} (v_{ij} - v^-{}_j)^2} \text{ where } i = 1, 2, 3, 4 \dots m$$

Tables 11 and **12** show the separation measures between the positive and negative ideal solutions.

5. Calculate the relative closeness of each alternative to the ideal solution (c_i^*) [17, 28, 29] using Eq. (11):

S1-S3	Positive Ideal
S1+ =	0.003
S2+ =	0.010
S3+ =	0.009

Table 11.
TOPSIS separation Mmasures to positive ideal solutions for IBS.

S1-S3	Negative Ideal
S1- =	0.012
S2- =	0.009
S3- =	0.009

Table 12.
TOPSIS separation measures to negative ideal solutions for IBS.

Position(s)	Organization(s)	Years of Experience
(1) Principal Logistics Specialist	DoD (NSWC Philadelphia)	+25
(2) Principal Logistics Specialist	DoD (NSWC Philadelphia)	+25
(3) DMSMS/Obsolescence Engineer	DoD (NSWC Philadelphia)	6
(4) Logistics Manager	DoD Contractor (ICI Services)	+35
(5) DMSMS/Obsolescence Analyst	NAVSEA SEA 21	+7
(6) ILS/Configuration Manager	DoD Contractor (ICI Services)	+35
(7) DMSMS/Obsolescence Team Lead	DoD (NSWC Port Hueneme)	+10
(8) ILS Program Manager	DoD (NSWC Port Hueneme)	+15
(9) ILS/Systems Engineer	DoD Contractor (LCE Inc.)	+30
(10) DMSMS/Obsolescence Manager	DoD (NSWC Philadelphia)	+20
(11) Obsolescence Engineer	DoD Contractor (Alion Science)	+30
(12) ILS Engineer	DoD Contractor (NDI Engineering)	+15
(13) Operations Engineer	DoD (NSWC Philadelphia)	+10
(14) ILS Program Manager	DoD (NSWC Philadelphia)	+15
(15) DMSMS/ILS Engineer	DoD (NSWC Port Hueneme)	4
(16) DMSMS/Obsolescence Engineer	DoD (NSWC Philadelphia)	+5
(17) DMSMS/Obsolescence Technical Rep.	DoD (NSWC Philadelphia)	+5
(18) DMSMS/Obsolescence Analyst	DoD (NSWC Philadelphia)	+4
(19) Systems Engineer	DoD Contractor (DDLOMNI Engineering)	+20

Table 13.
Experts' demographics.

$$c_i^* = S_i^- / (S_i^- + S_i^+),\ 0 < c_i^* < 1, i = 1, 2, 3, 4 \ldots, m \tag{11}$$

$$A_i \text{ equals } (A^+) \text{ if } c_i^* \text{ equals } 1; A_i \text{ equals } (A^-) \text{ if } c_i^* \text{ equals } 0$$

6. Sort the order of preference alternatives by the descending order of c_i^*: The nearer c_i^* is to one indicates a higher importance of the alternative [17, 28, 29].

3.3 Delivery mechanism

Before administering the research survey, each research participant was provided an information sheet and consent form to complete and instructions on how to complete the survey. Once retrieved, the survey files were password protected and saved. The experts' participation in the study was voluntary and anonymous. The breakdown of the experts' demographics is shown in **Table 13**.

4. Results

100 runs of data that were collected from the SABANP model using the IBSs on DDG-51, CG-47 and CVN-68 were aggregated. The results revealed that the DDG-51 IBS has a 52% probability of being the best system among the systems examined

in the trade-off analysis as shown in **Table 14**. The CG-47 IBS is the second best with a 51.78% probability, shown in **Table 15** and the CVN-68 IBS is the third best with a 51.56% probability as shown in **Table 16.** The sensitivity analysis conducted on the result over ten thousand times shows that the DDG-51 IBS is less susceptible to obsolescence than its counterparts.

The results of the SABANP model also revealed that in the 100 runs with respect to the best system, Procurement (PR), which includes Vendor Assembly and Installation support, at 79.1% is a critical criterion path that could have the most adverse effect on a system's lifecycle operations, and it should be prioritized with respect to the design, development, testing, maintenance. This is followed by the TRL at 76.1%, O&SR at 75%, and DR&TD at 72.1%. The least adverse effect is the availability of OA&S at 16.5%. **Table 17** show the breakdown of the likelihood of an impact for each obsolescence criterion across the systems that were selected.

Runs	Worst	Best
1	62.2	37.8
2	50.8	49.2
3	48.5	51.5
4	32.3	67.7
5	67.5	32.5
•	•	•
•	•	•
•	•	•
99	72.9	27.1
100	49.6	50.4
Aggregated Values:	**47.99**	**52.01**

Table 14.
SABANP runs DDG-51 IBS.

RUNS	Worst	Best
1	63.7	36.3
2	49.2	50.8
3	48.5	51.5
4	32.3	67.7
5	67.5	32.5
•	•	•
•	•	•
•	•	•
99	35.1	64.9
100	57.7	42.3
Aggregated Values:	**48.22**	**51.78**

Table 15.
SABANP runs CG-47 IBS runs.

RUNS	Worst	Best
1	66.5	33.5
2	49.2	50.8
3	48.5	51.5
4	32.3	67.7
5	67.5	32.5
•	•	•
•	•	•
•	•	•
99	35.7	64.9
100	57.7	42.3
Aggregated Values:	**48.44**	**51.56**

Table 16.
SABANP runs CVN-68 IBS runs.

		Rank (1)	Rank (2)	Rank (3)
Criteria	Measure	IBS DDG-51 Class	IBS CG-47	IBS CVN-68
(1) P&F	HIGH	43.40%	79.90%	22.1%
	LOW	56.60%	20.10%	77.9%
(2) Cost	HIGH	51.40%	49%	50.2%
	LOW	48.60%	51%	49.8%
(3) PT	NOT HIGHLY REQUIRED	49%	74.8%	61.7%
	HIGH REQUIRED	51%	25.2%	38.3%
(4) RAM	HIGH	28.60%	17.8%	92.4%
	LOW	71.40%	82.2%	7.62%
(5) PR	SUPPORTED	79.10%	72.8%	34.4%
	UNSUPPORTED	20.90%	27.2%	65.6%
(6) CM	NOT AVAILABLE	55.10%	58.2%	59.9%
	AVAILABLE	44.90%	41.8%	40.1%
(7) DR&TD	NOT PROVIDED	72.10%	61.3%	62.4%
	PROVIDED	27.90%	38.7%	37.6%
(8) OA&S	NOT AVAILABLE	16.50%	42.2%	75.4%
	AVAILABLE	83.50%	57.8%	24.6%
(9) TRL	HIGH	76.10%	67.4%	37.2%
	LOW	23.90%	32.6%	62.8%
(10) O&SR	HIGH	75%	42.2%	75.4%
	LOW	25%	57.8%	24.6%
Aggregated Result	**Worst Case Probability**	47.99%	48.22%	48.44%
	Best Case Probability	52.01%	51.78%	51.56%

Table 17.
Likelihood of impact for each obsolescence criterion across the selected systems (N = 100).

Systems	TOPSIS "S"	TOPSIS "R"
DDG-51 =	0.795	1
CG-47 =	0.473	3
CVN-68 =	0.494	2

Table 18.
IBS ranking of the result (TOPSIS) solutions. "S" score and "R" ranking.

4.1 Validation

To validate the results, comparative analyses were done using TOPSIS. Whereas for SABANP, the weight data were not required since normalization was the only required parameter. The result shows that TOPSIS ranked the DDG-51 IBS as the best system, which follows the results provided by the SABANP model. The results of the ranking and comparisons to TOPSIS is found in the **Table 18**.

5. Conclusions

The use of SABANP for obsolescence management and as a method for selecting the system or technology that could potentially mitigate obsolescence early in the design stage of a system was successfully demonstrated. The results also indicate that systems should be designed with a proactive obsolescence approach in mind. MCDM that is deterministic (TOPSIS) model was also applied and demonstrated similar results in identifying the best systems among alternatives that mitigate obsolescence. The proposed model is shown to successfully combine quantitative and qualitative expert judgment data that incorporate attributes such as risk and training criteria using SABANP in order to efficiently propagate the evidence of obsolescence.

The analysis conducted in this chapter can serve to provide a holistic analysis of obsolescence in systems. The results of the data analysis were presented to the experts, and concluded that the IBS on DDG-51 was the best system for mitigating obsolescence. Future research should be focused on conducting systems engineering trade studies with the use of SABANP in decision making. This allows for the documentation of early decisions in a program and reducing long-term waste. Notwithstanding, it is recommended that all identified criteria in this work be prioritized equally in the design, development, testing, and maintenance.

This chapter recommends the use of SABANP in obsolescence management in order to conduct trade studies for systems during the design stage. The chapter does not intend to be an authoritative decision mechanism nor provide a recommendation for the best MCDM to use for the normalization technique. Rather, it serves as a new tool, approach, or guidance in obsolescence decision management. Additionally, future research can evaluate the normalization of other MCDM techniques in comparison to the SAW that was utilized in the SABANP model.

Author statement

This chapter is an extension of the author's original published research article. The views that are conveyed in this article are those of the author and do not represent the official policy or position of NSWC Philadelphia, the DoD, and its contractors, or the U.S. Government.

Acronyms

BBN	Bayesian Belief Network
CG-47	USS Ticonderoga
CM	Configuration Management
COTS	Commercial Off-the-Shelf
CVN-68	USS Nimitz
DDG-51	USS Arleigh
DMSMS	Diminishing Manufacturing Sources and Material Shortages
DR&TD	Data Rights and Technical Documentation
IBS	Integrated Bridge System
MCDM	Multi-Criteria Decision Making
NETICAL	NETICAL Software Tool for modeling system criteria dependence
RAM	Reliability, Availability, and Maintainability
SABANP	Simple Additive Bayesian Allocation Network Process
SAW	Simple Additive Weighing
SME	Subject Matter Expert
OA&S	Open Architecture and Standards
O&SR	Obsolescence Schedule Risk
P&F	Performance and Functionality
PR	Procurement
PT	Personnel Training
TOPSIS	Technique for Order of Preference by Similarity to Ideal Solution
TRL	Technology Readiness Level

Author details

Oluwatomi Adetunji
The George Washington University, USA

*Address all correspondence to: tomie_20@gwu.edu

References

[1] Geng, F., Dubos, G. F., & Saleh, J. H. (2016). Spacecraft obsolescence: Modeling, value analysis, and implications for design and acquisition. *2016 IEEE Aerospace Conference*. doi: 10.1109/aero.2016.7500642

[2] Herald, T., Verma, D., Lubert, C., & Cloutier, R. (2009). An obsolescence management framework for system baseline evolution-Perspectives through the system life cycle. *Systems Engineering*, *12*(1), 1–20. doi:10.1002/sys.20106

[3] Sandborn, P. (2007). Designing for technology obsolescence management. In *IIE Annual Conference. Proceedings* (p. 1684). Institute of Industrial and Systems Engineers (IISE).

[4] Pecht, MG and Diganta Das. 2000. "Electronic Part Life Cycle." *IEEE Transactions on Components and Packaging Technologies* 23 (1): 190–192.

[5] Romero Rojo, F. J., Roy, R., & Shehab, E. (2009). Obsolescence management for long-life contracts: state of the art and future trends. *The International Journal of Advanced Manufacturing Technology*, *49*(9–12), 1235–1250. doi:10.1007/s00170-009-2471-3

[6] Adetunji, O., Bischoff, J., & Willy, C. J. (2018). Managing system obsolescence via multicriteria decision making. *Systems Engineering*, *21*(4), 307–321. doi: 10.1002/sys.21436

[7] Adams C. (2005). Getting a handle on cots obsolescence. *Avionics Magazine*.

[8] Sandborn, P. (2008). Strategic management of DMSMS in systems. *DSP Journal*, 24–30.

[9] Roy, R., Stark, R., Tracht, K., Takata, S., & Mori, M. (2016). Continuous maintenance and the future – Foundations and technological challenges. *CIRP Annals*, *65*(2), 667–688. doi:10.1016/j.cirp.2016.06.006

[10] Trabelsi, I., Zolghadri, M., Zeddini, B., Barkallah, M., & Haddar, M. (2020, July). FMECA-based risk assessment approach for proactive obsolescence management. In *IFIP International Conference on Product Lifecycle Management* (pp. 215–226). Springer, Cham.

[11] Verma, D., & Johannesen, L. H. (1999). Supportability engineering and logistics optimization/planning trends and challenges: a system integrator's perspective. In *Proceedings of the International Logistics Congress, University of Exeter*.

[12] Verma, D., Powers, T., Blanchard, B. S., Giffin, R. G., Webb, R., & VanBuskirk, D. (1996). COTS/NDI ASSESSMENT AND SELECTION METHODOLOGY. *INCOSE International Symposium*, *6*(1), 123–128. doi:10.1002/j.2334-5837.1996.tb01993.x

[13] Department of Defense, United States (US DoD). (2011). Technology Readiness Assessment (TRA) guidance, *Assistant Secretary of Defense of Research and Engineering*. https://www.acq.osd.mil/chieftechnologist/publications/docs/tra2011.pdf

[14] Boudali, H., & Dugan, J. (2005). A discrete-time Bayesian network reliability modeling and analysis framework. *Reliability Engineering & System Safety*, *87*(3), 337–349. doi: 10.1016/j.ress. 2004.06.004

[15] Salih Geduk & İlkay Ulusoy (2021) A practical analysis of sample complexity for structure learning of discrete dynamic Bayesian networks, Optimization, DOI: 10.1080/02331934.2021.1892105

[16] Kabir, S., & Papadopoulos, Y. (2019). Applications of Bayesian

networks and Petri nets in safety, reliability, and risk assessments: A review. *Safety Science*, *115*, 154–175. doi: 10.1016/j.ssci.2019.02.009

[17] Georgiadis, D. R., Mazzuchi, T. A., & Sarkani, S. (2012). Using multi criteria decision making in analysis of alternatives for selection of enabling technology. *Systems Engineering*, *16*(3), 287–303. doi:10.1002/sys.21233

[18] Afshari, A., Mojahed, M., & Yusuff, R.B. (2010). Simple additive weighting approach to personnel selection problem, *International Journal of Innovation, Management and Technology 1*, 511–515.

[19] Fishburn, P. C. (1968). Utility Theory. *Management Science*, *14*(5), 335–378. doi:10.1287/mnsc.14.5.335

[20] Triantaphyllou, E., Shu, B., Sanchez, S. N., & Ray, T. (1998). Multi-criteria decision making: an operations research approach. *Encyclopedia of electrical and electronics engineering*, *15* (1998), 175–186.

[21] Triantaphyllou, E., & Mann, S. H. (1989). An examination of the effectiveness of multi-dimensional decision-making methods: A decision-making paradox. *Decision Support Systems*, *5*(3), 303–312. doi:10.1016/0167-9236(89)90037-7

[22] Heerkens, H. (2006). Assessing the importance of factors determining decision-making by actors involved in innovation processes. *Creativity and innovation management*, *15*(4), 385–399.

[23] Olson, D. (2004). Comparison of weights in TOPSIS models. *Mathematical and Computer Modeling*, *40*(7–8), 721–727. doi:10.1016/j.mcm.2004.10.003

[24] Weber, M., & Borcherding, K. (1993). Behavioral influences on weight judgments in multiattribute decision making. *European Journal of Operational Research*, *67*(1), 1–12. doi:10.1016/0377-2217(93)90318-h

[25] Nydick, R. L., & Hill, R. P. (1992). Using the Analytic Hierarchy Process to Structure the Supplier Selection Procedure. *International Journal of Purchasing and Materials Management*, *28*(2), 31–36. doi:10.1111/j.1745-493x.1992.tb00561.x

[26] Ustinovichius, L., Zavadkas, E. K., & Podvezko, V. (2007). Application of a quantitative multiple criteria decision making (MCDM-1) approach to the analysis of investments in construction. *Control and cybernetics*, *36*(1), 251.

[27] Yoon, K. (1980). Systems selection by multiple attribute decision making [Ph. D. thesis]. *Manhattan (KS): Kansas State University.*

[28] Hwang, C., & Yoon, K. (1981). Methods for Multiple Attribute Decision Making. *Multiple Attribute Decision Making*, 58–191. doi:10.1007/978-3-642-48318-9_3

[29] Wang, R. (2001). "Performance Evaluation Method-Technique for Order Preference by Similarity to Ideal Solution (TOPSIS)." *Researcher.Nsc.Gov.tw/public/caroljoe/Data/02182133671.Ppt.*

[30] Kahraman, C. (2008). Multi-Criteria Decision Making Methods and Fuzzy Sets. *Springer Optimization and Its Applications*, 1–18. doi:10.1007/978-0-387-76813-7_1

Chapter 10

Political Leadership and Financial Emoluments: A Case of Developing Countries

Daniels Aide Okun and Osama Ose Iyawe

Abstract

The theoretical concept of political leadership would have to be the most elusive and fluid concept of leadership. It has within its authority dominated policies, influenced security- intelligence, shaped intellectual-cultures, inspired citizens-aspirations and has directed the trajectory of nation-states and sovereignties within international governance and global affairs. The political behaviors of developing nations through foreign policies, national interests and diplomacy have been a reflection of the authority of their political leadership; regime after regime. There are no best-kept secret to the fundamental strengths and weaknesses of political Leadership other than the influential impact of the political leader's self-empowerment, self-leadership and self-legacy. Political Leadership is fundamentally controlled by the polices of choices where decisions meet actions and authoritarian powers redefines humanity. The elusive extent, and fluid depth of political influence through the impact of governance does not measure -up to the assurance of humanity in most developing countries around the world. The political consciousness and idiosyncrasies of most individuals over the years have contributed none or fewer interests to the study, the justification, and the analytical reasoning of the influence of political leadership. This new study and the assertive findings on this chapter are aimed to pragmatically educate, inspire, and reignite the zealousness of visionary leadership, through the consciousness of humanity. The intellectual assertions in this chapter are envisioned to create, expand and illuminate the distinctive reality between of our profound empirical knowledge, theoretical beliefs and interpretive researches on the conceptual understanding of political leadership. The topics in this chapter are aimed to create an endless stream to the consciousness of political leadership and financial gains to the betterment of humanity. It expands the understanding of political leadership through psychological lens beyond the titles, offices and political display of power. Political leadership in developing countries can improve and offer better outcomes in todays world, when humanity meets the consciousness of political leadership in financial prosperity. The societal divisions of ethnicity, wealth and the polarization of political ideologies into sets of beliefs, questions the influential impact of political leadership. As political leaders govern and navigate through their leadership goals, aspirations and visions more often than not, the traits of their ethnic identity, individuality and beliefs constantly create struggles with their understanding and acceptance of humanity as a whole.

Keywords: individuality, nationality, opportunity, corruptibility, profitability, political consciousness, loyalty, humanity, service, legacy

1. Introduction

The theoretical concepts of political leadership creates an in-depth understanding of the societal consciousness of the political processes and the outcomes of the quality of leadership; retrospectively classical writers like; Niccolo Machiavelli, Robert Michels and Max Weber explored theoretical ideas, arguments, and definitions of the authority of political leadership. Political leadership has always had a great influence and an impact on the empowerment of the nation-building process of countries. The never-ending challenges and struggles that political leaders are faced with is the economic reality of their nations which have always been the question that dictates the achievements of the leadership quality of a political leader.

Political Leadership is the patriotic state of consciousness that ignites the spirit of nationalism, and the pride of citizenship that unifies ethnic diversity.

Political Leadership is the act of governance that distinguishes: leadership from politics, integrity from loyalty, and humanity from prosperity.

Political Leadership centers on the duties of social responsibilities, nation-building, cultural capital, and the welfare-betterment of humanity.

Political Leadership does not symbolize nor define left wing - right wing political competition against ideologies, positions, and party dominance on the political spectrum. It represents, justifies and validates the essence and advancement of togetherness through communal systems in the presence and acceptance of diversity.

The accountability demands, credibility measures and aspirational heights of political leadership ought to be grounded in their profound values and beliefs on humanity, capacity development, life and security. Conversely more often than not; these measures of expectations are solely directed to economics, financial gains, wealth creation and individual wealth appropriation which clearly never answers the deeper questions to the efficiency of political leadership.

Political Leadership avails a fundamental social responsibility for the unification of social cohesion in the presence of diversity, divides and conflicts in order to achieve a collective human-capital force that assures economic growth, prosperity, survival and protection. Pragmatically, these assertions do not resonate with the political realities of most developing countries; it is conversely on the opposite, state of affairs were political leadership disregards, excludes humanity from governance through the tactics of politics which hardly represents the ideals of leadership but utilizes the rustiness of power through authority.

The theoretical understanding of Political Leadership is not as elusive and fluid as presented overtime it is the trust-given responsible to serve, lead and advance the betterment of humanity harmoniously through prosperity, humanity capacity development and cooperation.

There a question in the developing countries that everyone dares and struggles to get an answer to which is:

"Why are the offices of political appointees, and leaders synonymous to the bank of wealth? ".

I believe pensively, that this question may never be answered as it references and represents a norm, a culture and a tradition that is systematically instituted to picture a reality. The inhibitions of political Leadership is found in the sensitivity and in the powerful pieces of decision making process and the execution of action that are constantly motivated by visionary leadership and inspired by the enthusiasm and compassion for humanity.

Political leaders are faced with the battle of consciousness between "Efficiency and Effectiveness". Confidently ensuring that their tasks and responsibilities are executed perfectly right apt enough to better welfare and ensuring that they are standing, endorsing and motivating the right actions that will justify the path of humanity towards peace, betterment and prosperity.

Political Leadership is not the absence of the quality, compassion and ideals of the other forms of leadership. But rather; it is indeed the collective accumulation of all the other forms of leadership aimed for a collective and mutual betterment and good for humanity. The stereotypical negative connotations of political leadership been associated and linked to corruption and wealth embezzlement has indeed created a social construct, a message of deceit and a norm which has hindered leadership accountability, credibility, selfless responsibilities, and expectations from the political leader.

Political Leadership is the given-responsibilities and authority by trust, belief, and assurance to an individual with the identification of patriotic loyalty, recognition of leadership, and compassion for humanity. Political leadership is not a game of politics, a display of wealth nor is it a competitive showcase of power and authority, it is the real business of putting humanity, first and above, policies, interests, ideological bents, beliefs and traditions. Political leadership is the combination of power, intelligence, security, wealth and authority into a force for enthusiasm and compassion for humanity.

Political leadership owes the people no greater speech, no greater promise, no greater policies, no greater agenda, no greater army, no greater bridges, no greater roads than the effective and efficient building of better, stronger and greater tomorrow that ensures and insures the harmonious -collective - consciousness of purpose, dedication to duty and the validation of the worthiness of humanity.

There will be no greater oath of office, affirmation of a strong-will dedication to office, than the one that specifically centers on the core fundamental values, principles and compassion for the greater good, advancement and prosperity of humanity in its worthiness and validation.

The swearing in to office of any appointed political leadership opportunity ought to be the-one-and-only social consciousness to duty that should exhilarate, justify and empower the interests, ambition and intentions to govern with political authority a leader can have.

The fear, anxiety and bravery to serve humanity through political leadership should be an oath of sacrifice, an allegiance to dedication of self and a pledge to better humanity with all the resources there is within or outside the sovereignty of nation states.

Political leadership creates the means and justifies the means to govern humanity towards the path of betterment by the people for the people and with the people. This does not make it a complicated mission to accomplish, it rather eliminates the space for self-interests, personal gains, personal agendas and competition of self-greatness. It reaffirms the truth bearing of faith and allegiance to serve humanity for a greater, better and a more harmonious life of creation that humanity is worthy of and validated for.

Political leadership is an authoritative responsibility that creates more for the people than it takes from the people. It is an office that benefits all, an opportunity that creates sustainable growth, progressive advancements and a harmonious culture for productivity. There is an endless path to the progressive advancement of political leadership in developing countries that ought to journeyed on, that path can only be traveled through with the human- capacity- development- investment- and- advancement as the only policies of change that should be demanded and gotten.

The theoretical concept of Political leadership is asserted to be an authority symbolic to parenthood. It carries on, upon it the responsibilities, the never ending

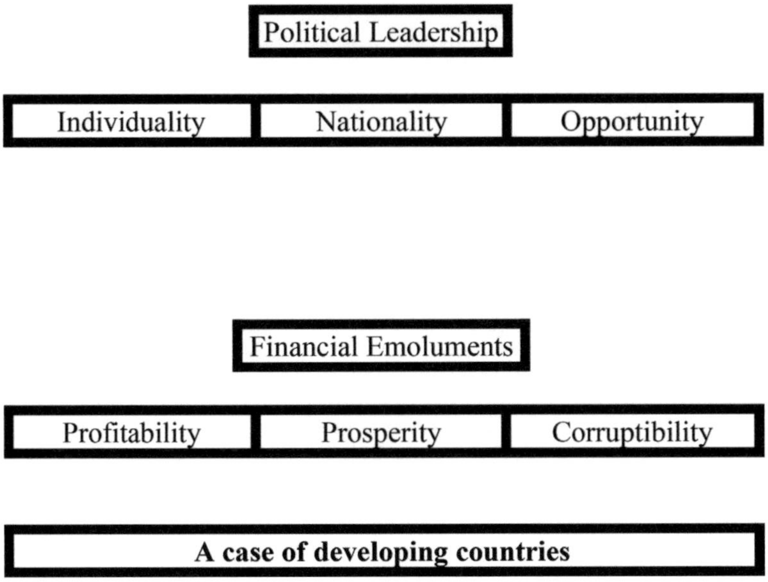

Figure 1.
Schematic Presentation of the title's core Components. Authors Compilation (2020).

duty of ensuring and insuring the betterment of humanity with which all the other means and agendas of prosperity is assured.

Political leadership in developing countries owes its humanity more than just the legal obligations of citizenry by means of identity but to the embracing of what it truly means, symbolizes, represents deeply, compassionately and emotionally to be a citizen of a country regardless of its political, socio-economic and moral status. Until the betterment of humanity as the only capital source of wealth is assured it is impossible to enrich or discover the wealth in any nation in the absence of slavery and exploitation.

Political Leadership is patriotically the social-political consciousness of the authority to utilize power to the ultimate advantage of the betterment of its humanity regardless of political realities, international regimes or competitive economic markets.

It is in the authenticity and intentions of purpose and the protection of citizenry that nation's competitive advantages are born. No nation could hardly excel productively, economically and intellectually without its citizenry. It is the putting first and above of its citizenry by political Leadership that puts a nation above other nations on the global map of relevance and power. No nation could journey without a strong-willed political Leadership that assures and insures the existence of its citizenry in a proud state of humanity (**Figure 1**).

1.1 Worthy of notice

The consciousness of individuality, the awareness of self worth, the embracing of nationality and the privileges of leadership opportunities are fundamental to the understanding and recognition of the influential authority of political leadership.

2. The S-E-L-F approach to political leadership

The theoretical practice of political leadership is structured in systematic processes and alignments that have become institutionalized norms, cultures,

The S-E-L-F Approach

S: Selflessness in the service of humanity

- The selflessness of service to humanity through political leadership defines and justifies the core values, driven-purpose, visionary inclinations, missions, goals and aim of office.
- A political leader truly assumes the affirmation of duty to serve when they are fully prepared to lay-off selfishness of interests, inhibitions, gains and agendas.
- Political leadership becomes the finest and most powerful form of leadership when it is without an iota of selfishness.

E: Enthusiastically apt enough to empower humanity

- Political leadership through authority, power, justice, institutions, structures and systems can invest in the humanity capacity development, advancement and betterment of its citizenry.
- Profoundly, it is through these investments, that individual are empowered, strengthened to create opportunities, hope, prosperity of peace and wealth in the country.
- Political leadership owes its citizenry the protection, security and assurance of wealth creation through human empowerment and capacity development. Political leadership ought to invest in the human capacity development of its citizenry.

L: Loyalty to the labor for humanity

- Political leadership has a meaningful purpose and an impactful mission when it is in alignment with humanity with the strongest feeling of support and allegiance to its betterment.
- This is when the harmony of purpose, collective consciousness, and oneness in purpose, the rule of law and a state of equality justifies the commonality of political leadership, authority and influence of power in the society.

F: Fundamental policies of Followership through humanity

- Political Leadership is the formulation of the fundamental values and polices on followership through humanity which broadens and deepens the duty of service through political leadership.
- The theoretical concept of followership is functional when political leadership is invested in the collective collaboration and strengthened relationship between political leaders and citizenry.
- The strength of followership is a political tool for collective consciousness, progressive prosperity and intelligence security. Followership on both sides; the citizenry to political leaders and political leaders to citizenry.

Figure 2.
Schematic Presentation of the concept of SELF. Authors Compilation (2020).

social constructs and beliefs that have either advanced or hindered the progress of political leadership.

Political Leadership is broader than an office or a position it is a functional duty, a political responsibility, a social responsibility, a patriotic duty, an oath of office and an allegiance to service. The huge shoulders of these responsibilities are sensitively influenced, motivated, controlled and manipulated by a holistic range of factors that directs the pace, the choices, the decisions and the impacts of political leadership duration the cause of time [1].

The situational reality of political leadership and the call to serve in developing countries is a unique case study one that involves a wider and deeper understanding of how individuality plays a huge role and creates a deep impact in social constructs and definition of political leadership (**Figure 2**).

3. The S-E-L-F approach

The S-E-L-F approach to political leadership is a psychological framework and a guiding-tool to the state of consciousness for political leadership. It serves as a leadership mantra for the formulation of political policies, fundamental structures and the institutionalization of systems that justifies and validates the efficiency and effectiveness of political leadership. Political Leadership therefore, becomes more effective and efficient when it serves humanity through its policies, interests, institutions, foreign policies, diplomacy, structures and systems.

4. The influential impact of individuality on political leadership

Political leaders are influenced by their personality traits, which creates an intellectual opening for them on how they view, see and assert the roles of political leadership. A visionary outlook on life's struggles, strives, successes and strengths is created from the persona of an individual. The mindset of an individual creates a map of imagination, dreams and visions which controls the levels expectations and ambitions that an individual can experience and birth. While it is important to define political leadership on the standards and principles of what it should be, what it is expected to accomplish and how it's expected to achieve much through humanity for humanity and by humanity; it is also fundamentally crucial to assert the influential impact of individuality on political leadership. The political tools needed to function effectively in office by a political leader is hugely influenced by the leader's character traits, behavioral strength, self-knowledge, and personality which builds and forms a mental strength that develops the leader's political skills, political intelligence, political strategy, and political approach to duties [2].

The understanding of the influential impact of individuality on the effectiveness of political leadership creates a broadened knowledge on how far a nation can journey and strive progressively under the regimes, policies and adopted systems of governance. The individuality of political leaders comes first in the direction and utilization of their political will and governing authority. What saves a political system from the collapse of individualistic anarchism is the consciousness of selfishness in humanity.

Pragmatically, the idiosyncrasies of most political leaders is clearly seen in the extent of how far they bring their own; ideologies, needs, wants, desires, responsibilities, goals, and targets to the political arenas during their regime; this then becomes fundamentally crucial to the state of success and advancement of their leadership role. While the Individuality of political leadership disregards and ignores the humanity of citizenry, it embezzles and plans to exploit excesses for selfishness through corruption and political isolation [3].

The executive actions of a political leader does not pose much an important question. The reason "why" the executive actions were carried out appears to be more crucial and worthy of understanding. Political leadership is crafted on the visionary path, mission and betterment of humanity, it is a selfless agenda aimed at ensuring the collective prosperity and advancement of humanity is assured. Compassionately, when individualism and collectivism compromises interests, needs and values for the purpose of advancement collective humanity, it brings alive the strengths and greatness of political leadership [4].

There is a greater possibility for political leadership to utilize profound individualism for compassionate collectivism for the betterment of humanity. Political leadership in the sovereign space of individuality where the rationality of self-interest prevails, show there is a recognition of true individualism. It is one that is associated and identifiable with compassion, consciousness and empathy for humanity.

Compassionate collectivism makes it possible for individualism in political leadership to collaborate interests, needs, desires and agendas into a submerged goal for the greater, mutual and collective good of humanity. This is indeed the greatest challenge of conflicting ideologies of interests that is socio-consciously reconcilable and achievable. Collectivism becomes an intellectual tool for security, prosperity and harmony, when individualism through political leadership perpetuates and creates systems that are powerfully apt enough to see humanity as the collective consciousness and influence of the individual [5].

The pursuits and interests of individuality can be birth in collectivism when it recognizes and validates the presence of humanity. Political Leadership strives stronger and greater through the influential impact of individuality, when its individuality is submerged in the security of collectivism for humanity. Political leadership through the impacts of individualism, collectivism and humanism makes it possible for effective and efficient governance to succeed in a struggling world. The psychological presence of individuality makes it possible for dreams to be envisioned and for inspiration to illuminate aspirations [6].

As individuality is key to self-leadership, so is it fundamentally present in political leadership. The recognition of the self-centered fulfillment of individualism in political leadership and the unresolved conflicts of division and the widened gap of poverty, makes is consciously sensitive for political leadership to find the strengths of individuality in collectivism for the betterment, advancement and prosperity of humanity [7].

5. The financial emolument of political leadership

Political Leadership has its payoffs, incentives as well as rewards just like every other endeavor and aspiration. All leaders in every sphere of influence, deserve to be honored respected and remunerated for work done and inputs made as a result of responsibilities tied to such leadership roles. From a political perspective, the benefits and returns for leadership responsibility varies. They include emotional, monetary, territorial, economic, physical and even legal. Motivations for leaders vary also, depending on personal traits, inclination and situation. The bottom-line is every political leader has a motivating factor that is tied to a reward whether it is positively or negatively aligned. Prolonged observation and evaluation has shown especially in developing climes that the monetary gain seems to be the highest motivating factor.

It must be understood at every point in time that every leader especially a political one, is just as human as any other individual. They have needs and desires just like everyone and have their emotions active accordingly. Their fundamental senses are at work just like all healthy humans. The preceding statement is vital, so as not to have overbearing expectations political leaders, even though more is required of them by virtue of the leadership positions they now occupy.

But then again, it behooves on us to assess political leaders on their true motive for taking up political positions and offering themselves for service. Evaluations of political leadership from developing countries in continents like Africa, have shown that more often than not, monetary benefits and self-aggrandizement are their primary focus.

Let us take into consideration a country like Nigeria for instance. Judging from her statistics and natural endowments, she ought to be the innovative driver for Africa. Is this the scenario at play currently? Apparently, it is not. A country richly endowed with natural resources and high quality human capital, but it is yet to find its rightful place among the comity of nations. A major reason that has been responsible for her socioeconomic stagnation is the element of corruption. Corruption rarely thrives were monetary benefits are not the major incentives attached to deliverables and accomplishments tied to job roles or positions.

6. What is financial emolument?

Emolument is the term used to describe payment for an office or employment; compensation for a job, which is usually monetary. It could also be in form of tangible items such as automobiles or houses but the emphasis in this work is on monetary payments.

7. Financial emoluments and the political leadership motivation

Over the years, money has been the major tool for individual and corporate transactions. It signifies empowerment, economic protection and supremacy. With such paradigm, financial hardship creates scenarios were individuals fall into the despondency from lacking the preceding attributes stated earlier and therefore will see themselves losing out economically, socially as well as territorially- the inability to dominate their sphere of influence. Hence, Political leadership seems to be the quickest route to achieving these aspirations and goals as it affords the political leader the opportunity to wield so much influence and control over vast financial resources by virtue of the scope of his position. One of the few institutional devices obtainable to regulate the action of politicians apart from elections is their remuneration structure [8].

Presently, the quest for political positions for the sake of financial gains, is highest in developing and underdeveloped countries. It is not so difficult to know why this is so. Such countries, have the weakest economies and inefficient institutions. Based on the foregoing, individuals in these nations see political leadership-because of the influence attached to it, as the fastest route to self-aggrandizement and acquisition of wealth. The emoluments attached to political positions in these countries are so humongous, that within months of being in office, the life and economic status of the office holders usually experience tremendous economic transformation. Critical evaluations shows that such benefits now make the contest for such positions a very intense one even to the risk of the lives of the participants.

Apparently, the nature of political leadership in such countries affects who vies for such offices and also who finally gets in.

8. The Maslow's hierarchy angle

The Maslow's hierarchy of needs is a motivational theory in psychology comprising a five- tier model of human needs, often depicted as hierarchical levels within a pyramid. Needs further south in the hierarchy must be satisfied before individuals can sort out needs northwards. From bottom-up, the needs are: physiological, safety, love and belonging, esteem and self-actualization.

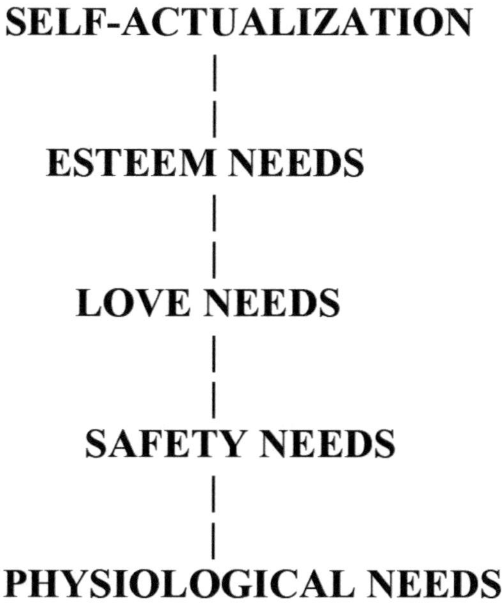

Maslow [9] using the above hierarchy of human need, stated that people are motivated to achieve certain needs and that some needs take precedence over others. From the list, he postulated that our most basic need is that of physical survival and this will be the first factor that motivates our behavior. Articulating that money is key to solving our physical needs, it therefore means that man gravitates quickly to wherever he can acquire funds with ease. Understanding the preceding fact, whatever positions have great monetary benefits attached usually will attract vehement but detrimental interest. Political Leadership is usually not an exception. The monetary emoluments attached to political positions; particularly in developing countries is enormous. As a result, the race to political offices are highly contested to critical levels such that it usually becomes a very risky affair. The acute poverty level in such countries ironically, is connected to the political leaders abysmal performance, creates an intense pursuit for political positions as an easy route to economic hardship.

9. Comparative analysis of emoluments in developing countries

To state that the pay packages of political office holders completely dwarfs that of civil servants/workers in developing countries is not an overstatement. From critical analysis and information sourcing, the civil servants remuneration is match for the average political leader in most countries in Africa. Citing scenarios from Nigeria, according to information captured from online tabloid-Pulse, the average Nigerian Senator earns a minimum of N32million monthly as pay package. And this is to represent a poverty-stricken people of whom most live on less than $1 a day. If we compare this with the earnings of the highest level researcher from the knowledge setup- a Professor, you will see the clear imbalance. The highest earning Professor in a country like Nigeria, with all emoluments put together earns nothing above the realms of N8million annually. Considering that they are the hope for the dissemination of new knowledge and discoveries as well as inventions, such pay in comparison with their political counterparts is appalling. This type of pay disparity will not encourage the youths and upcoming professionals to develop interest in other areas as much as politics. This what will bring all sorts on individuals into the political terrain. Rather than come for service, they will come in for wealth gain which never makes for productive leadership.

10. The profitability and corruptibility of political leadership

Political leadership represents the hope of the citizenry for societal progress and advancement. When political leadership is gotten right, no one misses out of the benefits. This calls for using crucial and well thought out processes to selecting such leaders. When the process is right, we can readily get the right political leaders in position. So also, when the process is flawed, we get to tolerate and endure flawed leadership. Political Leadership must be laced with the right leadership ingredients so as to get profitable outcomes for the citizens, location notwithstanding. Ingredients such as empathy, vision, uprightness, accountability, hard work, charisma, integrity honesty, mentorship, inter-relationship skills, conflict resolution capacity and so on.

There must be stringent laws, ethics and ordinances to guide all political office holders not to fall below the minimum expectation when it comes political positions. The outcomes of their political leadership must be made serious by way of regular accountability and consequences by law enforcement agencies for erring parties. This is crucial, as were the laws concerning political office becomes weak the political leader is at liberty to go overboard with his excesses. In the words of William Pitt "*Unlimited power is apt to corrupt the minds of those who posses it; and this I know, my lords: that where laws end, tyranny begins*". This preceding act has been the bane of unprofitable leadership in developing countries.

To make laws weak or impotent, is to indirectly empower corruption. The weakness of laws and the justice system of any nation is what empowers corruption. Once corruption can thrive within a political leadership space, the productivity of such leadership begins to erode. Consequently, when the political leadership class of a country espouses corruption, it becomes difficult for it to act positively to the benefit of the state and its citizens [10].

11. Case analysis on the corruption effect

As defined simply by Lewis [11] the phenomenon of corruption is referred to as "an impairment of virtue and moral principles".

Because the scenario as obtained in developing countries has painted a picture were political leadership is the path to easy wealth accumulation, corruption has become a systemic and institutional issue in most of these countries. Take for instance the continent of Africa where you have a large proportion of developing countries, a detailed investigation analysis will reveal that most of its leaders (rulers) have occupied those positions for an average of not less than fifteen (15) years. Were the period is less than this, it is possible to have a leader who has lead sometime in the past but has again returned to power. More often than not, this insatiate disposition stems from the quest to acquire possessions inordinately using such office. They forget that they were voted in or appointed to be good custodians of the nation's resources. As regards the above scenario, the case of Zimbabwe comes to mind. There, you had a man who had ruled a nation for 30 years and counting, but was unwilling to relinquish power. What could make a man so stuck on a political position after three decades, if not corrupt practices. This does not totally exempt the developed nations of corrupt political leadership, but we can deduce that it is not to the degree found in developing and underdeveloped nations.

A country like Nigeria who at present, ought to be the economic and industrial giant of Africa, has failed to assume this position for no other reason than highly institutionalized and syndicated corruption. Right from the pre-colonial (before 1960) era till now, the phenomenon has kept rearing its ugly head unchecked. From laws that give immunity coverage to political office holders to skewed election outcomes in favor of those with large treasure chest and in control of the treasury, the spate of corruption in high places has gone on unabated. A survey on the level of corruption in Nigeria carried out in 2003 by the Institute of Development Research of the Ahmadu Bello University, Zaria ranked political parties in the country third in the list of thirty most corrupt public institutions in Nigeria [12].

It therefore means that if there is be any meaningful change in the political leadership outcomes of developing nations, there must be a head on approach to corruption; financial corruption as a matter of fact.

12. The 21 pensible principles of political leadership

Political Leadership transcends through humanity the very powerful capital that influences and justifies the pathways, actions, policies and decisions of governance.

While in the absence and disregard of humanity political leadership assumes a different position and duty in regimes of most developing countries.

When it is not in the interests of political leaders to serve humanity through progressive policies of actions and in their political willingness to better the humanity of their citizenry; political leadership becomes exploitation, suppression and oppression.

The 21 pensible principles of political leadership represents the fundamental truths to the consciousness that ought to provide, protect and govern humanity in a striving world of survivals:

1. Political Leadership ought to serve humanity selflessly.

2. Political Leadership ought to inspire the creation of prosperity for its citizenry.

3. Political Leadership ought to collaborate and partner with its citizenry.

4. Political Leadership ought to be accountable for the welfare and betterment of its citizenry.

5. Political Leadership ought to have the credibility and integrity of office.

6. Political Leadership ought to be symbolic to parenthood.

7. Political Leadership ought to assure, and ensure the prosperity of humanity in the insurance of wealth and health.

8. Political Leadership ought to have compassionate knowledge on "what to do for" humanity.

9. Political Leadership ought to have the leadership structural skills on "how to serve" humanity.

10. Political Leadership ought to have the visionary inclinations and intellectual capacity to achieve a desirable future for its citizenry.

11. Political Leadership ought to have the mental intelligence to lead humanity.

12. Political Leadership ought to have the emotional intelligence to defend humanity.

13. Political Leadership ought to have a high-level of spiritual intelligence apt enough to illuminate humanity.

14. Political Leadership ought to have the cultural intelligence to unity the diversity in humanity.

15. Political Leadership ought to have the political willingness and bravery to protect and secure humanity.

16. Political Leadership ought to have protection, provisions, and an advancement for humanity to heights of excellence and security.

17. Political Leadership ought to formulate policies that protects the advancement of human capital, economic capital, social capital and natural capital.

18. Political Leadership ought to have the consciousness of empathy, sympathy and compassion for humanity.

19. Political Leadership ought to give more and take less from humanity.

20. Political Leadership ought to invest, collaborate, educate, enlighten and build humanity.

21. Political Leadership ought to lead through the social-cultural dynamics and diversity of humanity harmoniously and compassionately.

These pensible principles of political leadership are trusted enough to ensure that political leadership can strive for more and excel effectively and efficiently in governance through the consciousness of these principles and compassion for humanity.

13. Conclusion

From the foregoing, it is obvious that Political Leadership must be inspired by acts and expectations beyond financial emoluments. Work has its rewards no doubt but because leadership is about people; particularly political leadership, the incentives attached to political positions as well as public office must not be so enticing. This is so as not to create a scenario, were the responsibilties done, are taken as a means to an end. Political Leadership is first for service to humanity and societal development before anything else. This chapter clarifies in summary that if the structures placed for political offices are not ones that call for service and sacrifice, then the true motive for it will never be achieved. This is most critical in developing countries, were there is so much lack and deprivation.

Author details

Daniels Aide Okun[1] and Osama Ose Iyawe[2*]

1 Antalya Bilim University, Antalya, Turkey

2 University of Benin, Benin City, Nigeria

*Address all correspondence to: osamaiyawe@gmail.com

References

[1] Frohlich, N., & Oppenheimer, J. A. (2015). Political leadership and collective goods (Vol. 1298). Princeton University Press.

[2] Bittner, A. (2011). Platform or personality: the role of party leaders in elections. OUP Oxford.

[3] Greasley S, Stoker G. Urban political leadership. Theories of urban politics. 2009:125-136

[4] Grindle MS. Good enough governance: Poverty reduction and reform in developing countries. Governance. 2004;**17**(4):525-548

[5] Mudde C, Kaltwasser CR. Populism and political leadership (pp. 376-388). Oxford: Oxford University Press; 2014

[6] Peele G. Leadership and politics: a case for a closer relationship? Leadership. 2005;**1**(2):187-204

[7] Lásźló É. Individualism, collectivism, and political power: A relational analysis of ideological conflict. Springer; 2013

[8] Duha, T., Altindag, Elif, S., Filiz & Erdal, T. (2017) "Does it Matter How Much Politicians are Paid? "Working Paper for National Bureau of Economic Research (NBER) Massachusetts, USA.

[9] Maslow A. A. Theory of Human Motivation Psychological Review. 1943;**50**(4):370-396

[10] Ogbeidi MM. Political Leadership and Corruption in Nigeria Since 1960: A Socio-Economic Analysis. Journal of Nigerian Studies. 2012;**1**(2)

[11] Lewis A. Corruption. In word web. Princeton: Princeton University; 2006

[12] Adekeye F. 30 Most Corrupt Public Institutions in Nigeria. *Newswatch*. 2003;(December 22)

Chapter 11

New Technologies and Decision-Making for the Military

Gérard de Boisboissel

"One should act as a man of thought and think as a man of action".

Henri Bergson

Abstract

This chapter aims at reviewing the concept of decision-making on the battlefield for military leaders. Thus, it intends to address the changes implied by the use of new technologies (such as Robots, AI) that will gradually invade the battlefield. The leader of tomorrow will have to quickly manage remote information and keep control of high performance automated systems integrating a certain form of autonomy, including lethal autonomous weapon systems. He must ensure that a global meaning is given to the military action taking place on the battlefield. He has to be able to command to achieve his goals.

Keywords: military, leader, decision-making, decision aid, technology, autonomy, AI

1. Introduction

If the qualities required of a leader to be a good commander and a good decision maker remain constant in human history in the face of the complexity of the battle, the leader of tomorrow will have to adapt to the uses of new technologies. This will allow him to be better informed, and consequently to be more reactive in order to keep the initiative in the manoeuvre, but also to carry his action further and delegate certain tasks to the machines he will have at his disposal. Such adaptations are not trivial, because they reconsider the existing military doctrines, and can call into question the very principle of the hierarchy that makes the strength of armies. It is therefore necessary for the military to know how to use these new technologies through training, but also to know how to keep control of the use of new systems integrating a certain form of autonomy. Above all, it is important for the military leader to preserve the very essence of his very identity: to give meaning to military action and command to achieve his goals.

2. Commandment

Primarily, a military leader must command, which implies legitimate decision-making authority and a responsibility towards the soldiers entrusted to him for the mission which he must ensure.

The command is the very expression of the personality of the leader. It depends on the tactical situation which includes the risk and the obligations of the mission to be carried out.

To be a good military leader implies several additional qualities: to be demanding, to be competent, to have a high moral strength in the face of the difficulties of war, to have confidence in his own abilities and in those put at disposal, to be in responsibility to assume his decisions and for that to put in responsibility his subordinates, and finally to be able to decide in complete freedom.

He is the one who decides and commands. He is the one to whom all eyes turn in difficulty [1], but the exercise of his command requires a demanding discernment between reflection and action.

3. Decision

The military world is very demanding and dangerous. Having to take into account the danger for his soldiers, the danger for himself and the responsibility of the mission he has been given, the military leader should:

- discern in complexity (deploy true situational intelligence);
- decide in uncertainty (have the strength of character to accept calculated risks);
- act in adversity (to unite energies, encourage collective action and make conscious decisions);

This forms the basis of the educational project of the Saint-Cyr Coëtquidan military academy, and perfectly synthesises the objectives of a training system adapted to the officers of the 21st century. However, this initial training must take into account the technological evolutions allowing military decision-makers of today and tomorrow to reduce the fog of war.

3.1 Military leader is accountable for the decision

What is decision-making for a military officer? It consists of choosing between different possibilities and opting for a conclusion among the different possible solutions, while having analysed all effects that this decision implies.

In order to decide, the leader must master the various areas listed below: a perfect knowledge of the mission entrusted to him, of the means at his disposal and of his troops. Nothing is worse than indecision when the lives of soldiers are in danger. His decision must call for moral and intellectual courage.

"The unknown is the governing factor in war" said Marshal Foch. However, the role of the leader is above all to be able to adapt and modify his analysis and the behaviour of his troop in order to respond to unforeseen situations. This ability to adapt is essential to maintain the freedom of action that allows for initiative on the battlefield, and to be able to innovate according to the constraints.

The leader must show discernment in action, to appreciate facts according to their nature and their fair value. This implies being cautious in his choices and the scope of his choices.

Finally, the leader must be lucid, and control his stress, pressure and emotions. These to preserve his "esprit d'initiative".

3.2 Information, the key to victory

To meet all these requirements, information is one of the major foundations for the exercise of the command of the chief. It is the keystone of all military action, to keep the initiative and maintain supremacy on the ground [2].

In fact, information allows the chief to plan the military action, taking into account the means at his disposal, ensuring the transport logistics, and confronting the possible friendly and enemy modes of action in order to determine the manoeuvre that he will conduct.

The management of the information received is reflected "en conduite[1]" by the regular rhythm of reports and situation updates to higher or subordinate levels, in order to anticipate threats and maintain a capacity to react as quickly and efficiently as possible in the face of adversity or any obstacle hindering the manoeuvre.

For the decision-making process to run smoothly, the information must be updated regularly because the situation can change very quickly and the leader will have to adapt his analysis accordingly.

Thus, there is no single decision of the military commander in operation, but a continuum of decisions, some of which are almost routine or implicit, while others require extensive analysis. Some decisions are ultimately critical, as they can result in a favourable or tragic outcome to a given situation.

4. What is fundamentally changing

This chapter addresses the change in the art of decision-making for a military officer, implied by the use of some technologies that will gradually invade the battlefield.

Indeed, some technologies will allow the leader to be better informed, but also to be more reactive in order to keep the initiative. Their management requires a mastery of new data management processes resulting from the digitisation of the battlefield, in particular the possible influx of operational data from the field and their synthesis for the military leader.

4.1 A more accurate and faster remote information acquisition

The one who sees further and before the others is the one who dominates the military manoeuvre. This is what enables him to gain a tactical advantage because the one who acts first with determination is most often the one who wins. Moreover, the ability to see further and more accurately thanks to remote sensors or cameras brings an undeniable advantage to the military leader, enabling him to react faster than his enemy.

Today, spaces are getting tighter, and information can be transmitted in a few milliseconds to any point on the planet, provided that the sensor capturing the information is available. This is done through cyberspace which must be secured for military forces so that they can be sure of the veracity of the data they use. This immediacy of information is a new parameter in the art of command. It forces the leader to make a quick analysis and to be reactive in his response.

It also raises the question of his capacity to process the information, if there is too much data to process. In this case, it will be necessary to process automatically the data as soon as it is received by the systems, to extract only the relevant

[1] "en conduite" is a French expression literally translated by " while driving " which means to decide while the military action is taking place.

information. And if these systems are unable to do this, the leader will have to be assisted in the analysis and decision-making by a third party, which may also be a machine. This raises the question of the control of these decision aids provided and which he must rely on.

4.2 Act remotely to remove the danger and increase the area of action

One of the major military revolutions that began at the start of the 21st century in the Iraq and Afghanistan wars is the robotisation of the battlefield. It is unavoidable and will gradually be introduced into the battlefield because the use of unmanned robots (UAV, USV, UUS and UGV) offers many advantages to the armies that will use them on the ground.

Firstly, it avoids exposing our own combatants, which is all the more important in our modern armies where the latter are a scarce and expensive resources to train.

Secondly, it extends the area of perception and action of a military unit. In a sense, they are the "5 deported senses" of the fighter, i.e. his eyes (camera), his ears (reception), his mouth (transmission), his touch (actuator arm) and even his sense of smell and taste (detection of CBRN products).

As tools placed at the disposal of the combatant, robots will allow him to control the battlefield by deporting effectors or sensors allowing a control of the various dimensions and spaces of the battlefield, on land, in the air, at sea and even electromagnetically. These will thus progressively move the combatant behind the contact zone, in order to move him away from the dangerous area and reduce the risks, or allow him to dive in with the maximum of means at his disposal, thus significantly reducing the vulnerability of the combatants [3].

Finally, the ability to act remotely while preserving the lives of his men will allow the leader to act even the enemy can even deploy his forces for his manoeuvre.

Robotic systems will thus become new tactical pawns that the military leader will now use to prepare his action, to facilitate his progress, allowing him new effects on the enemy, the terrain, the occupation of space and on the rhythm of the action. Especially since these machines will eventually be more efficient, more precise and faster for specific tasks than a human being can be. This is currently evident in industrial manufacturing and assembly plants.

4.3 The disruption of autonomy

This military revolution of deporting action with robotic systems is accompanied by another, no less disruptive, that of the autonomy of these systems. Autonomy will allow for omnipresence of action in the area, 24 hours a day, subject to energy sufficiency. It will allow the machines to adapt to the terrain and its unforeseen events in order to carry on the mission entrusted to them by the military leaders. Autonomous systems will allow them to react to complex situations by adapting their positioning strategy, and even adapting the effects it produces on the battlefield. For example, it may be an automatic reorganisation of the swarm formation adopted by a group of robots to follow an advancing enemy, followed by the decision to block an axis of progression with smoke or obstacles to hinder enemy progression.

However, autonomy is not fundamentally new for a leader. A section or a platoon leader has combat groups under his command, whose group leader who receives a mission has full autonomy to carry it out. The new fact is that if robots are tactical pawns at the disposal of the combatant, and if they can have a certain form of autonomy in the execution of their action, they do not have and will never have the awareness of their action and the capacity of discernment which are characteristics of the human being. This opens up a number of ethical questions regarding the opening of fire that will not be addressed in this chapter (See [3]).

5. The contribution of new technologies to military decision-making

These upheavals are based on technologies that create new opportunities in military decision-making processes.

5.1 All deployed systems are interconnected

The digitisation of the battlefield stems from the constant trend towards the integration of electronic components in all future military equipment, which, coupled with a means of transmission, allow for their interconnection and the dissemination of the information collected. It affects all systems deployed in the field (from weapons systems to military vehicles), right down to the disembarked combatant who, just like any civilian with a smartphone, will be connected to the great digital web of the battlefield and therefore traceable and reachable. Just like every individual in the civil society, every actor on the battlefield is traceable and able to communicate.

5.2 Enriched information

As explained above, technology will enable a faster detection of threats on the battlefield. The Law of Moore has sometimes been used to describe the increase in the capabilities of digital cameras, according to a ratio of "twice as far" or "twice as cheap" or "twice as small" every 3 years. In fact, each innovation allows to see further for a smaller footprint. The digital zoom allows high magnifications but at the cost of algorithmic processing of the image which causes lesser definition quality. It is often paired with the optical zoom, which consists of adapting the focal length to the target you want to look at. Cameras can now merge data from multiple sensors of different types. In particular, thermal imaging allowing you to see a large fraction of the spectrum and to view and measure the thermal energy emitted by an equipment or a human. To which one can add light intensification processes to amplify the existing residual light to recreate an image usable by the human eye, in low light conditions.

All of this fused data can enrich the field of vision of the combatant by superimposing additional data that completes his knowledge of the tactical situation. This is the principle of augmented reality.

5.3 The immediacy of information processing

If data acquisition and transmission is possible, the information should nevertheless be processed. However processing it requires easily accessible hardware and software resources offering the necessary computing capacity to react as quickly as possible, particularly in order to be extremely reactive in situations where the analysis time is too short for a human to do it by himself. Embedded computer software can provide such capacity at the core of deployed systems, but this capability can also be moved to a secure cloud, which can be both a tactical cloud, i.e. a cloud deployed on the battlefield in support of the manoeuvre, or to a further away, highly sovereign and secure cloud.

5.4 To the detriment of human decision-making

This immediacy of information processing allows a hyper-reactivity of systems, foreshadowing the concept of "hyperwar" formulated by General John Allen & Amir Hussain Allen in 2019, which puts forward the idea that the advent of hyperwar is the next fundamentally transformative change in warfare.

"What makes this new form of warfare unique is the unparalleled speed enabled by automating decision-making and the concurrency of action that become possible by leveraging artificial intelligence and machine cognition... In military terms, hyperwar may be redefined as a type of conflict where human decision-making is almost entirely absent from the observe-orient-decide-act (OODA) loop. Consequently, the time associated with an OODA cycle will be reduced to near-instantaneous responses. The implications of these developments are many and game changing[2]".

5.5 A support for information processing

For information processing, the volume of data produced increases exponentially and the accuracy and granularity of the data produced by sensors grows. This trend will become more and more pronounced over time [4].

Military experts usually process observation data retrieved from the battlefield by satellites, reconnaissance aircraft, drones or sensors abandoned on the ground. However, as human resources are scarce and the volume of data is constantly increasing, it will be necessary to delegate the processing of this amount of data to AI algorithms in support of the human being, at the risk of not being able to process all of them without this technology.

On the ground, the deployed combatant will be increasingly charged cognitively by the complexity of the systems to operate and the amount of information to process. It will be vital to automate the processing of certain information in order to unload it, so that only what is really necessary will be presented. This needs to be done in an extremely ergonomic way. This requires defining which data can be subjected to artificial processing, and up to what hierarchical level their processing can be automated.

5.6 The contribution of artificial intelligence

Automated management of routine, repetitive and time-consuming procedures could emerge. In a headquarters, for example, reports management and automatic production of summaries adapted to the level of command would immediately make the chain of command more fluid. The AI could take the form of a dashboard to stimulate the reflection of the commander and his advisers by dynamically delivering relevant information and updated statements [5].

During operational preparation, depending on the tactical situation, the leader must confront the possible modes of action he envisages with the reference enemy situation and the possible enemy modes of action. Very often he does not have the material time to confront his action with several enemy modes of action, and he only anticipates certain non-compliant cases that he considers probable. Artificial intelligence could be more exhaustive in confronting more possible modes of action of the enemy, and thus present a more complete analysis of possible options to the military leader who could then decide accordingly.

---

[2] https://www.fifthdomain.com/dod/2017/08/07/emerging-hyperwar-signals-ai-fueled-machine-waged-future-of-conflict/

The field is wide, and even more infinite. A new question then arises: for new technologies, is a new way of command needed?

6. Reduction of the OODA decision cycle

The technologies listed above have a direct effect on the OODA decision cycle, which will be profoundly impacted by the new technologies.

This concept was defined in 1960 by an American military pilot by the name of John Boyd to formalise the decision cycle in air combat. It has since been used to schematise any decision cycle. The author will use it here in the light of the potential offered by the technologies detailed above (**Figure 1**).

6.1 Observe: a better detection

"Seeing without being seen" is essential in military operations, and remains a common adage. Technology is helping, with the extended distances made possible by long-range cameras and their deportation to robotic systems. It can now also help to overcome several natural detection constraints such as night, fog or walls.

Moreover, digitised systems can operate 24 hours a day with great consistency, where humans are subject to fatigue and inattention, avoiding the risk of missing information.

For surveillance or patrol missions, where human resources are often lacking, the leader can delegate to systems the analysis of images of the area for the detection of movements and the potential presence of enemies. It should be noted that this detection should filter out false alarms as much as possible, such as the movement of leaves in the trees when the wind picks up.

6.2 Orient: a better analysis

Remotely seeing will make it possible to identify a potential target from afar, to discriminate it (is the target a combatant) and to characterise its behaviour (is it hostile or not). If these criteria are met, the target becomes a potential target that can easily be geolocated, this information will then be transmitted to the

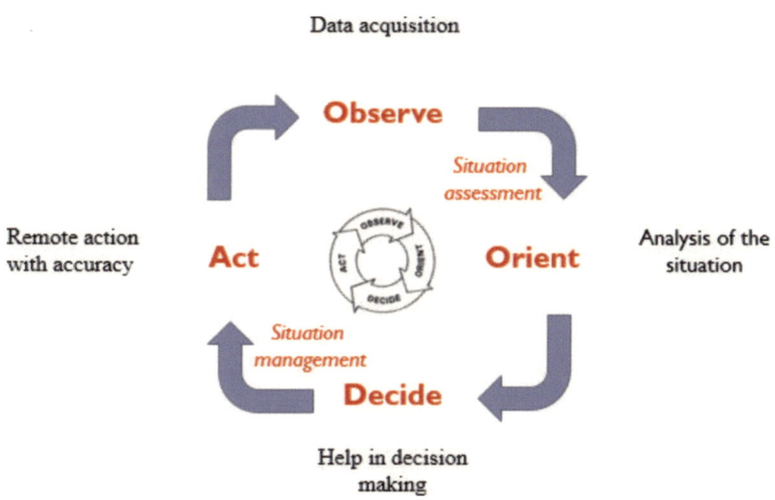

Figure 1.
OODA cycle time reduction: A better reactivity.

decision-making levels. The gain here is that of anticipating the analysis for better decision-making.

The leader will also be able to rely on the automatic processing of data acquired within the digital environment of the battlefield. Faced with the potential 'infobesity' of the battlefield, artificial intelligence will enable massive data processing, subject to the availability of a computing capacity directly embedded in remote robotic platforms, or by remote processing of information via long-distance communications. It will allow constant monitoring of the analysis of captured images or sounds, a task that the best human experts can only supervise because they are subject to fatigue and inattention. This is particularly the case with satellite images or images captured by surveillance drones, which can monitor an area 24 hours a day. Finally, it will also enable the detection of weak signals that would be invisible to humans, by correlation between several distinct events, or by cross-checking.

There are still two essential components to the analysis of the situation that a machine can never integrate. Firstly, instinct and intuition, which a machine cannot have and which are the fruit of a life-long learning of human experience, and secondly, the transcendence of military action which only a metaphysical dimension in the literal sense can provide.

6.3 Decide: a better reaction

The military commander is the decision-maker for military action. It is therefore up to him to take the decision according to the information at his disposal. He can of course rely on a deputy or on operational advisers who help him analyse the situation, if time permits.

For example, France is intervening in Mali and the Sahara as part of the *Barkhane* military operation to combat Salafist jihadist armed groups infiltrating the entire Sahel region. Launched on 1 August 2014, this operation replaces operations *Serval* and *Épervier*. The following scenario is fictitious: an armed Reaper drone of the French army flies over a region of the Malian desert at night and its cameras (incorporating AI for automatic motion detection processing of the captured images) detect a suspicious movement. The sensor operator of the drone is alerted and zooms in on the area to detect a jihadist 4x4 occupied by armed personnel via its Infrared camera. This vehicle is moving towards a village 20 kilometres away. Setting up an operation with Special Forces is not possible because they are not in the area, and there is a great risk that the occupants of the 4x4 will disperse once they reach the village. The legal advisor on duty quickly confirms the possibility of the drones firing on the target because no collateral damage is possible in this desert area. The head of the operation decides to give the order to fire the drone.

This example clearly shows the drastic reduction in the OODA decision cycle offered by the new technologies: the chief detects and is informed as soon as possible by an automatic detection of a suspicious movement of an enemy vehicle. He confirms with his image operator the Positive identification (PID) of the target as an enemy. He then reports it to his hierarchy and receives the order to open fire. He can thus, in compliance with IHL, open fire from a distance. The enemy has not even spotted him.

There are still situations where time is critical and the leader will not have time to make a decision due to the rapidity of the attack. The automation of response processes then becomes a possible option, i.e. he can delegate to a machine the possibility of giving an appropriate response to a situation by itself. This is already the case with missiles or ballistic threats, which require armies to use automatic systems to counter them. This requires automatic systems that are faster and more precise than human beings (e.g. coupling weapons and radar). Tomorrow, faced with future systems that will develop unpredictable trajectory strategies (enemy missiles with AI), faced with saturating threats that risk overwhelming our defences, faced with swarms of offensive robots, our systems will have to adapt in real time to counter the threat. Only a certain autonomy of the defensive systems will make it possible to face them, an autonomy which will have to remain under the control of the leader having these systems at his disposal.

6.4 Act: a quicker and more accurate reaction

A quicker reaction: A man reacts in a few seconds, the machine in a few milliseconds or less. Where a human thinks in a few seconds for the best, the machine will analyse parameters in a few milliseconds and propose a response in near real time.

A more accurate action: A human shooter who moves, breathes and shakes is less accurate than a machine that does not move, breathe or shake because it is not subject to emotion. Precision in action will therefore increasingly be the prerogative of the machine.

The outcome of a fight or a counter-measure may depend on these factors 10 or 100 seconds to a thousand seconds.

7. Technology as a decision aid for the leader

Military decision-making is centred on the military leader, because he is at the heart of the command situation. He takes responsibility for military action, a mission given to him by the legitimately elected political power.

The leader must therefore control the decisions taken within the framework of military action because he is the guarantor and he assumes the consequences.

What lessons can one learn from the opportunities offered by new technologies for military decision-making and the possible resulting changes in the art of command?

7.1 To reduce the "fog of war"

The leader must rely on technology to reduce the uncertainty and fog of war. It will allow him to be more aware of his tactical situation by searching for intelligence. Furthermore, it will enable him to delegate to machines the management of repetitive tasks that do not require constant situational intelligence.

Depending on the circumstances and if he has time to reflect, the digitisation of battlefield information will also allow the leader to replay certain possible scenarios before taking a decision. Finally, it will give him the possibility to select the information he has received that he deems important, to view it several times (especially if the information is imprecise) before making a decision.

7.2 For decision support

A digital aid will be welcome to synthesise the multiplication of digital actors on the ground with whom he is in contact, or whom he must command or coordinate as a leader.

One of the consequences of the digitization of the battlefield is that it may lead to information overload for the leader who is already very busy and focused on his tasks of commanding and managing. It is already accepted in the military community that a leader can manage a maximum of seven different information sources at the same time, and even less when under fire.

Delegating is one way to avoid cognitive overload. Thus, one possible solution is to create a "digital assistant" who can support the leader in the information processing steps.

His digital deputy can be a digital assistant, an autonomous machine that will assist the leader in filtering and processing information, which will help the leader in the decision-making process.

Nevertheless, the leader will have to fight against the easy way out, take a step back, allow himself time to reflect, and reason with a critical sense when faced with machines that will think for him. This process will help him fight against a possible inhibition of human reasoning. Artificial intelligence does not mean artificial ignorance if it is used as an intellectual stimulant, although it can have this flaw.

7.3 For an optimization of its resources

The chief will be able to entrust machines with the execution of certain time-consuming and tedious tasks, such as patrols or the surveillance of sectors, and thus conserve his human resources for missions where they will have a higher added value.

The same applies to missions that require reactivity and precision, especially if there is a need to be extremely quick to adapt to the situation. For example, it will be useful in the case of saturating threats, where targeted destruction or multi-faceted and omnipresent threats such as swarms of drones must be dealt with.

8. But technology as a decision aid subject to control and confidence

Delegation of tasks to increasingly autonomous machines raises the question of the place of humans who interface with these systems and should stay in control.

8.1 The leader must always control execution of an autonomous system

At first, the military will not use equipment or tools that they do not control, regardless of the army in the world. Every military leader must be in control of the military action, and for this purpose, must be able to control the units and the means at his disposal. He places his confidence in them to carry out the mission, which is the basis of the principle of subsidiarity.

For this reason, it is not in his interest to have a robotic system that governs itself with its own rules and objectives. Moreover, this system could be disobedient or break out of the framework that has been set for it. Thus, machines with a certain degree of autonomy must be subordinate to the chain of command, and subject to orders, counter orders, and reporting [6].

8.2 Operators must have confidence when delegating tasks to an autonomous system

The military will never use equipment or tools that they do not trust. This is the reason why a leader must have confidence in the way a machine behaves or could behave. For that, military engineers should develop autonomous systems capable of explaining their decisions.

Automatic systems are predictable, thus, one can easily anticipate how it will perform the task entrusted to it. However, this becomes more complex with autonomous systems, especially self-learning systems where one may well know the objective of the task to be performed by the machine, but has no idea how it will operate. This raises a serious question of trust in this system. As an example, when I ask an autonomous mowing robot to mow my lawn, I know my lawn will be mowed, but I do not know exactly how the robot will proceed.

The best example to focus on are the expectations of the soldier about Artificial Intelligence embedded in autonomous systems.

AI should be trustable. This means that adaptive and self-learning systems must be able to explain their reasoning and decisions to human operators in a transparent and understandable manner;

AI should be explainable and predictable: one must understand the different steps of reasoning carried out by a machine that delivers a solution to a problem or an answer to a complex question. For this, a human-machine interface (HMI) that explains its decision-making mechanism is needed.

One must therefore focus on more transparent and personalised human-machine interfaces for the operator and the leader [6].

9. The risks inherent in the use of new technologies for military decision-making

9.1 Tunnel effect

Easy access to information or possible information overload both favour a possible tunnel effect. This effect, due to a sudden rise in adrenaline, causes a failure in the analysis of signals and data received by a brain that is no longer able to step back and analyse the situation. For the military, this tunnel effect is clearly the enemy of the soldier who has to concentrate on a screen, on a precise task, forgetting to look at the enemy threat around him and thus exposing himself seriously. It is also the enemy of the leader who, because he focuses on a piece of information that he finds crucial, becomes unable to step back and fulfil his role as a leader, which is to take into account the globality of the military action, and not one of its particular aspects highlighted by this information. Too much information should not prevent the commander from stepping back and reflecting.

The question of the gender of the soldier operator may be an avenue of exploration here, as women may have the capacity to manage several tasks simultaneously better than men.

9.2 Inhibit the action

Easy access to information encourages another possible flaw in decision-making. That of not deciding anything until one has all the information at his disposal. This flaw can probably become a major concern in the future. With the responsibility of the soldier at stake, he may hesitate until the last moment to take a decision because he lacks information that he can hope to recover by technological means. This is the death of daring, of manoeuvre by surprise, which often ensures a victory for the leaders who dare to practice them.

9.3 AI will influence the decision of the leader

Stress is an inherent component of taking responsibility. It is common for a military leader to have the feeling of being overwhelmed in a complex (military) situation. In such contexts, the leader will most often be inclined to trust an artificial intelligence because it will appear to him, provided he has confidence in it, as a serious decision-making aid not influenced by any stress, having superior processing capabilities, and able to test multiple combinations for a particular effect.

9.4 Too much predictability in operational decision-making patterns

The modelling of human intelligence by duly validated but very fixed algorithmic processes can lead to the inhibition of human intelligence. In particular, there will be a risk that military thinking will be locked into decision-triggering software. In other words, the formatting of military thought into controlled and controllable decision-making processes, developed by the need to respect the rules of engagement and international rules, particularly those of the decision to open fire. The processes will certainly be validated, but once activated, these processes may become completely rigid technological gems, admirably designed, but incorporating doctrinal biases that cannot be challenged in the face of unpredictable enemy behaviour [7]. By the time, these systems and their uses are adapted, it will be too late and the battle will be lost.

Another major risk is the predictability of the behaviour of these systems by the enemy. As these systems are known, their vulnerability will also be known. It will therefore be easy for the enemy to circumvent them by manoeuvres combining cunning and opportunity, with victory only reflecting the inability of these highly technical systems to adapt to an unpredictable or simply illegal conflict.

The leader must therefore anticipate these pitfalls and use the means at his disposal with intelligence. On these aspects, the French army has developed the concept of "major effect" to be achieved. This major effect conceptualises the way in which the leader intends to seize the initiative in the execution of his mission and which makes it possible to adapt the means and methods of execution to the final effect sought [8].

9.5 A principle of subsidiarity undermined

As a corollary to the extraordinary potential of the digitisation of the battlefield, namely to allow all levels of the hierarchy to access information in real time and simultaneously, there is also a new risk at every level of the military hierarchy: that of the leader having the possibility of directly accessing 'target information', thus breaking the principle of subsidiarity, which requires him to delegate to his subordinates the responsibility for and the use of the means made available to him. The temptation to interfere in the decisions of subordinates and to decide in their place will be great, given his experience and his position. In order to avoid this possible risk, it will be necessary to define precisely the right level of information to be communicated for the right strategic level, in order to respect the freedom of action of each level and to avoid a general and systematic dissemination of information without intermediate processing and filtering.

10. Conclusion

"The philosophy of war does not change. It will not change as long as it is men who make war" said General Charles de Gaulle.

In spite of everything, new technologies bring new equipment to the forces in operation. They are transforming the art of waging war through the opportunities they offer and by the new uses they bring to the battlefield.

With these new means at his disposal, the leader must continue to ensure the delicate balance between reflection and action. Without real and concrete

DOI: http://dx.doi.org/10.5772/intechopen.98849

commitment, there can be no good understanding of the situation, and without hindsight, there can be no good decisions [9].

This balance can only be achieved through advanced training. Firstly, human learning, to know how to command his men and respect the opponent. Secondly, intellectual learning, because he must understand the technologies he will use on the battlefield. Military training, because war is an art that leaves no room for the unexpected and requires skills and qualities that are acquired through effort, courage and performance training.

It is this leader of tomorrow that the French Military Academy of Saint-Cyr Coëtquidan is training in Brittany, in the western part of France.

Glossary

AI	Artificial Intelligence
CBRN	Chemical, Biological, Radiological and Nuclear
HMI	Human-Machine Interface
OODA	Observe-Orient-Decide-Act
PID	Positive Identification
UAV	Unmanned Aerial Vehicle
UGV	Unmanned Ground Vehicle
USV	Unmanned Surface Vehicle
UUS	Unmanned Underwater Vehicle

Author details

Gérard de Boisboissel
Challenges of Emerging Technologies for the Armed Forces, Military Academy Saint-Cyr Coëtquidan Research Centre, France

*Address all correspondence to:
gerard.de-boisboissel@st-cyr.terre-net.defense.gouv.fr

References

[1] French Army Staff. L'exercice du commandement dans l'armée de Terre, 2016 ; Available from: https://www.defense.gouv.fr/content/download/467991/7465134/Exercice_commandement.pdf [Accessed: 2021-05-28]

[2] Gérard de Boisboissel. Special edition DSI magazine n° 45, Le soldat augmenté, 2016, p. 54.

[3] Gérard de Boisboissel. Special edition Revue Défense Nationale, déc. 2018 : Autonomie et létalité en robotique militaire, p.45; and Available from: https://www.defnat.com/pdf/cahiers/Cahier%20CREC%202018%20-%20Autonomie%20et%20l%C3%A9talit%C3%A9%20en%20robotique%20militaire.pdf [Accessed: 2021-05-28]

[4] Cédric Villani. Donner un sens à l'intelligence artificielle, 2018, p. 220; and Available from: https://www.aiforhumanity.fr/pdfs/MissionVillani_Report_ENG-VF.pdf [Accessed: 2021-05-28]

[5] Major Sauget. Special edition DSI magazine n° 65, IA & Défense, 2019, p. 30.

[6] Gérard de Boisboissel. The contribution of human work to safety in high-hazard industries in the future, editors Foundation for an industrial safety culture (FonCSI); 2021.

[7] Benoit Bihan. Special edition Guerres & Histoire magazine n°60, 2021, p. 14.

[8] general Michel Yakovleff. Theoretical Tactics, 2nd ed. Économica, 2018.

[9] Ivan Morel. L'Hyper-conscience du chef militaire : moteur ou frein pour l'action ?, editors revue Inflexions, 2006/2, p. 115 et 124.